ᵁᴱᴿSITYᴼF

The Psychology of Doping in Sport

This is the first book to draw together cutting-edge research on the psychological processes underlying doping use in sport and exercise, thereby filling an important gap in our understanding of this centrally important issue in contemporary sport. Covering diverse areas of psychology such as social cognition, automatic and controlled processes, moral decision-making, and societal and contextual influence on behavior, the book also explores methodological considerations surrounding doping assessment in psychological research as well as future directions for evidence-based preventive interventions and anti-doping education.

Written by a team of leading international researchers from countries including the US, Canada, Australia, the UK, Greece, Germany, Italy, Denmark, and Ireland, the book integrates empirical findings with theoretical guidance for future psychological research on doping, and illuminates the challenges, needs, and priorities in contemporary doping prevention. It is important reading for advanced students and researchers in sport and exercise science, sport management, and sport policy, and will open up new perspectives for professional coaches, sports administrators, policymakers, sport psychologists, and sport medicine specialists looking to better understand the doping behaviors of athletes in sport.

Vassilis Barkoukis is Assistant Professor of Teaching in Physical Education in the Department of Physical Education and Sport Science at the Aristotle University of Thessaloniki. His research interests involve the application of social-cognitive approaches in physical education, physical activity, and sports. He has authored several articles and book chapters on the psychological processes underlying doping use. He has participated in several international research projects on doping funded by the WADA, EU, and other funding bodies.

Lambros Lazuras is Senior Lecturer in Psychology at the International Faculty of the University of Sheffield, and research associate in the Department of Social and Developmental Psychology at "La Sapienza" University of Rome. His research is focused on the social-cognitive predictors of substance use and health-related behaviors. He has authored research articles, books, and chapters in edited books about doping use, and participated in several research projects about doping, funded by the World Anti-Doping Agency, and the European Commission.

Haralambos Tsorbatzoudis is Professor of Applied Sport Psychology in the Department of Physical Education and Sport Science at the Aristotle University of Thessaloniki. His research interests focus on the applications of social-cognitive theories in sport and physical education. He has authored more than 150 articles in sport psychology, physical education, and physical activity, and has authored, translated, and edited ten books relevant to psychology, education, research methods, and sport science in Greek. He served as principal investigator in three WADA-funded projects.

Routledge Research in Sport and Exercise Science

The *Routledge Research in Sport and Exercise Science* series is a showcase for cutting-edge research from across the sport and exercise sciences, including physiology, psychology, biomechanics, motor control, physical activity and health, and every core sub-discipline. Featuring the work of established and emerging scientists and practitioners from around the world, and covering the theoretical, investigative and applied dimensions of sport and exercise, this series is an important channel for new and ground-breaking research in the human movement sciences.

Available in this series:

The Psychology of Doping in Sport

Edited by Vassilis Barkoukis,
Lambros Lazuras and
Haralambos Tsorbatzoudis

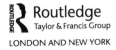 Routledge
Taylor & Francis Group

LONDON AND NEW YORK

First published 2016
by Routledge
2 Park Square, Milton Park, Abingdon, Oxon OX14 4RN

and by Routledge
711 Third Avenue, New York, NY 10017

Routledge is an imprint of the Taylor & Francis Group, an informa business

© 2016 V. Barkoukis, L. Lazuras and H. Tsorbatzoudis

British Library Cataloguing-in-Publication Data
A catalogue record for this book is available from the British Library

Library of Congress Cataloging in Publication Data
The psychology of doping in sport / edited by Vassilis Barkoukis, Lambros Lazuras and Haralambos Tsorbatzoudis.
    pages cm. – (Routledge Research in Sport and Exercise Science)
    Includes bibliographical references and index.
    1. Doping in sports. 2. Doping in sports–Psychological aspects.
    3. Athletes–Drug use. I. Barkoukis, Vassilis.
    RC1230.P79 2015
    362.29′088796–dc23   2015002442

ISBN: 978-1-138-79347-7 (hbk)
ISBN: 978-1-315-76110-7 (ebk)

Typeset in Times New Roman
by Wearset Ltd, Boldon, Tyne and Wear

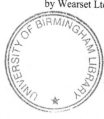

To my children, Yannis and Efthimia, and my wife, Despoina, for their continuous support and understanding

Vassilis Barkoukis

The two most important sources of inspiration in my life: My 9-year-old daughter Elizabeth and my life partner Chryssi

Lambros Lazuras

To Yannis, Stella and Helen for their love and unconditional support

Haralambos Tsorbatzoudis

Contents

Figures

Tables

Contributors

Susan Backhouse is Full Professor and Head of the Centre for Sports Performance in the Institute of Sport, Physical Activity and Leisure (ISPAL) at Leeds Beckett University, UK. She leads an established team of researchers focused on developing understanding of the psychosocial factors influencing doping and nutritional supplement behaviors in sport and society. Her expertise has been sought by the European Union (EU), as a member of the ad-hoc Expert Group on Doping in Sport and as a member of UK Anti-Doping's Research Steering Committee. Her research expertise is complemented by her applied experience in the field of anti-doping education. She is the Education representative on the UK Athletics Anti-Doping Policy and Sport Support Team and a UK Anti-Doping Agency (UKAD) National Trainer. As a result of her researcher–practitioner approach, Susan convened the British Association of Sport and Exercise Sciences Clean Sport Interest Group in 2013.

Vassilis Barkoukis is Assistant Professor of Teaching in Physical Education in the Department of Physical Education and Sport Science at the Aristotle University of Thessaloniki, Greece. His research interests involve the application of social cognitive models in physical education, sport, and physical activity. His research on doping involves the investigation of social cognitive approaches, the development of integrative models in better understanding doping behavior, and the integration of this information in the development of effective anti-doping prevention interventions. He has co-authored more than 120 Greek and international research articles and book chapters, and edited three books. Vassilis has received grants from World Anti-Doping Agency, Australian Research Council, and European Union to study doping in competitive and amateur sports.

Franz Baumgarten is Research Assistant at the Division of Sport and Exercise Psychology at the University of Potsdam. His research focus is primarily on doping in sports. He is interested in the adaption of behavior models and the development of methods to evaluate precedents and antecedents of these performance-enhancing behaviors. He has been part of several international research projects and gained experience as lecturer.

Ralf Brand is Full Professor of Sport and Exercise Psychology at the University of Potsdam, Germany. His research is characterized by a social cognition approach to motivated behavior and often emphasizes processes related to one's automatic evaluations of this behavior. His studies refer to the use of performance enhancing substances in sport and everyday life as well as to health behavior change and maintenance, especially exercise. He serves as the Editor-in-Chief of the *German Journal of Sport Science.*

Paige Clarke received a B.A. from Kenyon College, an M.A. in Developmental Psychology from Columbia University Teacher's College, and is pursuing a Ph.D. in Applied Social Psychology at George Washington University in Washington, DC. Her research focuses on the study of risky health behaviors such as anabolic steroid misuse, prescription stimulant misuse, and alcohol consumption. Her research explores how social-psychological theories such as implicit theory and game theory can influence judgments about the acceptability of misuse of performance-enhancing substances in the academic and athletic domains. Furthermore, she is interested in understanding the relationship between physical activity, sport type, and risky health behaviors.

Lea Cleret first developed her interest in the humanities of sports through the application of bio-ethics to the issue of doping and pursued it to studying the values of sport for her Ph.D. After working within a French multi-sport governing body, she moved to the World Anti-Doping Agency for close to a decade and was the manager of the Education department. Through the management of the Social Science Research Grant Program and the coach education program, and seeing an exponential growth of the evidence base for the development of effective prevention programs, she was keen to develop education programs first for coaches then athletes which would combine the latest findings in social sciences, anti-doping psychology, education and learning technology, whilst taking into account the realities of the field. She has now joined the fight against match-fixing with the International Center for Sport Security and is working on a comprehensive education program which aims to cater to all issues of sport through combined activities.

Tonya Dodge, Ph.D., is Associate Professor of Psychology in the Department of Psychology at George Washington University. Her research is focused generally on attitude formation and decision-making in the context of health. Current work in her lab seeks to better understand how health communication and social contexts shape or change attitudes toward health behaviors. Studies that focus on health communication are designed to understand how individuals interpret and respond to health information. While attitudes reflect a relatively personal aspect of decision-making, work by Dr. Dodge and her research team also focuses on how the social context (e.g., peers, sports participation) can affect health behavior directly and indirectly (e.g., through attitudes).

Robert J. Donovan, Ph.D., is Professor of Behavioural Research in the Faculty of Health Sciences at Curtin, Adjunct Professor in the School of Sport and Exercise Science at the University of Western Australia, and principal of Mentally Healthy WA's Act–Belong–Commit campaign. After a career in commercial marketing he returned to academia in the early 1990s. He has conducted research and program development across a broad range of areas, including alcohol, tobacco and drugs, physical activity and the built environment, child abuse, domestic violence, racism, doping in sport, suicide prevention and mental health. He chairs the World Anti-Doping Agency's Social Sciences Research Sub-Committee.

Anne-Marie Elbe, Ph.D., is an Associate Professor for sport psychology at the University of Copenhagen, Denmark. Her publications and research interests focus on motivational and self-regulatory aspects of athletic performance, recovery, sport psychological diagnostics, doping and cross-cultural aspects. She is section editor for the *International Journal of Sport and Exercise Psychology* and the *Zeitschrift für Sportpsychologie*. She is Vice-President of FEPSAC, the European Federation of Sport Psychology.

Daniel Gucciardi is Senior Research Fellow in the School of Physiotherapy and Exercise Science, Curtin University. His research interests are in applied psychology with a particular focus on personal and contextual factors related to high performance, health behaviors, and well-being in contexts such as sport, education, and the workplace. Within this broad spectrum of research, he is currently involved in several projects that span topics such as doping in sport, mental toughness, life skills development, workplace well-being, and motivational factors in health behaviors (e.g., knee pain, cardiac rehabilitation) and teaching and learning contexts. Some of his research is currently supported by a Curtin Research Fellowship, and funding from the Australian Research Council. He currently serves as an Associate Editor (*Journal of Sport Psychology in Action*) and Section Editor (*European Journal of Sport Science*) for two international scholarly outlets.

Suzanne Guerin is Senior Lecturer in Research Design and Analysis at the School of Psychology, University College Dublin. Her research activity spans a broad range of topics in the area of applied psychology, including bereavement and aging in intellectual disability, knowledge transfer in palliative care, and evaluation research. Given her expertise in qualitative and quantitative research methods she has contributed to a number of studies in sport psychology, such as cheating and doping in sport and the performance environment of elite athletes.

Twan Huybers is Associate Professor in the School of Business at UNSW-Canberra. His research interest and expertise are the innovative application of choice experimental research methods. The areas in which he has applied such methods are wide ranging and include tourist destination choices, student evaluations of university teaching, and sport related applications. He has been involved in doping and sport related research since 2007 which has included best–worst-scaling based studies of the spirit of sport and a choice experiment of athlete doping decisions.

Geoffrey Jalleh is Associate Professor in the School of Public Health, Faculty of Health Sciences at Curtin University. His primary research interests are in health communication and social marketing. He has been involved in formative research, intervention development and evaluation over a broad variety of health areas including doping in sport, tobacco control, alcohol, illicit drugs, physical activity, nutrition, mental health promotion, cancer control, and injury prevention.

Maria Kavussanu is Senior Lecturer in Sport and Exercise Psychology at the University of Birmingham, UK. Her main area of research is morality in sport, which she has been studying for the past 20 years. She is trying to understand why some athletes cheat, whereas others play by the rules, and what are the psychosocial factors that facilitate prosocial and reduce antisocial behavior in sport. Her latest work focuses on socio-moral predictors of doping intentions and the mediating role of moral disengagement and guilt. She has published over 80 journal articles and book chapters. She has received funding for her research from the Economic and Social Research Council (ESRC), the Nuffield Foundation, and the World Anti-Doping Agency, and research awards from the North American Society for the Psychology of Sport and Physical Activity and the European College of Sport Science. Currently, she serves on the ESRC peer review college, is Associate Editor of the *Journal of Applied Sport Psychology*, and sits on the Editorial Board of *Psychology of Sport and Exercise, Sport, Exercise and Performance Psychology*, and *International Review of Sport and Exercise Psychology*.

Kate Kirby completed her Ph.D. at University College Dublin on the psychosocial factors associated with doping. This work was co-funded by the World Anti-Doping Agency and the Irish Sports Council, and contained the first published peer-reviewed research involving interviews with elite athletes who had admitted to doping for performance enhancement. Since then, her work has taken on a more applied sport psychology focus. She was a member of the Team Ireland support staff for the London 2012 Olympics, and more recently, has been employed as a player development manager with the Irish Rugby Union Players' Association.

Lambros Lazuras is Senior Lecturer of Psychology at the International Faculty of the University of Sheffield, CITY College, and a researcher at the University of Rome "La Sapienza." His research focuses primarily on the application of psychological theories of decision-making and goal-setting in health-related and substance use behaviors, and has been funded by Cancer Research UK, the World Anti-Doping Agency, and the European Commission. He has authored research articles, book chapters, and books about the psychological drivers of doping use in elite and amateur sports and participated in several research grants from World Anti-Doping Agency and European Union in relation to doping behavior in sport and other unhealthy behaviors.

Fabio Lucidi is Full Professor in Psychometrics at the Faculty of Medicine and Psychology, Sapienza, University of Rome, where he also earned his Ph.D. degree in 1996. He was Assistant Professor in Psychometrics from 1999 to 2001 and Associate Professor in Psychometrics from 2001 to 2010. He is the President of Italian Psychological Association and member of the Managing Councils of International Society of Sport Psychology. His research interest focuses on the areas of health and sport psychology, with special attention to the processes involved in people's "self-regulation" of health behavior with an emphasis on the psychological variables associated to doping use. He has co-authored more than 200 publications and scientific communications in research areas related to sport psychology, psychometrics, the and health psychology. In these research areas, he led and coordinated national and international research programs and he has developed research collaborations in Australia, Estonia, Finland, Germany, Greece, the United Kingdom, and the United States.

Luca Mallia is Senior Ph.D. Research Assistant, currently working at the University of Rome "Foro Italico." He earned his Ph.D. degree at the Sapienza, University of Rome in 2007, with which he actively collaborated in these years. His research interests are focused on the analysis of the belief systems and decision-making processes underpinning risky behaviors in young people. Over the years, this research focus has been pursued in the context of risky driving and doping use. In this research field, he participated in international research programs, he was co-author of several international publications, and received scientific awards.

James Matthews is College Lecturer in the School of Public Health, Physiotherapy and Sport Science at University College Dublin, Ireland. He is a registered Psychologist who provides psychological support services to international athletes and has additional consulting experience designing mental skills training programms for teams that work in high risk environments. His current research interests and publications focus on the motivational and social cognitive aspects of sport and exercise, and the development of theory-based interventions to enhance sport performance and increase exercise behavior.

Jason Mazanov is Senior Lecturer with the School of Business, UNSW-Canberra. He has been working towards expanding the social science of drugs in sport issues since 2005. This has resulted in publications exploring the role of drugs in sport across the breadth of social science disciplines, including his home discipline of psychology, sociology, economics, ethics, and the law. This work has seen him become a prominent commentator on drugs in sport, having been interviewed over 100 times for Australian and international television, radio, and print media. To ensure little spare time, he is also the founding Editor of the journal *Performance Enhancement and Health*.

Aidan Moran is Professor of Cognitive Psychology and Director of the Psychology Research Laboratory in University College Dublin, Ireland. A Fulbright Scholar, he is the Editor-in-Chief of the *International Review of Sport and Exercise Psychology* and co-author (with John Kremer) of *Pure Sport: Practical Sport Psychology* (2nd edn, Routledge, 2013). A former psychologist to the Irish Olympic Squad, he has advised many of Ireland's leading professional athletes and teams. His research investigates mental/motor imagery, attention (eye-tracking), and the cognitive processes underlying expertise in skilled performance.

Andrea Petróczi is Professor of Public Health at Kingston University, London. Her research is centered on behavioral choices with public health implications, where short-term gains are traded off for potential health consequences later in life; and method development. With a strong commitment to multidisciplinary research spanning across disciplines allied to medicine and psychology, her research explores the various forms of human enhancements (performance, appearance, and experience), reasons that justify and the mental representations of such practices in the broader context of human enhancement. She is an internationally recognized expert in social science doping and anti-doping research. She provides consultancy to the World Anti-Doping Agency, serves as an advisor for the Commonwealth Scholarship Commission in the UK and as a member for the Editorial Boards of *Psychology of Sport and Exercise* (Elsevier); and *Substance Abuse, Treatment, Prevention and Policy* (BMC). Her research has attracted funding from the World Anti-Doping Agency, the National Prevention Research Initiative/Medical Research Council, the British Academy, and the European Council. Recently, in collaboration with Professor Paul Norman, she contributed to the World Anti-Doping Agency's preventive online educational tool (*Athlete Learning Program about Health & Anti-Doping, ALPHA*).

Werner Pitsch is an Interdisciplinary Sports Scientist who works in the Department of Sport Sciences at Saarland University, Saarbrücken, Germany. His research is focused on the methodology of research on deviant behavior but covers other topics from the sociology, psychology, and economics of sport as well. His published work on doping in sport encompasses different perspectives like prevalence studies, predictive values of doping tests, and unintended effects of doping and anti-doping.

Steffi Renninger received a B.A. from the University of the South, and is in pursuit of her doctoral degree in Applied Social Psychology at George Washington University in Washington, DC. Her research interests are in how communication can be used to promote health. Most recently, she has applied this interest to developing an intervention to increase physical activity among college students. These interests extend to the topic of performance enhancing substance use where she is interested in understanding how different types of health communication can affect use of performance enhancing substances.

Haralambos Tsorbatzoudis is Professor of Applied Sport Psychology at the School of Physical Education and Sport Sciences, Aristotle University of Thessaloniki, Greece. He graduated from the University of Athens and received his Ph.D. from the Sport University of Cologne. He served as consultant to a number of elite athletes in track and field, swimming, tennis, shooting, archery, and wrestling. His major research interests are motivation, anxiety, stress, aggression, bullying, ethics, and doping including behavioral interventions for physical activity and generalization of treatment effects in sport and physical activity. He has published more than 150 scientific articles and book chapters, and he has authored or co-authored ten books on sport psychology and physical education.

Lisa Whitaker is a Researcher working as part of the Centre for Sports Performance in the Institute of Sport, Physical Activity and Leisure (ISPAL) at Leeds Beckett University, UK. Her main research interest lies within the anti-doping domain. Specifically, she is interested in developing an understanding of the psychosocial factors influencing doping and nutritional supplement use in sport. She is a member of the British Association of Sport and Exercise Sciences (BASES) Clean Sport Interest Group, and the International Network of Humanistic Doping Researchers (INDHR).

Wanja Wolff is Associate Researcher at the University of Potsdam and works in the Division of Sport and Exercise Psychology. His main interest is understanding and predicting functional substance (ab)use. Specifically, he is interested in peoples' use of psychoactive substances as a means to enhance performance. He is also interested in understanding such enhancement behavior in a broad sense through theories of Self-Regulation and Dual Process Models of Information Processing. He finds it fascinating to investigate how reaction times (e.g., in an Implicit Association Test) might actually be linked to the automatic parts of behavior. Therefore, he is working on the development and testing of reaction time based measures to assess performance-enhancing substance related cognitions.

Arnaldo Zelli is Full Professor of Psychology, currently working at the University of Rome "Foro Italico." He earned his Ph.D. degree at the University of Illinois at Chicago in 1992 and worked in the United States for several years as Senior Research Scholar in several research institutions, including the Center for Child and Family Policy, Sanford Institute of Public Policy Studies (Duke University), and the Vanderbilt University's Department of Psychology and Human Development. His research interests are in the fields of social and personality psychology, and he broadly is interested in belief systems and social judgment processes that may account for differences in social behavior.

Over the many years, this research focus has been pursued in the context of youth antisocial behavior as well as in the context of sport performance. He has been one of the leading scholars in a series of funded research programs focusing on doping substance use conducted among Italian and European professional and amateur sport athletes.

Preface

Since the conception of the Olympic Games in ancient Greece, sports have been promoted as the demonstration of excellence, success, elitism, and competence. The evolution of doping use witnessed in the past four decades poses a threat to the athletes' health and hurts the image of sports and the Olympic Spirit. Starting with the foundation of the World Anti-Doping Agency (WADA) in 1999, there has been an ongoing systematic effort to tackle doping use in sport. A few years ago, in 2005, WADA initiated a shift in the doping prevention paradigm by supporting social science research, in order to identify the psychological mechanisms underlying doping use across all levels of sports. This was expected to help policymakers and anti-doping organizations better understand the reasons why athletes decide to engage in illegitimate performance enhancement methods, and accordingly develop educational and early prevention campaigns to minimize doping use in the future.

A search in the international databases (e.g., EBSCO, ScienceDirect, Scopus, ERIC) revealed that prior to 2005 approximately 30 studies were published on psychological aspects of doping use. From 2005 to 2015 this number has increased to more than 150 published articles. This indicates a growing interest in the psychological study of doping use, and signifies a dynamically developing interdisciplinary field that incorporates psychology, sociology, ethics, and sport science. This book provides a summary of existing research and offers theoretical guidance for future psychological research on doping use. The research presented herein covers a wide range of topics in the psychological study of doping use including: decision-making and action-initiation, dual processes and automaticity, ethical and moral aspects of doping use and anti-doping policies, the role of nutritional supplements, methodological considerations and limitations in measurement and assessment, and the theoretical foundation for preventive interventions against doping use.

So far, a considerable number of published books have dealt with the medical, ethical, and socio-policy aspects of doping. Nevertheless, none of the existing books has addressed the psychological processes underlying doping use in sport and exercise by summarizing the extant research in this area. This book focuses on the psychological processes underlying doping use and discusses: (1) the state-of-the art and future trends in doping research from diverse areas of psychology, including social cognition, automatic, and controlled processes, moral decision-making, and societal/contextual influences on behavior; (2) the methodological considerations surrounding doping assessment in psychological research, including accounts of novel measurement methods (e.g., implicit attitudes); and (3) the implications and future directions for evidence-based preventive interventions and anti-doping education.

The book provides an ideal compendium for researchers involved in the study of doping behavior, especially those interested in the psychosocial processes that explain doping in sports. Academics and higher education students (undergraduate and postgraduate) in the behavioral and sport sciences will also find this book useful in supplementing their studies, and gaining broader knowledge of the doping problem. Finally, professionals that may constitute the athletes' entourage (e.g., physical educators, coaches, sport psychologists, and sports medicine specialists) and policymakers involved in anti-doping education will find useful information about current challenges, needs and priorities in doping prevention.

Overall, the book comprises four parts, and each part has been selected carefully to present a specific, key area of contemporary psychological research on doping. More specifically, Part I taps social psychological processes underlying doping use. In Chapter 1, Kirby, Guerin, Moran and Matthews provide an overview of attitudes and discuss how the Theory of Planned Behavior has been applied in doping research. Zelli, Mallia, and Lucidi discuss, in Chapter 2, the theoretical underpinning and current research on interpersonal appraisals. In Chapter 3, Brand, Wolff, and Baumgarten present the basic tenets of dual process thinking processes and decision-making, and their application in the study of doping use. In the last chapter of this part, Lazuras provides an overview of integrative models of behavioral prediction and discusses the different dimensions (e.g., personal, social/contextual, institutional) that are relevant to the study of doping use.

In Part II readers interested in undertaking research in doping will have the opportunity to read about existing methodological approaches and gaps, and novel applications in doping measurement. Lucidi, Mallia, and Zelli summarize research evidence from the main quantitative approaches, discuss the qualitative methods used so far in the study of doping use, and offer suggestions for mixed-method designs that can be implemented in future doping research. In Chapter 6, Gucciardi, Jalleh, and Donovan provide an overview of the literature on social desirability in doping research and offer suggestions to overcome socially desirable responding. Petróczi, in Chapter 7, provides an overview of the direct and indirect measurements utilized in psychological research of doping, and their potential to "reveal" honest responses about doping use and beliefs in future studies. In the last chapter of Part II, Pitsch provides an outline of the development of randomized response methods and their capacity to generate reliable responses in doping research.

Part III tackles the psychological study of ethical and moral issues in doping research. Cleret discusses the nature and origin of the basic concepts of sport and sport values, and provides the philosophical basis for the moral reasoning that is inherent in the current anti-doping paradigm. In Chapter 10, Mazanov and Huybers critically discuss the Spirit of Sport concept and address the role of morality. Kavussanu, in Chapter 11, presents relevant theory and empirical evidence pertaining to the study of moral disengagement in sport, and its relevance to doping behavior. Finally, in Chapter 12, Elbe and Brand discuss the role of moral reasoning in the context of anti-doping prevention, and present the first intervention that was developed to tackle doping use by improving athletes' moral reasoning.

Finally, Part IV provides a roadmap for future doping research and the development of evidence-based interventions. Backhouse and Whitaker, in Chapter 13, discuss the risks stemming from nutritional supplement use, athletes' reasons for using nutritional supplements, and the hypothesis that use of nutritional supplements can act as a gateway to doping use. In Chapter 14, Dodge, Clarke, and Renninger discuss the potential utility of parent-based interventions in preventing doping use among adolescent athletes. In the next chapter, Barkoukis presents evidence about the anti-doping interventions employed so far and critically discusses how the existing empirical research on doping can inform future anti-doping interventions. In the last chapter of the book, Tsorbatzoudis, Lazuras, and Barkoukis highlight the ten most important questions for future psychological research on doping.

We truly hope that readers will find the book timely, useful and thought-provoking, and incorporate the ideas presented herein in their research endeavors.

Vassilis Barkoukis, Lambros Lazuras, and Haralambos Tsorbatzoudis

Acknowledgments

This book is the culmination of endless meetings, arguments, and creative discussions among the editors about the very nature of doping use, and the driving forces that lead athletes to the use of various prohibited performance enhancement substances and methods. We set sail for a journey in doping research almost a decade ago, when the foundations of the research presented in this book were first established. Skype meetings, conference presentations, and round-table discussions in interesting places across Europe, Asia, and Australia set the scene for exchange of ideas and fruitful collaborations amongst researchers interested in the study of doping use. Most of these researchers are the contributing authors in this book, and we would like to acknowledge their effort, commitment, and dedication in realizing this joint endeavor. This book would never have been realized without their valuable input. We are also grateful to the anonymous reviewers who also did an excellent job by providing timely, detailed, and constructive feedback within tight deadlines.

Part I

Psychosocial processes underlying doping use

1 Doping in elite sport

Linking behavior, attitudes, and psychological theory

Kate Kirby, Suzanne Guerin, Aidan Moran, and James Matthews

Recent years have witnessed an upsurge of research interest in the psychosocial factors associated with competitive athletes' propensity to use prohibited performance-enhancing drugs (PEDs; e.g., see Barkoukis *et al.* 2013; Hauw and Mohamed 2015; Hodge *et al.* 2013; Morente-Sánchez and Zabala 2013). This practice is commonly known as "doping" and typically refers to athletes' proclivity to use "illegitimate performance enhancement substances and methods" (Lazuras *et al.* 2010: 694). Although the problem of doping in sport may appear to be a relatively new phenomenon, it has a surprisingly long history. For example, prohibited substances such as caffeine and cocaine were used by cyclists in a bid to enhance competitive performance as far back as the 1890s (Hoberman 1998). Unfortunately, studies on doping in elite athletes are afflicted by at least two unresolved issues. First, the links between doping attitudes and doping behavior have not received sufficient research attention to date. Second, the role of psychological theory in elucidating these links has not been addressed adequately. Therefore, the purpose of the present chapter is to address these two issues. We shall proceed as follows. Following an overview of "attitudes" and approaches to attitude measurement, we shall consider the measurement of attitudes to doping in sport. After that, we shall explain how the Theory of Planned Behavior (TPB; Ajzen 1991) has been applied to studies of doping in sport. Finally, we shall explore some potentially fruitful new directions for research in this field.

The nature of attitudes

In psychology, the term "attitudes" refers to the preferences and evaluations (or likes and dislikes) that people form in relation to specific objects of their thought (Banaji and Heiphetz 2010). Reflecting this view, Eagly and Chaiken defined an attitude as "a psychological tendency that is expressed by evaluating a particular entity with some degree of favour or disfavour" (1993: 1). Attitudes can be formed to groups of people (e.g., athletes), phenomena (e.g., social media), situations (e.g., competitions), and even to abstract ideas (e.g., sportspersonship), and social practices (e.g., doping in sport). Regardless of the particular target involved, however, attitudes are multidimensional in structure, with cognitive (i.e., beliefs about the target of the attitude), affective (i.e., positive or negative feelings toward such targets), and behavioral (i.e., whether or not any actions occur as consequences of one's evaluations) components. To illustrate how these components may interact, one might believe that athletes who engage in doping are "cheats" (cognitive component) who deserve scorn (affective component) and who should be banned from the sport in which they participate (behavioral component). Historically, many theorists have traditionally regarded attitudes as relatively stable and enduring personal dispositions that are stored in memory and can be "pulled out" and used when required. On the other hand, more recent researchers such as Schwartz (2007) favor the view that attitudes are adaptive reactions to environmental demands – and hence, are temporary, context-specific judgments constructed from currently accessible information. In attempting to resolve this disagreement, Bohner and Dickel proposed that researchers should "take into account both stable and situationally variable aspects of attitudes" (2011: 394).

The assumption that attitudes predict behavior accurately is highly questionable. For example, a seminal review by Wicker (1969) of 42 relevant studies found that the correlation between attitudes and behavior ranged between 0.15 and 0.30. He concluded that overall "it is considerably more likely that attitudes will be unrelated or only very slightly related to overt behaviors than that attitudes will be closely related to actions" (1969: 64) because "only rarely can as much as 10% of the variance in overt behavioral measures be accounted for by attitudinal data" (1969: 65). After Wicker's (1969) review, social psychologists identified a host of variables moderating the relationship between attitudes and behavior. This line of research led to the conclusion that people's behavior is influenced by many factors (such as situational constraints and peer pressure) other than attitudes.

Approaches to attitude measurement: from explicit to implicit

Scientific approaches to attitude measurement began in the 1920s (e.g., Thurstone 1928) and 1930s (e.g., Likert 1932) with the use of verbal self-report scales designed to assess people's beliefs, opinions, and values. The rationale underlying this self-report approach is that people are both willing and able to accurately introspect on, and subsequently report, the contents of their own thoughts. Until the late 1970s, the use of such explicit self-report scales was the most popular approach in this field. However, around that time, two problems occurred which prompted researchers to shift from explicit to *implicit* (i.e., not accessible to conscious awareness) attitude measurement (Bohner and Dickel 2011; Banaji and Heiphetz 2010). First, response biases such as "social desirability" emerged with the discovery that people tend to hide their true attitudes in an effort to present themselves in a positive light (e.g., by suppressing negative attitudes to groups such as immigrants). Second, the assumption that attitudes are open to introspective access was challenged by evidence (see review by

Nisbett and Wilson 1977) that people often do not know – and hence cannot report reliably on – the reasons for their own behavior. In an effort to address these problems, certain implicit strategies for measuring attitudes (Fazio and Olson 2003) have been developed (see Chapters 3 and 7). According to Bohner and Dickel (2011), the objectives of these strategies are not only to counteract people's response biases but also to explore those aspects of people's attitudes that are not open to conscious introspection and control. Briefly, both of these approaches assume that evaluative associations in a respondent's mind should produce different response times to categorical stimuli that represent the attitude object in question. These differences in response time may be used to infer implicit attitudes on the part of the respondent.

The measurement of attitudes to doping in sport – from athletes to entourage

Numerous studies have measured explicit attitudes to doping among a variety of athletic populations. Among the topics investigated in this largely atheoretical research literature are attitudes to doping in different sports (Alaranta *et al.* 2006), attitudes to doping and supplementation (Bloodworth *et al.* 2012), projected motives for doping in sport (Laure and Reinsberger 1995; Özdemir *et al.* 2005; Scarpino *et al.* 1990), and attitudes to drug testing and education (Striegel *et al.* 2002; Waddington *et al.* 2005). In such studies, researchers typically developed custom-built, doping-related questionnaires. Unfortunately, given the lack of psychometric detail available in this research, definitive conclusions regarding athletes' attitudes to doping are not possible (Backhouse *et al.* 2007).

Fortunately, descriptive, "one-shot" studies of attitudes of doping have been increasingly supplanted by theoretically driven research. For example, Sas-Nowosielski and Swiatkowska (2008) found that athletes who were high in ego orientation and low in task orientation displayed significantly more positive (permissive) attitudes to doping than those who displayed a low ego, high task orientation. Similarly, Kirby (2011) reported that certain subscales significantly predicted more lenient attitudes to doping, namely: coach criticism, unequal recognition, and ego orientation. These studies also determined that males tended to have significantly more favorable attitudes toward doping than females – a finding that has been replicated in other studies on doping in sport (Alaranta *et al.* 2006; Lucidi *et al.* 2008). The cornerstone of such research is the proposition that anti-doping education and deterrence methods cannot be fully effective unless athletes' attitudes toward doping and their motives for banned substance use are more clearly understood (Lucidi *et al.* 2008).

In addition to the preceding research, some studies have explored the knowledge and attitudes of coaching staff in relation to doping in sport (Fung and Yuan 2006; Laure *et al.* 2001; Shirazi and Tricker 2005). Whereas Shirazi and Tricker (2005) set out to explore athletic directors' policies on drug testing, Laure *et al.* (2001) investigated the frequency with which coaches are asked for information about doping by their athletes. Unfortunately, little effort has been made to determine the factors that shape the coaches' attitudes to doping, or to examine the factors that predicted coaches' intentions to promote anti-doping among their athletes (Backhouse and McKenna 2013). Interestingly, according to Waddington and Smith (2009), "if we wish to understand the use of drugs in elite sport then it is crucial that we understand the centrality of the relationship between elite level athletes and practitioners of sports medicine" (2009: 82). However, surprisingly few studies have attempted to understand the doping-related knowledge and attitudes of sports physicians. Indeed, as Backhouse *et al.* concluded, "the literature in relation to doping and the medical population is weak" (2007: 74). The earliest studies that examined attitudes to doping using physicians as participants focused on estimations of the prevalence of doping (Scarpino *et al.* 1990). This study by Scarpino *et al.* was significant because it was the first of its kind in Europe to assess the knowledge, attitudes, and perceived prevalence of doping among people involved in sport. However, very little information is provided about the characteristics and specific responses of the 102 physicians surveyed, except that 21 percent of them (compared to 30 percent of coaches, managers, and athletes) indicated that athletic performance can be enhanced by doping. Laure and colleagues examined attitudes to, and knowledge of, doping in sport among 202 French physicians (Laure *et al.* 2003) and retail pharmacists (Laure and Kriebitzsch-Lejeune 2000).

Unfortunately, as mentioned previously, researchers investigating the attitudes to doping of athletes, coaches and support staff have typically used custom-built measures rather than systematically validated ones. Indeed, many of the preceding studies did not report the rationale underlying their scale development process or provide adequate information on the psychometric adequacy of the scales used (Backhouse *et al.* 2007) – problems which hamper accurate interpretation of the results of the studies. Accordingly, Backhouse *et al.* (2007) concluded that direct comparisons across such studies are difficult to make. Furthermore, as the psychometric properties of these scales are rarely reported, doubts exist about the validity and generalizability of findings in this domain. Addressing this issue, Petróczi and Aidman (2009) argued that when test scores are interpreted as attitudes and inferences are made about athletic populations based on these scores, adequate reliability and validity are essential requirements. Unfortunately, many of the studies that report athletes', coaches', and physicians' attitudes to doping fail to adequately define the term "doping" itself – or to give sufficient detail on the development or content of the questionnaires employed. In fact, Backhouse *et al.* (2007) suggested that the term "doping attitude" had been so poorly defined that frequently the doping *knowledge* of athletes rather than their *explicit attitudes* has been surveyed.

An interesting addition to the research literature on doping has been the "Performance Enhancement Attitude Scale" (PEAS; Petróczi and Aidman 2009), which is a self-report measure examining *generalized doping attitude* (defined as "an individual's predisposition toward the use of banned performance enhancing substances and methods" Petróczi 2007: 7) (see also Moran *et al.* 2008). A positive association with elevated PEAS score and self-admitted doping has been reported (Petróczi and Aidman 2008). Although this finding does not demonstrate conclusively that permissive attitudes to doping predict doping behavior, it does provide preliminary evidence that the two concepts are related.

Nevertheless, self-report scales (such as the PEAS) are marred by problems of response bias – or the tendency of participants to answer questions that reflect what they think the investigator wants to hear rather than as an index of their true beliefs. Recently, Morente-Sánchez and Zabala noted that "there could be a significant difference between what athletes say and what they really think" (2013: 410). Interestingly, this issue of the validity of athletes' self-reported attitudes to doping was examined by Gucciardi *et al.* (2010), who showed that, as expected, favorable attitudes to doping were associated with greater susceptibility to doping. However, the strength of this relationship between attitudes to doping and doping susceptibility was moderated by social desirability – a finding that highlights the importance of controlling for this latter variable when conducting self-report studies of doping in athletes.

To conclude this section, a promising new direction in doping measurement reflects the move toward the use of *implicit* rather than explicit assessment techniques (see also Chapters 3 and 7 of this volume). This move has been prompted by a desire to circumvent the biases afflicting explicit attitude assessment (for a review see Fazio and Olson 2003). Reflecting this new approach, Brand *et al.* (2014) argued that *indirect* attitude measures could prove valuable in studies of doping in sport. However, implicit measures are not unanimously favored. For example, Petróczi (2013) provided a critical consideration of the use of response times in the indirect measurement of doping attitudes.

As psychological research in the field of doping has evolved, researchers such as Lucidi *et al.* (2008) and Barkoukis *et al.* (2013) have attempted to explain theoretically, rather than simply describe, key issues. More generally, recent studies have moved away from descriptive accounts and turned increasingly to social psychological theories (e.g., self-determination theory, Deci and Ryan 2000; achievement goal theory, Nicholls 1984) in their quest to understand the relationship between athletes' attitudes to, and engagement in, doping behavior. Of the various psychological theories available to doping researchers, perhaps the most influential (e.g., see Lucidi *et al.* 2008; Goulet *et al.* 2010) is the Theory of Planned Behavior (TPB; Ajzen 1991). This theory, which was developed in order to explain behaviors which are not fully under volitional control, has been used extensively to predict health risk behaviors such as self-harm, driving behavior and substance abuse (see Ajzen 2014; Armitage and Conner 2001). Given this latter application, the TPB offers researchers a useful theoretical perspective from which to investigate doping behavior in sport.

Applying the Theory of Planned Behavior to doping in sport

The TPB has exerted a seminal influence on recent studies of doping in sport (e.g., Barkoukis *et al.* 2013; Chan *et al.* 2015). Although space limitations preclude a detailed explanation of the TPB, one of its central tenets is the idea that the most proximal determinant of behavior is a person's intention to engage in that behavior (i.e., the conscious decision to perform a behavior in the future). This theory also postulates that behavioral intentions are determined by three other factors – the individual's attitude toward the behavior, his or her subjective norms (i.e., the perceived social pressures the person feels to perform the behavior) and perceived behavioral control (PBC; the extent to which a person believes the behavior is under their active control). Attitudes, subjective norms, and PBC are thought to be underpinned by corresponding salient beliefs, namely behavioral, normative, and control beliefs. The TPB suggests that these beliefs not only reflect the underlying cognitive structure of these variables but also that behavior is ultimately a function of salient beliefs regarding the behavior. Specifically, attitudes are held to be determined by behavioral beliefs which, in turn, reflect the perceived likely consequences of engaging in the targeted behavior, weighted by an evaluation of these consequences. Normative beliefs are thought to influence subjective norms and comprise the expectations of important others and the extent to which an individual is motivated to comply with such expectations. Finally, "perceived behavioral control" is underpinned by control beliefs which refer to the factors that can enable or inhibit performance of the targeted behavior and the perceived impact these factors may have on the behavior (Ajzen 1991; Armitage and Conner 2001). The components of the TPB and how they interact can be seen in Figure 1.1. Typically, behavioral intention is reported as the strongest predictor of behavior, while attitude has the largest effect on behavioral intention (Armitage and Conner 2001). From this brief synopsis of TPB, an important implication is that attitudes, subjective norms, and PBC may serve as proxy indices of behavior through their *direct* relationship with behavioral intention and their *indirect* relationship with behavior.

Building on the preceding assumption, researchers guided by the TPB have reported how variables such as doping attitudes and subjective norms can predict doping intention and behavior (Ntoumanis *et al.* 2014). Consequently, some doping researchers have argued that it is not necessary to collect data on actual

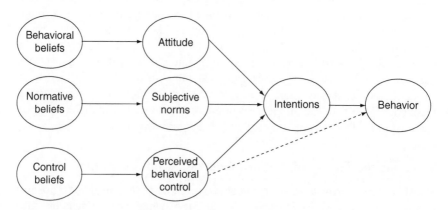

Figure 1.1 Overview of the TPB (source: adapted from Armitage and Conner 2001).

doping behavior from competitive athletes. Instead, assessing an athlete's behavioral intention to dope and other TPB variables such as attitudes toward doping may be sufficient to better understand doping behavior and its antecedents. This assumption is the cornerstone of several early models of PED use in sport (e.g., those of Donovan *et al.* 2002; Petróczi and Aidman 2008) and has also influenced more recent models (e.g., Whitaker *et al.* 2014). However, caution must be applied when considering this type of approach, as troubling issues remain. First, there are concerns regarding self-reporting and social desirability when exploring athletes' attitudes toward doping and doping intentions. Therefore, the effects of social desirability must be accounted for in future studies (Lazuras *et al.* 2010). Second, there is a lack of empirical evidence to support the assumption that doping-related attitudes can reliably predict doping behavior. As a result, future research should consider using experimental studies to examine the causal relationships between these theoretical variables (Ntoumanis *et al.* 2014).

Overall, however, there are distinct advantages in the TPB assumption that attitudes can serve as proxies of behavior. For example, at a methodological level, it is helpful because it enables researchers to collect data from large samples of athletes conveniently and systematically. These data can then be included in multiple regression models, thereby increasing the statistical power of the analysis and allowing greater confidence in study results. A further advantage of measuring attitudes to doping – as opposed to doping behavior – is that it facilitates the recruitment of samples of elite athletes rather than those of students and/or recreational gym users.

In summary, the TPB has been used frequently in doping research, and related theoretical variables such as attitudes toward doping and doping intentions are believed to predict doping behavior. However, researchers have begun to use variables outside of the TPB to enhance the predictive value of this theoretical framework, and some of these variables will be considered in the next section of this chapter. This leads to the intriguing question as to whether or not an extended TPB or integrated theoretical frameworks as proposed by Barkoukis *et al.* (2013; see also Chapter 4) may further develop our understanding of doping behavior.

Empirical research on doping in sport influenced by the Theory of Planned Behavior

One of the earliest applications of the TPB on the study of doping in sport was that undertaken by Tricker and Connolly (1997). These researchers investigated the attitudes to doping of a large (over 500 respondents) sample of student athletes and succeeded in identifying athletes "at risk" of doping based on their stated behavioral intention to use steroids, human growth hormone, amphetamines, cocaine, and marijuana. However, the way Tricker and Connolly's (1997) items were generated in order to measure attitude, subjective norm, and behavioral control variables was unclear so, in the absence of data on questionnaire reliability and validity, their findings need to be evaluated cautiously. With that caveat in mind, these authors reported that the most significant factors influencing the decisions of their participants in relation to PED use were subjective norms that related to the impact of drug testing, peer influence, and a fear of detection. Despite some conceptual confusion,[1] the studies by Tricker and colleagues were valuable because they provided some initial empirical insights into the complex relationship between attitudes, subjective norms, perceived behavioral control, and behavioral intent. Interestingly, these studies also showed that the decisions of at-risk athletes *not* to use drugs were determined primarily by perceived *external* rather than internal influences – a discovery that yielded useful information for the future development of drug education programs. More recently, Wiefferink *et al.* (2008) surveyed 144 gym users to identify the social psychological determinants underlying PED use among bodybuilders, powerlifters, and combat-sport athletes. They examined numerous variables including behavioral intention, attitudes to doping, personal norms, social influences, background characteristics, and self-efficacy. About a third of the respondents had used PEDs in the past, and 29 percent reported an intention to use them in the future. The strongest predictors of future doping intentions were previous PED use, followed by personal norms and beliefs about the performance outcomes of drug use. Non-users had a more restrictive morality toward drug use than current or ex-users. This abstinence group also estimated the number of significant others who were drug users as lower than did current or ex-PED users, who tended to attribute greater advantages to the use of banned substances, and minimized the risks involved.

Based on their results, Wiefferink *et al.* (2008) concluded that the decision by a gym population to use PEDs may not be due to a rational individual choice. Instead, it may reflect norms and past behaviors. So, Wiefferink *et al.* (2008) argued for the inclusion of a "personal norms" variable in the TPB. Unfortunately, although they did publish some of the items that made up the personal norm subscale of their questionnaire, they did not adequately define the term.

Additional doping research spawned by the TPB was conducted by Lucidi *et al.* (2004, 2008) and Zelli *et al.* (2010). To illustrate, Lucidi *et al.* (2004) aimed to evaluate whether behavioral intention to use doping substances can be predicted by TPB variables. In order to improve the predictive power and relevance of the TPB to the specific, ethically questionable behavior under observation, they also added the variable *moral disengagement*. This study was strengthened by the large population employed ($n=952$), 3.1 percent of whom reported doping use in the preceding three months. Attitude toward doping use was the strongest predictor of intention to dope, followed by subjective norms. Perceived behavioral control showed a small but significant relationship to doping intent. This finding is unusual, since subjective norms are very often the weakest predictor of intentions in TPB testing (Armitage and Conner 2001). Just like Wiefferink *et al.* (2008), Lucidi *et al.* (2004) explained this unexpected finding by highlighting the crucial role played by significant others (e.g., peers, coaches, and athlete support staff) in an individual's decision to engage in doping. Moral reasoning and past use of ergogenic aids each made a significant contribution to adolescents' intentions to engage in doping. Although Lucidi *et al.*'s (2004) findings are promising in identifying the various determinants of intentions to engage in doping, they are limited in their application to elite-level sport, since less than one-third of the respondents were classified as "competitive athletes." Furthermore, the authors highlighted the need to establish a relationship between the intention to engage in doping and subsequent actual use of PEDs to definitively test the determinants of doping *behavior* using a longitudinal research design, rather than simply relying on evidence of doping intent.

In a follow-up study, Lucidi *et al.* (2008) attempted to overcome the preceding limitations by surveying a very large (*n*=762) sample of adolescent students and repeating the process again after three months. The aim of this longitudinal research was to analyse the effects of social-cognitive mechanisms on adolescents' substance use over time. Just like Wiefferink *et al.* (2008), Lucidi *et al.* (2008) measured doping-specific, self-regulatory efficacy (i.e., participants' beliefs in their ability to withstand pressure to engage in doping) and their levels of moral disengagement.

Testing at time 1 showed that strong positive doping attitudes, beliefs that others would approve of doping, convictions that doping can be justified and a low capacity to resist situational pressure were related to positive *intentions* to engage in doping. Intentions to engage in doping behavior significantly predicted differences between doping users and nonusers, even if this effect was quite small (0.17) and over a short time period of three months. However, this study provided preliminary evidence supporting the value of measuring doping intent in the absence of reliable and objective data on doping behavior. Specifically, at time 2 participants with stronger moral disengagement scores were more likely to *have* doped or used supplements. Favorable attitudes toward doping and strong subjective norms also predicted doping use. In contrast, adolescents with strong self-regulatory efficacy were more likely to resist PED use. In this study the final model accounted for 55 percent of the variance, and all psychological factors measured, with the exception of perceived behavioral control, exerted significant effects on behavioral intentions to dope.

Influenced by Lucidi *et al.*'s (2008) findings, Zelli *et al.* (2010) examined the additional contribution of *social influences* as potential moderators of the relationship between personal beliefs and doping intentions and behavior. They reported that adolescents who were more inclined to assign positive meaning to someone's motives for soliciting substance use also held stronger favorable attitudes toward doping, assigned a stronger value to significant others' approval for using PEDs, and expressed stronger intentions to engage in doping in the future. For example, athletes who considered that solicitation to use doping substances was motivated by a concern for their welfare showed stronger intentions to dope than those who interpreted such solicitations as being motivated by the counterparty's personal interest. Unfortunately, the participants who held problematic appraisals of doping situations did not report any *actual* doping use during the longitudinal study, so the prediction model was only applied to doping intent and not to doping behavior.

Overall, Zelli *et al.* (2010) found that doping beliefs accounted for about 50 percent of the variance in doping intentions. Longitudinal analysis revealed that intentions accounted for nearly 75 percent of the variation in adolescents' actual doping behavior, again providing evidence for the suitability of the TPB in social and psychological research on doping in sport. However, by selecting as participants a cross section of adolescents (rather than exclusively competitive athletes), the study assumed that either performance enhancement *or* physical appearance motives characterize possible doping use.

A more recent study by Lazuras *et al.* (2010) examined other contextual factors in the doping process by extending beyond the traditional TPB variables to include "situational temptation." This latter construct was defined as an external control mechanism which reflects people's eagerness to endorse behaviors under specific circumstances. Lazuras *et al.* (2010) also extended the measurement of subjective norms (beliefs about what *ought to be* happening) to include the concept of "descriptive norms" (beliefs about what *is* happening). These authors recruited impressive participant numbers of elite adult athletes ($n=750$) for their study. However, athletes' classification as "elite" is questionable. Overall, their model predicted 69 percent of the variance in doping intentions. Traditional TPB variables, as well as descriptive norms and situational temptation, significantly predicted doping intentions. The strength of the relationship between doping intentions and behavior was not reported due to the cross-sectional nature of the research design. However, the overall significance of the model justifies the inclusion of these additional variables in research on doping with elite athletes, and highlights the relative importance of contextual, as well as individual, factors in influencing athletes' doping decisions.

In one of the few studies attempting to understand the predictors of coaches' doping-related behaviors, Fung and Yuan (2006) tested the relationships between perceived and actual knowledge, subjective norms, attitudes and behavioral intent of over 100 "community coaches" in Hong Kong. Partial support for the TPB was reported, in that coaches' behavioral intent was significantly related to their attitudes to doping. However, the relationship between subjective norm and behavioral intent was not found to be significant. One of the clear limitations of the study may account for this finding. Specifically, the questions relating to subjective norm explored the notion of international sport and world records, but the population tested were described as "community coaches." Therefore, the questionnaire items may not have adequately captured their "recreational" sport experience. The subjective norm subscale was also criticized by Backhouse *et al.* (2007), as being more about what *is* happening (descriptive norms), than about what *ought to be* happening (subjective norms). Unfortunately, the basic correlational statistics employed in the study also precluded any inferences about *predictors* of coaches' behavioral intent.

As outlined above, research using the TPB has provided some encouraging evidence to support certain factors that are predictive of doping behavior in sport. However, as a large proportion of the variance in PED use among elite athletes remains unexplained, there is clearly a need to extend beyond the traditional TPB variables and to develop a more comprehensive doping explanatory theory. The addition of individual psychological variables such as motivational profiles, morality, and efficacy beliefs, as well as the inclusion of additional situational and systemic variables, should further enhance our understanding of the problem.

New directions for research on doping in sport

At least four new directions may be identified for future research on doping in sport. To begin with, a major limitation of current research on doping behavior is the lack of theoretically driven studies using elite athletes as participants. Although psychological theories such as the TPB provide a fertile framework for hypothesis testing in doping research, there is a dearth of elite athlete participants in studies in this field. Existing studies of doping behavior have struggled to elicit information about athletes' experiences with PEDs, even when anonymity is assured (Petróczi *et al.* 2010; Uvacsek *et al.* 2009). Accordingly, many studies on doping in sport use participants sampled from proxy populations such as recreational gym users, bodybuilders and/or student athletes. Acknowledging this limitation, Quirk (2009) urged doping researchers to try to recruit more elite athletes for their studies in order "to confirm or disconfirm results from amateur or collegiate sporting contexts" (2009: 389). Unfortunately, even when athletes are persuaded to participate in doping research, sample sizes are invariably small. To illustrate, assuming a doping prevalence rate of approximately 2 percent (Petróczi *et al.* 2008) researchers would need to survey about 2,500 athletes in order to obtain an actual sample of 50 suitable participants. Clearly, such large-scale surveys are prohibitive for financial and logistical reasons. Overall, however, it is essential that researchers should continue to recruit elite athletes for studies of doping in sport. Second, a major challenge facing doping researchers is the issue of how to establish the degree to which doping-related attitudes and intentions can reliably predict doping behavior. In this regard, one promising strategy (see Barkoukis *et al.*'s 2013 "meta-theory" perspective) is to develop integrated theoretical models designed to explore the risk factors that might help to explain doping intentions. Another strategy could involve the use of longitudinal research designs to test the relationship between doping-related attitudes and intentions (e.g., see Lucidi *et al.* 2008). Such studies suggest that athletes' beliefs and intentions *can* predict their actual doping behaviors. However, the strength of this relationship is unclear. Third, in the light of recent research by Chan *et al.* (2015), it would be interesting to explore the nature of doping *avoidance* intentions and behavior among elite athletes. Changing the target behavior under investigation from doping behavior to doping avoidance behavior in TPB studies would also further facilitate better quality, theoretically driven research with athlete support staff, given that questions on personal consumption of PEDs are irrelevant to them. Finally, future research on doping in sport could benefit significantly from developments in neuroscience. Specifically, as brain regions such as the amygdala are known to be activated during evaluative judgments (Banaji and Heiphetz 2010), it would be intriguing to investigate the patterns of cortical activation elicited among athletes during tasks that require rapid responses to doping-related scenarios/dilemmas.

Note

1 Tricker and Connolly defined subjective norms as the students' "perception of the norms within his/her social environment" (i.e., of the penalties for using) (1997: 116). Curiously, however, this definition seems at odds with Ajzen's definition of the same variable: "the perceived social pressure to perform or not to perform the behaviour" (1991: 188). In fact, Ajzen's definition of perceived behavioral control, "perceived ease or difficulty of performing the behaviour ... assumed to reflect past experience as well as anticipated impediments and obstacles" (1991: 188), seems to better reflect Tricker and Connolly's (1997) interpretation of subjective norms.

References

Ajzen, I. (1991). The theory of planned behaviour. *Organizational Behavior and Human Decision Processes*, *50*, 179–211.

Ajzen, I. (2014). The theory of planned behaviour is alive and well, and not ready to retire: A commentary on Sniehotta, Presseau, and Araújo-Soares. *Health Psychology Review*. Epub ahead of print http://dx.doi.org/10.1080/17437199.2014.883474.

Alaranta, A., Alaranta, H., Holmila, J., Palmu, P., Pietilä, K., and Helenius, I. (2006). Self-reported attitudes of elite athletes towards doping: Differences between type of sport. *International Journal of Sports Medicine*, *27*, 842–846.

Armitage, C. J. and Conner, M. (2001). Efficacy of the theory of planned behaviour: A meta-analytic review. *British Journal of Social Psychology*, *40*, 471–499.

Backhouse, S. H. and McKenna, J. (2013). Reviewing coaches' knowledge, attitudes and beliefs regarding doping in sport. *International Journal of Sports Science and Coaching*, *7*, 176–175.

Backhouse, S. H., Atkin, A., McKenna, J., and Robinson, S. (2007). *International literature review: Attitudes, behaviours, knowledge and education. Drugs in Sport: Past, present and future*. Montreal, Canada: World Anti-Doping Agency (WADA). www.wada-ama.org/en/resources/social-science/international-literature-review-attitudes-behaviours-knowledge-and (accessed March 4, 2007).

Banaji, M. R. and Heiphetz, L. (2010). Attitudes. In S. T. Fiske, D. T. Gilbert, and G. Lindzey (eds.), *Handbook of social psychology*, Volume 1 (353–393). New York: John Wiley.

Barkoukis, V., Lazuras, L., Tsorbatzoudis, H., and Rodafinos, A. (2013). Motivational and social cognitive predictors of doping intentions in elite sports: An integrated approach. *Scandinavian Journal of Medicine & Science in Sports*, *23*, e230–e240.

Bloodworth, A. J., Petróczi, A., Bailey, R., Pearce, G., and McNamee, M. J. (2012). Doping and supplementation: The attitudes of talented young athletes. *Scandinavian Journal of Medicine & Science in Sports*, *22*, 293–301.

Bohner, G. and Dickel, N. (2011). Attitudes and attitude change. *Annual Review of Psychology*, *62*, 391–427.

Brand, R., Wolff, W., and Thieme, D. (2014). Using response-time latencies to measure athletes' doping attitudes: The brief implicit attitude test identifies substance abuse in bodybuilders. *Substance Abuse Treatment, Prevention, and Policy*, *9* (*36*), 1–10.

Chan, D. K. C., Hardcastle, S., Dimmock, J. A., Lentillon-Kaestner, V., Donovan, R. J., Burgin, M., and Hagger, M. S. (2015). Modal salient belief and social cognitive variables of anti-doping behaviours in sport: Examining an extended model of the theory of planned behaviour. *Psychology of Sport and Exercise, 16,* 164–174.

Deci, E. L. and Ryan, R. M. (2000). The "what" and "why" of goal pursuits: Human needs and the self-determination of behaviour. *Psychological Inquiry, 11,* 227–268.

Donovan, R. J., Egger, G., Kapernick, V., and Mendoza, J. (2002). A conceptual framework for achieving performance enhancing drug compliance in sport. *Sports Medicine, 32,* 269–284.

Eagly, A. H. and Chaiken, S. (1993). *The psychology of attitudes.* Orlando, FL: Harcourt Brace Jovanovich.

Fazio, R. H. and Olson, M. A. (2003). Implicit measures in social cognition research; Their meaning and use. *Annual Review of Psychology, 54,* 297–327.

Fung, L. and Yuan, Y. (2006). Performance enhancement drugs: Knowledge, attitude and intended behaviour among community coaches in Hong Kong. *The Sport Journal, 9* (*3*). Unpaginated.

Goulet, C., Valois, P., Buist, A., and Côté, M. (2010). Predictors of the use of performance-enhancing substances by young athletes. *Clinical Journal of Sports Medicine, 20,* 243–248.

Gucciardi, D. G., Jalleh, G., and Donovan, R. J. (2010). Does social desirability influence the relationship between doping attitudes and doping susceptibility in athletes? *Psychology of Sport and Exercise, 11,* 479–486.

Hauw, D. and Mohamed, S. (2015). Patterns in the situated activity of substance use in the careers of elite doping athletes. *Psychology of Sport & Exercise, 16,* 156–163.

Hodge, K., Hargreaves, E. A., Gerrard, D., and Lonsdale, C. (2013). Psychological mechanisms underlying doping attitudes in sport: Motivation and moral disengagement. *Journal of Sport & Exercise Psychology, 35,* 419–432.

Hoberman, J. (1998). A pharmacy on wheels – the tour de France doping scandal. Available at https://thinksteroids.com/articles/festina-tour-de-france-doping-scandal/ (accessed November 24, 2014).

Kirby, K. (2011). *Doping in sport: An empirical investigation of influential psychological, social and contextual factors.* Unpublished Doctoral Dissertation, University College Dublin, Ireland.

Laure, P. and Kriebitzsch-Lejeune, A. (2000). Retail pharmacists and doping in sports: Knowledge and attitudes. A national survey in France. *Science and Sports, 15,* 141–146.

Laure, P. and Reinsberger, H. (1995). Doping and high-level endurance walkers. Knowledge and representation of a prohibited practice. *Journal of Sports Medicine and Physical Fitness, 35,* 228–231.

Laure, P., Bisinger, C., and Lecerf, T. (2003). General practitioners and doping in sport: Attitudes and experience. *British Journal of Sports Medicine, 37,* 335–338.

Laure, P., Thouvenin, T., and Lecerf, T. (2001). Attitudes of coaches toward doping. *Journal of Sports Medicine and Physical Fitness, 41,* 132–136.

Lazuras, L., Barkoukis, V., Rodafinos, A., and Tzorbatzoudis, H. (2010). Predictors of doping intentions in elite-level athletes: A social cognition approach. *Journal of Sport and Exercise Psychology, 32,* 694–710.

Likert, R. (1932). A technique for the measurement of attitudes. *Archives of Psychology, 140,* 1–55.

Lucidi, F., Grano, C., Leone, L., Lombardo, C., and Pesce, C. (2004). Determinants of the intention to use doping substances: An empirical contribution in a sample of Italian adolescents. *International Journal of Sport Psychology, 35*, 133–148.

Lucidi, F., Zelli, A., Mallia, L., Grano, C., Russo, P. M., and Violani, V. (2008). The social-cognitive mechanisms regulating adolescents' use of doping substances. *Journal of Sports Sciences, 26*, 447–456.

Moran, A., Guerin, S., Kirby, K., and MacIntyre, T. (2008). *The development and validation of a doping attitudes and behaviour scale (DABS)*. World Anti-Doping Agency. Available at www.wada-ama.org/en/resources/social-science/the-development-and-validation-of-a-doping-attitudes-and-behaviour-scale (accessed December 15, 2014.

Morente-Sánchez, J. and Zabala, M. (2013). Doping in sport: A review of elite athletes' attitudes, beliefs, and knowledge. *Sports Medicine, 43*, 395–411.

Nicholls, J. G. (1984). Achievement motivation: Conceptions of ability, subjective experience, task choice, and performance. *Psychological Review, 91*, 328–346.

Nisbett, R. E. and Wilson, T. D. (1977). Telling more than we can know: Verbal reports on mental processes. *Psychological Review, 84*, 232–259.

Ntoumanis, N., Ng, J. Y., Barkoukis, V., and Backhouse, S. (2014). Personal and psychosocial predictors of doping use in physical activity settings: A meta-analysis. *Sports Medicine, 44 (11)*, 1603–1624.

Özdemir, L., Nur, N., Bagciva, I., Bulut O., Sümer, H., and Tezeren, G. (2005). Doping and performance enhancing drug use in athletes living in Sivas, Mid-Anatolia: A brief report. *Journal of Sports Science and Medicine, 4*, 248–252.

Petróczi, A. (2007). Attitudes to doping: A structural equation analysis of the relationship between athletes' attitudes, sport orientation and doping behaviour. *Substance Abuse Treatment, Prevention, and Policy, 2*. doi: 10.1186/1747–597X-2–34.

Petróczi, A. (2013). The doping mindset – Part II: Potentials and pitfalls in capturing athletes' doping attitudes with response-time methodology. *Performance Enhancement and Health, 2*, 164–181.

Petróczi, A. and Aidman, E. (2008). Psychological drivers of doping: The life-cycle model of performance enhancement. *Substance Abuse, Treatment, Prevention, and Policy, 3*. doi: 10.1186/1747–597X-3–7.

Petróczi, A. and Aidman, E. (2009). Measuring explicit attitude toward doping: Review of the psychometric properties of the Performance Enhancement Attitude Scale. *Psychology of Sport and Exercise, 10*, 390–396.

Petróczi, A., Aidman, E. V., and Nepusz, T. (2008). Capturing doping attitudes by self-report declarations and implicit assessment: A methodology study. *Substance Abuse, Treatment, Prevention and Policy, 3*, 9.

Petróczi, A., Aidman, E. V., Hussain, I., Deshmukh, N., Nepusz, T., Uvacsek, M., Tóth, M., Barker, J., and Naughton, D. (2010). Virtue or pretence? Looking behind self-declared innocence in doping. *PLoS ONE, 5*, e10457. doi: 10.1371/journal.pone.0010457.

Quirk, F. H. (2009). Health psychology and drugs in sport. *Sport in Society, 12*, 375–393.

Sas-Nowosielski, K. and Swiatkowska, L. (2008). Goal orientations and attitudes toward doping. *International Journal of Sports Medicine, 29*, 607–612.

Scarpino, V., Arrigo, A., Benzi, G., Garattini, S., La Vecchia, C., Rossi Bernadi, L., Silvestrini, G., and Tuccimei, G. (1990). Evaluation of prevalence of "doping" among Italian athletes. *The Lancet, 336*, 1048–1050.

Schwarz, N. (2007). Attitude construction: Evaluation in context. *Social Cognition, 25*, 638–656.

Shirazi, A. and Tricker, R. (2005). Current drug education policies in NCAA institutions: Perceptions of head athletic trainers. *Journal of Drug Education, 35*, 29–46.

Striegel, H., Vollkommer, G., and Dickhuth, H. H. (2002). Combating drug use in competitive sports: An analysis from the athletes' perspective. *Journal of Sports Medicine and Physical Fitness, 42*, 354–359.

Thurstone, L. L. (1928). Attitudes can be measured. *American Journal of Sociology, 33*, 529–554.

Tricker, R. and Connolly, D. (1997). Drugs and the college athlete: An analysis of the attitudes of student athletes at risk. *Journal of Drug Education, 27*, 105–119.

Uvacsek, M., Nepusz, T., Naughton, D. P., Mazanov, J., Ránky, M. Z., and Petróczi, A. (2009). Self-admitted behaviour and perceived use of performance-enhancing vs. psychoactive drugs among competitive athletes. *Scandinavian Journal of Medicine and Science in Sports, 21*, 224–234.

Waddington, I. and Smith, A. (2009). *An introduction to drugs in sport. Addicted to winning?* London and New York: Routledge.

Waddington, I., Malcolm, D., Roderick, M., and Naik, R. (2005). Drug use in English professional football. *British Journal of Sports Medicine, 39*, e18.

Whitaker, L., Long, J., Petróczi, A., and Backhouse, S. H. (2014). Using the prototype willingness model to predict doping in sport. *Scandinavian Journal of Medicine and Science in Sports, 24*, e398–e405.

Wicker, A. W. (1969). Attitudes versus actions: The relationship of verbal and overt behavioural responses to attitude objects. *Journal of Social Issues, 25*, 41–78.

Wiefferink, C. H., Detmar, S. B., Coumans, B., Vogels, T., and Paulussen, T. G. W. (2008). Social psychological determinants of the use of performance-enhancing drugs by gym users. *Health Education Research, 23*, 70–80.

Wright, S., Grogan, S., and Hunter, G. (2001). Body-builders' attitudes towards steroid use. *Drugs: Education, Prevention and Policy, 8*, 91–98.

Zelli, A., Mallia, L., and Lucidi, F. (2010). The contribution of interpersonal appraisals to a social-cognitive analysis of adolescents' doping use. *Psychology of Sport and Exercise, 11*, 304–311.

2 *"I am not sure what you mean…"*

The possible contribution of interpersonal appraisals to social-cognitive accounts of doping use

Arnaldo Zelli, Luca Mallia, and Fabio Lucidi

The theoretical and research considerations presented in this chapter overall are guided by the assumption that doping behavior partly depends on the dynamic interplay between an individual's beliefs and the appraisals he or she makes in evaluating self-relevant interpersonal experiences. The chapter focuses on a particular form of interpersonal appraisals, namely, one's interpretations of others' intentions in situations which have personal relevance. Relatedly, this chapter introduces the general hypothesis that these forms of interpersonal appraisals are of particular importance in contributing to the scientific understanding of doping use, as they might help account for individual differences in doping intentions and doping use. In so doing, it will first introduce broad theoretical and research frameworks that indirectly support this general view and will subsequently address the value of a research focus on interpersonal appraisals in doping research. The chapter will finally describe a research program that has moved its initial steps to inquire and find empirical support to the hypothesized linkages between interpersonal appraisals and doping use in various sport contexts.

Appraisal processes, psychological functioning, and individual differences in behavior

In the field of personality psychology, the study of personality and behavioral functioning has broadly established and converged on some basic fundamental points concerning appraisal processes and their role in regulating psychological experiences and social actions (Caprara and Cervone 2000; Cervone and Shoda 1999; David *et al.* 2002). First, both emotional experiences and behaviors are elicited by the subjective meaning people assign to events and arise in response to the meaning structures of given situations (Frijda 1988; Lazarus 1991; Gendron and Feldman Barrett 2009). Different meanings of a single situation or event may thus trigger different psychological and behavioral experiences in different individuals. Second, appraisals are and can be conceptualized as "relational" at their core, as they are not merely forms of cognitions concerning features of the environment in isolation but, instead, express the meaning and relevance of events for one's personal well-being. It is the perceived relation between environmental events and personal goals, capabilities, and norms for behavior that triggers and shapes psychological and behavioral experiences (David *et al.* 2002; Scherer *et al.* 2004; Smith and Pope 1992).

These broad views are consistent with a social-cognitive analysis of psychological and behavioral experiences, in which the basic tenet is that appraisals give form to persons' meanings of social features, events, and situations. With this in mind, the fundamental scientific task consists in the definition of the social-cognitive units of analysis of appraisal processes (Caprara and Cervone 2000). There are ample and distinct examples of this scientific goal in classical and existing literature. For instance, Lazarus and colleagues over the years articulated a model of emotional experiences in which one's appraisals of the relevance of events for one's personal concerns and goals (i.e., the importance of events for personal well-being), as well as distinct appraisal dimensions concerning one's personal capabilities to cope with events regulate and account for different emotions (Lazarus 1991; Smith and Pope 1992). Still in the field of emotional work, Scherer and colleagues (e.g., Scherer 1997; Scherer and Wallbott 1994; Scherer *et al.* 2004) showed that the link from particular appraisals to particular emotions might hold across cultural contexts (e.g., an event or circumstance that is appraised in violation of moral standards elicits guilt or shame in European as in Asian countries). At the same time, though, these authors' work also suggests that cultural or national differences exist in the particular contribution that distinct appraisal dimensions may have on emotional experiences (e.g., people from different countries or cultures may vary in the degree of unfairness that may assign to a given event).

At the outset of this chapter, it is important to mention a useful heuristic, namely, the distinction between appraisals and knowledge. Appraisals are evaluations of *particular* encounters or events and, more specifically, they are evaluations of the *relevance* of encounters to one's personal well-being (e.g., the evaluations an adolescent may make with respect to a friend who solicits doping use to gain muscle mass). Knowledge, in contrast, refers to belief systems, that is, enduring mental representations about isolated features or facts about oneself, other persons, or the physical and social world (e.g., the beliefs an adolescent may hold about the advantages of doping use on one's own body or, rather, about its negative health effects) (Cervone 2005; Cervone and Shoda 1999). People bring their general beliefs and convictions with them into situations but their psychological and behavioral experience in a particular situation or at a given moment depends on the extent to which and the ways this situation is evaluated as relevant to one's personal life. This fundamental distinction has helped psychological research in various fields. For instance, long-standing developmental research on child and adolescent aggression or antisocial behavior has demonstrated that individuals who lack clear beliefs about the understanding of others' emotions tend to evaluate others' intentions as hostile in social situations, and that these interpersonal appraisals more directly contribute to differences in aggressive behaviors (Dodge 1993; Dodge *et al.* 2002). According to a similar theoretical framework, we have recently investigated one's willingness to report crimes to law enforcement authorities among nearly 4,000 Italian adolescents residing in high-risk regions of the country. In that study, adolescents imagined to be the witnesses in a series of hypothetical crime situations and rated the likelihood to file a police report, thus providing an indirect measure of behavioral individual differences in crime reporting (Zelli *et al.* 2013). The study showed that adolescents' willingness to file a police report depended on their interpersonal appraisals of the hypothetical crime situations (e.g., the evaluation of the severity of the hypothetical unlawful act; the evaluation of the benefits for the hypothetical victim in filing a report to police authorities). Furthermore, the study also showed that these interpersonal appraisals partially mediated the contribution that personality and belief characteristics (e.g., prosocialness; views or beliefs about appropriate codes of social conduct) would have on individual differences in crime reporting (Zelli *et al.* 2013).

Thus, knowledge or beliefs, alone, do not seem to be sufficient to trigger psychological and behavioral experiences, and interpersonal appraisals stand as a more proximal antecedent, mediating and accounting for the influence knowledge may exert on one's psychological and behavioral experiences in social situations. In addressing the topic of doping research, the following section will call upon this key distinction in presenting various theoretical and research models and in offering a rationale for the integration of interpersonal appraisals into well-established doping research hypotheses.

Beliefs systems and interpersonal appraisals processes in doping research

As in the case of other complex health-related behavioral phenomena, the understanding and the treatment of doping use necessarily must rely on firm theoretical grounds and on the research-based evidence that clear theoretical considerations possibly generate. This principle has guided scientific work on doping use in the last decade or so, and much of this work seems to be well positioned within the broad framework of social-cognitive theorizing (Donovan 2009; Lazuras *et al.* 2010). This framework characterizes a great deal of current psychological research and offers, in many respects, the most systematic and explicit theoretical outlet for addressing behavioral phenomena in terms of the dynamic interplay between one's belief systems and appraisals of ongoing social situations, events, or interpersonal encounters.

Broadly speaking, much recent doping research shares the assumption that doping use is a volitional behavior that often depends upon individuals' explicit intentions to use illegal substances. Coherently with this general view, doping research has addressed whether knowledge or belief systems stand as critical social-cognitive determinants of doping behavior and, in doing so, this research also has reached a consensus on what types of beliefs are most relevant (Dodge and Jaccard 2007; Laure *et al.* 2004; Wiefferink *et al.* 2008). For instance, traditional doping research, embedded and consistent with the explicit hypotheses of the "Theory of Planned Behavior" (Ajzen 1991), has clearly demonstrated that doping intentions and adoption partly are influenced by one's positive attitudes about doping use (e.g., Mallia *et al.* 2013) on the expected social approval from significant others (i.e., social norms), and on one's perceived sense of behavioral control, that is, personal beliefs about the ease or difficulty of using doping substances and about the degree of personal control over situational or social contingences (Dodge and Jaccard 2007; Laure *et al.* 2004; Lucidi *et al.* 2004). Additional research has extended these findings by also including other relevant and more explicit social-cognitive belief constructs (Lucidi *et al.* 2004, 2008, 2013). Thus, doping intentions and actual use also might be uniquely influenced by one's perceived capacity to withstand social pressure or solicitations from others to use doping substances (i.e., self-regulatory efficacy), as well as by an individual's moral disengagement, that is, the justifications one personally considers to bypass the legal and moral implications of doping use (e.g., believing that "it is not right to condemn those who use illicit substances since many do the same" – diffusion of responsibility, one of the eight mechanisms of moral disengagement theorized by Albert Bandura) (Bandura *et al.* 2001).

Interestingly, these belief systems and constructs conceptually call upon individuals' social and situational experiences, a key element of interpersonal appraisals. For instance, the notion of social norms and one's beliefs about the expected social approval from significant others necessarily calls upon the interpersonal contexts and encounters within which one may seek support for his or her intention to use or for the actual use of doping substances. Likewise, self-regulatory efficacy beliefs about one's own capacity to resist social pressure or others' solicitations to use doping substances plausibly matter within the particular interpersonal contexts and encounters one may typically experience. More importantly, one's psychological or mental experience at the time of endorsing certain beliefs (e.g., during a self-report assessment of belief measures) may directly, at least in part, rely on individuals' capacity to mentally anticipate the consequences for the self of specific, real or imagined, interpersonal encounters concerning doping use.

These possible, conceptual and psychological, linkages between beliefs and interpersonal appraisals imply, for instance, that individuals' beliefs about significant others' approval of doping use, their personal confidence in resisting social pressure or solicitations, and, more generally, their attitudes or intentions toward doping use might be mentally associated with the personal ways these individuals evaluate potentially risky interpersonal encounters. Thus, illustratively, individuals who may show relatively low efficacy beliefs about resisting social pressure from others in using doping substances may also be those who more readily foresee (i.e., mentally appraise) personal benefits, rather than risks, for the self in a situation where someone else solicits doping use, be it the byproduct of real or, rather, imagined experiences.

In the doping literature of the last two decades or so, Donovan and his colleagues' "Sport Drug Control Model" (SDCM) has perhaps offered the most explicit theoretical paradigm for the study of the relations between appraisals and doping use in sport (Donovan 2009; Donovan *et al.* 2002). It also provided, albeit indirectly, a clear supporting framework for many of the above considerations. These authors propose that athletes' attitudes and intentions toward the use of performance-enhancing substances are sustained by a system of six input factors, among which two classes of appraisals are particularly important, namely "threat" and "benefit" or incentive appraisals. Broadly speaking, the former class of appraisals refers to an athlete's evaluations of the possible threats implicitly embedded both in the enforcement rules concerning doping use (e.g., the perceived likelihood of being tested in and out of competition or the perceived likelihood of a specific drug to be detected during drug controls) and in the ill-health effects of doping use (e.g., the perceived likelihood of succumbing to the ill-health effects of doping use). Likewise, the "benefit" or incentive appraisals refer to a set of evaluations through which an athlete carefully considers the costs/benefits of using performance-enhancing substances. Within this class of appraisals, an athlete, for instance, may evaluate a series of possibly important factors ranging from the extent to which substance use may actually and effectively help in reaching one's own desired competition level, to whether such an achievement would have considerable and tangible rewards, or to the extent to which adverse effects or economic considerations may undo or counteract the benefits of using performance-enhancing substances (Donovan 2009; Donovan *et al.* 2002).

The SDCM model is consistent with much of the core elements of appraisal processes introduced earlier in the chapter. Both threat and incentive appraisals refer to an athlete's evaluation of the *self-relevance* of information, facts, or events concerning doping use. Both types of appraisals also are clearly embedded in a system of relations with forms of knowledge or beliefs, as in the case – for instance – of the expectations an athlete may hold with respect to the tangible rewards coming from personally reaching high sport achievements or other personal views sustaining positive doping attitudes. Along and consistent with these considerations, the SDCM model treats threat and incentive appraisals, along with other dispositional or belief variables (e.g., self-esteem, optimism, or personal morality), as input factors acting onto doping attitudes and intentions.

Donovan and colleagues' system of input factors has very recently been supported by research evidence (Gucciardi *et al.* 2011; Jalleh *et al.* 2014). The 2013 study by Jalleh and colleagues, for instance, supported the basic tenets of the SDCM by showing that morality, threat appraisals (i.e., perceived threats for health and from law enforcement and regulations), and benefit appraisals showed the largest unique prediction of athletes' doping attitudes and use. This study is quite relevant as it provides relatively independent measurements of different types of social-cognitive variables implicated in doping attitudes and intentions, including threat and incentive appraisals. Similarly, Overbye *et al.* (2013) focused on the possible deterrents and incentives influencing elite athletes' decisions to use doping substances and examined the specific circumstances which male and female athletes say would affect their (hypothetical) use of doping substances. In Overbye and colleagues' study, athletes evaluated and rated a series of social, personal, emotional, and situational reasons or motives at the time of imagining themselves in situations in which they had to decide whether to use doping substances. Reasons or motives that could hypothetically make them refuse to use doping substances were classified as "potential deterrents" (e.g., peers or family members would disapprove; unwillingness to do anything illegal). Likewise, reasons or motives that could hypothetically make the athletes use doping substances were classified as "potential incentives" (e.g., qualified medical supervision; financially secured after career; ensure a gain in muscle mass). The study findings suggested that fewer incentives than deterrents would affect elite athletes' decisions about doping use, even though this finding does not necessarily mean that deterrents are more effective than incentives (Overbye *et al.* 2013: 127). All in all, the studies by Overbye and colleagues (2013) and by Jalleh and colleagues (2014) confirm, along with other research using a variety of methodologies (e.g., Huybers and Mazanov 2012; Mazanov and Huybers 2010; Strelan and Boeckmann 2006), that sport athletes may evaluate the pros and cons of a variety of reasons or motives at the time of deciding whether to use doping substances, and that these reasons and motives may differentially represent deterrents or, on the contrary, incentives to dope.

This notwithstanding, there are some issues concerning the investigation of appraisal processes implicated in doping use that may move research forward. Donovan and colleagues' SDCM model, as well as the doping appraisal research reviewed above, overall support the possibility that an athlete may rely on the appraisals of social, personal, and self-relevant situations and information. Quite consistent with this approach, it also is plausible that an athlete's decision to use doping substances may also come from the particular ways he or she evaluates and interprets specific interpersonal encounters (e.g., the ways an athlete interprets the intention of a teammate who approves or suggests doping use). In other words, the above research may find further evidence from addressing a particular and specific form of situational appraisals, namely, an athlete's appraisals of interpersonal encounters he or she may face.

In addressing this possibility, there are theoretical and methodological issues that come to the foreground. Theoretically, as also mentioned in an earlier section of this chapter, interpersonal appraisals are construed as the proximal determinants of one's psychological and behavioral responses to a specific situation at hand. This means that, within a given single situation, interpersonal appraisals theoretically mediate any influence a person's dispositional or belief characteristics exert on his or her psychological and behavioral responses. Methodologically and empirically, these theoretical hypotheses would require complex research designs to be correctly tested. Illustratively, a researcher interested in testing a belief-to-interpersonal appraisal doping use study should first assess some athletes' dispositional and belief characteristics, then sequentially assess – within given (classes of) situations – these athletes' interpersonal appraisals, their intentions to use doping substances, and actual doping use. In other words, interpersonal appraisals theoretically call upon a sort of situational specificity in behavioral assessment. More broadly, however, it is plausible to presume that, over time, people's beliefs and interpersonal appraisals influence each other and jointly account for relatively stable individual differences in behavior.

The above considerations elicit additional and specific methodological and measurement issues. A first issue is concerned with the development of ecologically valid situational stimuli representing doping-related interpersonal encounters. In this regard, individual and team sports may contextually refer to distinctly different types of interpersonal situations. For instance, while in individual sports an athlete and his/her coach may represent the key dyad in many of the interpersonal situations they both face, team athletes may in principle face a variety of interpersonal situations perhaps only involving another teammate, some teammates together or, rather, the team coach.

A second issue is concerned with the choice of the dimensions to be used to measure athletes' interpersonal appraisals. As mentioned earlier, appraisals theoretically express the relevance of social events for one's personal well-being, and measurements should elicit self-relevance evaluations. A broad class of interpersonal appraisals that may serve this purpose refers to the ways athletes may interpret the intentions of others they deal with. From a measurement standpoint, it may then become critical to assess whether others' intentions are interpreted as benign or, rather, as malevolent, for the self. For instance, an athlete who is solicited by others to use doping substances may interpret this solicitation benignly, viewing it as a sign others care about him or her. Alternatively, another athlete may interpret the same solicitation as a sign that others seek to benefit from it, more than a sign they care about the athlete's personal well-being.

A third issue is concerned with the possibility of measuring reliable individual differences in athletes' interpersonal appraisals. It is plausible that athletes, at the time of evaluating others' intentions in a series of interpersonal encounters or situations concerning doping use, may show relatively stable tendencies to perceive benign or, alternatively, malevolent intentions in others. These tendencies may, in other words, reflect athletes' past experiences with real or imagined interpersonal situations concerning doping use, as well as be the expression of beliefs or convictions about significant others athletes have come to form or endorse.

Finally, a fourth and related issue is concerned with the modeling of the relations linking doping-related beliefs, interpersonal appraisals, and variables such as attitudes, intentions, and actual use. As anticipated earlier, a research investigation focusing on these relations might consider one of two complementary design choices. The first would call for specificity in the assessment of interpersonal appraisals and behaviors, that is, the possibility of measuring athletes' interpersonal appraisals, relevant doping beliefs, doping intentions, and doping use within a given class of situations. This design choice would then legitimately permit to verify the "mediation" hypothesis that interpersonal appraisals intervene and give meaning to any relation linking one's beliefs to doping intentions and actual use. In the second design choice, instead, the assessment of doping-related interpersonal appraisals could be qualitatively distinct from behavioral assessment, that is, interpersonal appraisals and doping use are measured across different classes of situations. In this design choice, a "moderation" hypothesis would then be tested in which interpersonal appraisals interact with beliefs in influencing doping intentions and actual use (i.e., a multiplicative influence in multiple regression terms). Illustratively, this latter hypothesis would, for instance, suggest that the strength of the relation between positive doping attitudes and doping intentions would be relatively stronger among those athletes who see no problem or presume good intentions in others who solicit or encourage them to use doping substances. Figure 2.1 depicts the general terms of this "moderation" hypothesis.

In a recent line of doping research, we attempted to address the above issues in an effort to integrate existing social-cognitive models of doping attitudes, intentions, and use with an explicit research focus on interpersonal appraisals among young amateur athletes, professional athletes, and young non-athletes. The remaining sections of this chapter will summarize this research program and the initial research findings that it has spawned.

A new research program on interpersonal appraisals and doping use

The basic notion guiding our research program is that athletes competing at a relatively high level in both individual and team sports possibly face social situations and interpersonal exchanges in which others may suggest, solicit, or support the use of doping substances for improving sport performance. If so, it is plausible that an athlete would evaluate these situations and judge their relevance for his-/herself by also interpreting others' guiding motives or intentions (e.g., by evaluating whether others care about the athlete's welfare). These assumptions offer the ground for two general research hypotheses. The first is that – across interpersonal situations eliciting self-relevant interpretations – an athlete may show a relatively stable tendency to perceive others' intentions either favorably for his-/herself (e.g., others' solicitations are guided by good

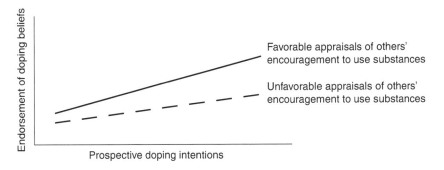

Figure 2.1 Diagram of the "moderation" of interpersonal appraisals in the relation between doping beliefs and prospective doping intentions.

intentions/they care about me) or unfavorably (e.g., others' solicitations are guided by personal interests/they do not care about me). The second general hypothesis is that those athletes who – across interpersonal situations – tend to interpret others' motives or intentions favorably, perhaps dismissing the possible threats associated with others' solicitation, are at a higher risk for endorsing doping attitudes and intentions and, ultimately, for doping use.

Our research program initially focused on the identification of distinct sets of interpersonal situations concerning doping use that could be ecologically valid for young amateur athletes, professional athletes, and young non-athletes. This focus on the general population, rather than solely on sport-specific contexts, was due to an initial interest in the possible array of motives and personality characteristics that could be associated with doping use such as, for instance, the desire or wish to improve physical appearance rather than to enhance sport performance. On these premises, the research program began by pursuing several empirical goals.

The first goal was the assessment of the ways athlete and non-athlete adolescents would evaluate the intentions of hypothetical counterparts who solicit them to use doping substances (i.e., a specific form of interpersonal appraisal). The second goal was the assessment of the longitudinal and possibly reciprocal relations linking adolescents' appraisals of others' intentions to the set of social-cognitive variables typically assessed in relevant doping research (e.g., doping attitudes, self-regulatory efficacy in resisting social pressure, moral disengagement). A third empirical goal was to statistically assess whether interpersonal appraisals would act as a *moderating* factor, along the lines of the hypothesis diagrammed earlier in Figure 2.1. This third goal, in other words, sought to establish whether the relations linking social-cognitive variables to – for instance – doping attitudes or doping intentions would be significantly stronger among adolescents interpreting others' solicitations favorably than among adolescents interpreting others' solicitations less favorably or unfavorably.

Details about this initial research, conducted with a relatively large sample of Italian high-school students, have been published elsewhere (Zelli *et al.* 2010), and this chapter only summarizes key methodological information and main findings. A relatively large sample of Italian high-school students across the country participated in two assessments within three/four consecutive months. Both assessments provided self-report data on students' doping and supplement use, as well as on their beliefs, attitudes, and intentions concerning doping use. Students also imagined being the protagonist in a series of eight hypothetical interpersonal situations in which someone else suggested or solicited them to use performance-enhancing substances. Students were asked to interpret the solicitors' intentions and, importantly, each scenario was formulated to keep the solicitor's "true" intentions as ambiguous as possible, therefore allowing interpersonal appraisal ratings to vary across students as much as possible. Scenarios presented situations occurring in a variety of sports contexts, and substance use was merely suggested or strongly encouraged by a coach, a peer, or a friend. A sample scenario goes as follows:

You regularly go to a fitness center and use body-building machines. You have been doing this for several months and like going also because you have become acquainted with the people and the personal trainers who follow you when you are there. One day, one of the instructors comes by and asks you to follow him as he wants to show you something. You do so and, after talking for a while about products that can enhance your performance and fitness in a couple of weeks, he strongly advises you to use some pills he has in his locker. He gives you a little bottle containing some pills and tells you that using them will be free of charge for the next couple of weeks.

For each of the eight hypothetical scenarios, students evaluated the counterpart's intentions on three distinct dimensions of interpersonal appraisals by using a 5-point likelihood scale. In particular, they rated the likelihood that the counterpart acted (1) in the protagonist's/student's interest or welfare; (2) for his own personal interest; and (3) to harm the protagonist/student. Students also provided a fourth rating by indicating the likelihood that they would do what the counterpart encouraged them to do, should the situations actually occur (i.e., a sort of behavioral prediction).

The analyses suggested that interpersonal appraisals may meaningfully contribute to doping research. As one would expect, on average, students thought that solicitors acted in their own interests and considered it quite unlikely that they would do what hypothetically they were asked to do (e.g., to take the performance-enhancing pills). The findings also suggested that students' interpersonal appraisals were measured reliably, that is, students interpreted the solicitors' intentions in systematic ways across the hypothetical scenarios (i.e., across scenarios, each type of appraisal rating was correlated significantly). There were, in other words, systematic individual differences in students' ratings, and this students' rating variability mattered in many respects.

It was linked in meaningful ways to the social-cognitive belief variables traditionally investigated in doping research (e.g., doping attitudes, social norms, self-regulatory beliefs). Furthermore, these patterns of relations linking doping beliefs to students' interpersonal appraisals were, as expected, an indication of reciprocal influences over time. Early students' appraisals predicted later doping beliefs. That is, high-school adolescents who early on interpreted hypothetical others' solicitation to use substances favorably (e.g., it is because he/she cares about me) later on showed a relatively stronger tendency to find justifications for doping use (i.e., stronger moral disengagement), lesser personal confidence in their capacity to resist social pressure, stronger doping attitudes, stronger perceived approval by significant others, and stronger intentions to use doping substances in the near future. The evidence of reciprocal influences emerged from the fact that the reverse pattern of predictions was also significant, that is, early students' beliefs predicted later interpersonal appraisals. All in all, these longitudinal and reciprocal relations were particularly meaningful in lieu of the fact that interpersonal appraisals and more traditional social-cognitive variables relied on qualitatively and semantically distinct measurements.

Individual differences in students' interpersonal ratings also provided a means for a thorough test of the "moderation" hypothesis mentioned earlier. As a reminder, one research goal was concerned with the possibility that the predictive relations linking doping beliefs to doping intentions and actual use would be relatively stronger among those students who interpreted favorably others' intentions or solicitations to use substances. To test this hypothesis we followed several steps. For each student, we first created four distinct scale scores of interpersonal appraisals (i.e., by averaging each type of rating across the eight interpersonal scenarios students evaluated). We then used these four scale scores, which were relatively uncorrelated with each other, to calculate a "Risk Index" score for each student. This index was a cumulative risk measure of the extent to which each student interpreted favorably the hypothetical solicitation to use substances, and its value could range from 0 to 4 (i.e., on the basis of a median-split categorization for each of the four appraisal scale scores, an index score of 4 indicated that a student interpreted favorably others' intentions on each appraisal). This index score was finally used to classify students who provided completed longitudinal data in three main groups, namely, those who showed "no risk" (i.e., an index score of 0), those who showed "moderate risk" (i.e., an index score of 1 or 2), and those who showed a "relatively high risk" (i.e., with an index score of 3 or 4).

The risk index seemed to be a valid measure of students' risk for doping use. None of the high-school students who were classified as "no risk" declared to have used doping substances or supplements in the past. Furthermore, among these "no risk" students, only doping attitudes ($\beta=0.28$) and personal confidence in resisting social pressure (i.e., self-regulatory efficacy, $\beta=-0.23$) significantly contributed to adolescents' intentions to use doping substances in the near future. However, in line with the above "moderation" hypothesis, the number and the strength of the factors predicting students' doping intentions increased with risk level. Among "moderate risk" adolescents, in addition to the effects of attitudes ($\beta=0.22$) and efficacy to resist social pressure ($\beta=-0.18$), subjective norms ($\beta=0.53$) also contributed significantly to adolescents' prospective intentions to use doping substances. Finally, for "relatively high risk" students, nearly all the social-cognitive factors predicted adolescents' prospective doping intentions, that is, attitudes ($\beta=0.33$), subjective norms ($\beta=0.16$), self-regulatory efficacy ($\beta=-0.32$), and moral disengagement beliefs ($\beta=0.18$). These differences in the number and magnitude of predictive social-cognitive effects corresponded to substantial differences in "explained variance" of adolescents' prospective doping intentions, with more than a fourfold increment in the "relatively high risk" group ($R^2=0.52$), as compared to the no-risk group ($R^2=0.13$).

In sum, our initial research (Zelli *et al.* 2010) overall confirmed that doping-relevant belief systems contribute to doping intentions and to doping use, and it did so by also showing that beliefs' contribution is particularly evident among those young adolescents who, in facing hypothetical interpersonal encounters, presumed good intentions in those who solicited them to use doping substances. However, this initial research focusing on high-school students was limited in several respects and spawned additional scientific and empirical issues. It lacked a systematic analysis of students' level of sport involvement, thus not permitting to ascertain whether beliefs and interpersonal appraisals would be particularly relevant to those who, presumably, are particularly concerned with or motivated by performance enhancement. Relatedly, this initial research was not designed to empirically compare individual sports versus team sports, thus limiting its findings' generalizability.

These issues have been addressed in a more recent two-year, cross-national research program that was funded by WADA in 2012. Broadly speaking, this research program integrated our focus on interpersonal appraisals with a parallel interest in young team athletes. This focus on team sport athletes and the cross-national effort of the investigation (i.e., Italy, Germany, and Greece) represented the novel elements of this funded research program. A first objective of this research was to develop assessment instruments that were sensitive and tailored to young athletes practicing team sports and that could be comparable across different national contexts. A second broad objective was to establish whether and to what extent young team athletes' beliefs (i.e., moral disengagement and self-efficacy) and their interpersonal appraisals – measured with respect to significant features of team interpersonal situations – would account for differences in team athletes' doping intentions.

This new research program represented a significant extension of prior doping research on interpersonal appraisals. For instance, it was of significant scientific value to examine whether the notion of "risk" interpersonal appraisals would also hold with respect to situational features and hypothetical encounters that could characterize team sports and teammates' typical interpersonal experiences. As in the initial research with high-school students (Zelli *et al.* 2010), young team athletes were asked to imagine being the protagonist of four hypothetical team interpersonal situations (identified through preliminary focus groups with different team athletes). Again, as in prior research, in each situation the protagonist was solicited or encouraged to use substances, but the solicitation more specifically came from either a coach or a teammate. Again, for each scenario, the young team athletes interpreted and rated the "true" intentions of their team counterpart by indicating the likelihood that the solicitation was in the athlete's interest, in the team's interest or, rather, it was due to the solicitors' personal gains or to the desire to hurt or get the team athlete/protagonist into trouble.

This research is underway and results are only preliminary. The team instruments measuring young team athletes' interpersonal appraisals seem reliable and do so across all three national contexts where the study is being carried out. In other words, these instruments seem to measure equally well the interpersonal appraisals of Italian, German, and Greek athletes. Furthermore, the preliminary results also show cross-national consistent patterns in the general finding that interpersonal appraisals of young team athletes are meaningfully related to their propensity to endorse positive doping attitudes and willingness to use doping substances in the future. More specifically, young team athletes who tend to interpret favorably others' hypothetical solicitations are also those who show relatively stronger prospective intentions to use substances, should the hypothetical situations really occur.

Conclusions

Overall, our research program focusing on interpersonal appraisals highlights the possibility that athlete and non-athlete adolescents who preemptively tend to foresee a positive meaning for the self in others' actions or intentions might be less inclined to acquire or utilize self-regulatory resources to deal with doping use. The study also suggests that preventive interventions should focus on the processes of social influence and, in particular, on the possibility of correcting adolescents' misperceptions of risky interpersonal situations soliciting doping use. As others have pointed out (Hubner and Kaiser 2006), intentions and enactment concerning behaviors that have moral implications, such as doping use, rely heavily on strong ties between attitudes and subjective norms. Factors that may weaken these ties may reinforce the role of moral considerations on behavior, thus promoting behavioral change. Consistent with these notions, and with the general recommendations of research on implementation intentions (Brandstatter *et al.* 2001), a focus of preventive interventions on reducing adolescents' misperceptions of risky interpersonal situations and on promoting desired behaviors in specific situations (e.g., *If someone offers me performance-enhancing drugs, then I will…*) may contribute to weaken the linkages between attitudes and subjective norms and the system of beliefs.

References

Ajzen, I. (1991). The theory of planned behaviour: Some unresolved issues. *Organizational Behaviour and Human Decision Processes*, 5, 179–211.

Bandura, A., Caprara, G. V., Barbaranelli, C., Pastorelli, C., and Regalia, C. (2001). Sociocognitive self-regulatory mechanisms governing transgressive behaviour. *Journal of Personality and Social Psychology*, 80 (*1*), 125–135.

Brandstatter, V., Lengfelder, A., and Gollwitzer, P. M. (2001). Implementation intentions and efficient action initiation. *Journal of Personality and Social Psychology*, 81, 946–960. doi: 10.1037//0022–3514.81.5.946.

Caprara, G. V. and Cervone, D. (2000). *Personality: Determinants, dynamics, and potentials*. Cambridge: Cambridge University Press.

Cervone, D. (2005). Personality architecture: Within-person structures and processes. *Annual Review of Psychology*, 56, 423–452.

Cervone, D. and Shoda, Y. (1999). Social-cognitive theories and the coherence of personality. In D. Cervone and Y. Shoda (eds.), *The Coherence of personality: Social-cognitive bases of consistency, variability, and organization* (3–33). New York: Guilford Press.

David, D., Schnur, J., and Belloiu, A. (2002). Another search for the "hot" cognitions: Appraisal, irrational beliefs, attributions, and their relation to emotion. *Journal of Rational – Emotive and Cognitive – Behavior Therapy*, 20 (*2*), 93–131.

Dodge, K. A. (1993). Social-cognitive mechanisms in the development of conduct disorder and depression. In L. W. Porter and M. R. Rosenzweig (eds.), *Annual Review of Psychology*, *44*, 559–584.

Dodge, K. A., Laird, R., Lochman, J. E., and Zelli, A. (2002). Multidimensional latent-construct analysis of children's social information processing patterns: Correlations with aggressive behavior problems. *Psychological Assessment*, *14* (*1*), 60–73.

Dodge, T. and Jaccard, J. J. (2007). Negative beliefs as a moderator of the intention-behavior relationship: Decisions to use performance-enhancing substances. *Journal of Applied Social Psychology*, *37* (*1*), 43–59.

Donovan, R. J. (2009). Towards an understanding of factors influencing athletes' attitudes towards performance enhancing technologies: Implications for ethics education. In T. H. Murray, K. J. Maschke, and A. A. Wasunna (eds.), *Performance-enhancing technologies in sport: ethical, conceptual and scientific issues* (283–317). Baltimore: Johns Hopkins University Press.

Donovan, R. J., Egger, G., Kapernick, V., and Mendoza, J. (2002). A conceptual framework for achieving performance enhancing drug compliance in sport. *Sports Medicine*, *32* (*4*), 269–284.

Frijda, N. H. (1988). The laws of emotions. *American Psychologist*, *50*, 69–78.

Gendron, M. and Feldman Barrett, L. (2009). Reconstructing the past: A century of ideas about emotion in psychology. *Emotion Review*, *1* (*4*), 316–339.

Gucciardi, D. F., Jalleh, G., and Donovan, R. J. (2011). An examination of the Sport Drug Control Model with elite Australian athletes. *Journal of Science and Medicine in Sport*, *14*, 469–476.

Hubner, G. and Kaiser, F. G. (2006). The moderating role of the attitude-subjective norms conflict on the link between moral norms and intention. *European Psychologist*, *11* (*2*), 99e109. doi: 10.1027/1016–9040.11.2.99.

Huybers, T. and Mazanov, J. (2012). What would Kim do: A choice study of projected athlete doping considerations. *Journal of Sport Management*, *26* (*4*), 322–334.

Jalleh, G., Donovan, R. J., and Jobling, I. (2014). Predicting attitude towards performance enhancing substance use: A comprehensive test of the Sport Drug Control Model with elite Australian athletes. *Journal of Science and Medicine in Sport*, *17* (*6*), 574–579. doi: 10.1016/j.jsams.2013.10.249.

Laure, P., Lecerf, T., Friser, A., and Binsinger, C. (2004). Drugs, recreational drug use and attitudes towards doping of high school athletes. *International Journal of Sport Medicine*, *25* (*2*), 133–138.

Lazarus, R. S. (1991). *Emotions and adaptation*. New York: Oxford University Press.

Lazuras, L., Barkoukis, V., Rodafinos, A., and Tzorbatzoudis, H. (2010). Predictors of doping intentions in elite-level athletes: A social cognition approach. *Journal of Sport and Exercise Psychology*, *32* (*5*), 694–710.

Lucidi, F., Grano, C., Leone, L., Lombardo, C., and Pesce, C. (2004). Determinants of the intention to use doping substances: An empirical contribution in a sample of Italian adolescents. *Journal of Sport Psychology*, *35* (*2*), 133–148.

Lucidi, F., Zelli, A., and Mallia, L. (2013). The contribution of moral disengagement to adolescents' use of doping substances. *International Journal of Sport Psychology*, *44*, 331–350. doi: 10.7352/IJSP 2013.00.000.

Lucidi, F., Zelli, A., Mallia, L., Grano, C., Russo. P. M., and Violani, C. (2008). The social-cognitive mechanisms regulating adolescents' use of doping substances. *Journal of Sport Sciences*, *26* (*5*), 447–456. doi: 10.1080/02640410701579370.

Mallia, L., Lucidi, F., Zelli, A., and Violani C. (2013). Doping attitudes and the use of legal and illegal performance-enhancing substances among Italian adolescents. *Journal of Child & Adolescent Substance Abuse, 22* (*3*), 179–190. doi: 10.1080/1067828X.2012.733579.

Mazanov, J. and Huybers, T. (2010). An empirical model of athlete decisions to use performance-enhancing drugs: Qualitative evidence. *Qualitative Research in Sport and Exercise, 2*, 385–402.

Overbye, M., Knudsen, M. L., and Pfister, G. (2013). To dope or not to dope: Elite athletes' perceptions of doping deterrents and incentives. *Performance Enhancement and Health, 2* (*3*), 119–134. doi: 10.1016/j.peh.2013.07.001.

Scherer, K. R. (1997). The role of culture in emotion-antecedent appraisals. *Journal of Personality and Social Psychology, 73*, 902–922.

Scherer, K. R. and Wallbott, H. G. (1994). Evidence for universality and cultural variation of differential emotion response patterning. *Journal of Personality and Social Psychology, 66* (*2*), 310–328.

Scherer, K. R., Wranik, T., Sangsue, J., Tran, V., and Scherer, U. (2004). Emotions in everyday life: Probability of occurrence, risk factors, appraisal and reaction patterns. *Social Science Information, 43* (*4*), 499–570.

Smith, C. A. and Pope, L. K. (1992). Appraisal and emotion: The interactional contribution of dispositional and situational factors. In M. S. Clark (ed.), *Annual Review of Personality and Social Psychology, Vol. 14: Emotion and Social Behavior* (32–62). New York: Sage.

Strelan, P. and Boeckmann, R. J. (2006). Why drug testing in elite sport does not work: Perceptual deterrence theory and the role of personal moral beliefs. *Journal of Applied Social Psychology, 36* (*12*), 2909–2934. doi: 10.1111/j.0021–9029.2006.00135.x.

Wiefferink, C. H., Detmar, S. B., Coumans, B., Vogels, T., and Paulussen, T. G. W. (2008). Social psychological determinants of the use of performance-enhancing drugs by gym users. *Health Education Research, 23* (*1*), 70–80. doi: 10.1093/her/cym004.

Zelli, A., Mallia, L., and Lucidi, F. (2010). The contribution of interpersonal appraisals to a social-cognitive analysis of adolescents' doping use. *Psychology of Sport and Exercise, 11*, 304–311. doi: 10.1016/j.psychsport.2010.02.008.

Zelli, A., Lucidi, F., Mallia, L., Giannini A. M., and Sgalla, R. (2013). Adolescents' legality representations and crime reporting. *Psychology, Crime and Law, 19* (*4*), 345–370. doi: 10.1080/1068316X.2011.639770.

3 Modeling doping cognition from a dual process perspective

Ralf Brand, Wanja Wolff, and Franz Baumgarten

From time to time we find ourselves doing things that we never actually intended to do. For example, although one makes a firm decision to avoid unnecessary calories, one may find oneself unable to resist "spontaneously" taking a piece of a delicious cheesecake. Is it possible and reasonable to suggest that something similar may take place in the context of doping behavior? From a more general psychological viewpoint there sometimes seem to be two forces at work, one that is very immediate and more or less uncontrollable and another that is more considered, i.e., based on reasoned thinking and a – possibly subjective – idea of what is rational. This distinction is at the core of psychological dual process approaches. At its most general, dual process theories assume that motivated behavior is rooted in two different kinds of thinking.

Nobel Prize winner Daniel Kahneman has stated the characteristic differences between the two types of thought in a clear, comprehensive manner and assigned them into two different cognitive systems:

> The operations of System 1 are typically fast, automatic, effortless, associative, implicit (not available to introspection), and often emotionally charged; they are also governed by habit and are therefore difficult to control or modify. The operations of System 2 are slower, serial, effortful, more likely to be consciously monitored and deliberately controlled; they are also relatively flexible and potentially rule governed.
>
> (Kahneman 2003: 698)

The issue of whether or not it is necessary to assume two separate systems is contentious (e.g., Kruglanski *et al.* 2006), but the distinction between more and less conscious information processing is one of the most widely recognized in social cognition (e.g., Evans 2008; Evans and Stanovich 2013; Hofmann *et al.* 2009).

We were motivated to write this chapter because it is our impression that the vast majority of published research on doping behavior (e.g., Ntoumanis *et al.* 2014) refers to what Kahneman (2003) has described as system 2 output; however very recently response time-based methods closely linked to system 1 began to be used in doping-related studies (Brand *et al.* 2014a; Brand *et al.*

2011; Brand *et al.* 2014b; Lotz and Hagemann 2007; Petróczi *et al.* 2010, 2011; Petróczi *et al.* 2008). It is the aim of this chapter to familiarize readers with central ideas from the dual process approach to the human mind and thinking, and to bring conceptual and terminological clarity to research efforts in doping research that are (sometimes unspoken) related to this approach. The respective studies are briefly reviewed and put into a dual process perspective. It is beyond the scope of this chapter to fundamentally reconsider empirical findings on the dual process approach from general psychology. This is done, for example, in Evans (2008) or in Evans and Stanovich (2013).

Theoretical frameworks for defining type 1 and type 2 process interplays

The *Reflective-Impulsive Model* (RIM; Strack and Deutsch 2004) provides a very general illustration of the relationship between the two types of thinking (Figure 3.1). The RIM proposes that situational cues (e.g., the prospect of a poor performance) trigger processes in a *reflective system* which is used to weigh information and evaluate it in the light of personal values (e.g., "doping is against the spirit of sport"), attitudes (e.g., "doping is nevertheless necessary to win"), norms (e.g., "doping is illegal"), or potential consequences (e.g., sanctions). This rather slow process may result in a decision or intention to refrain from doping, which can be used to activate appropriate behavioral schemata (e.g., avoid tempting situations).

The situational cue simultaneously initiates a parallel automatic process in the *impulsive system* based on activation of associative networks. These activations generate affectively toned states (e.g., "doing this feels wrong") that are capable of generating approach/avoidance motivation for the relevant behavioral schema. Both systems provide information that influences the other system, but the impulsive system plays a more central role in behavior regulation as it is always

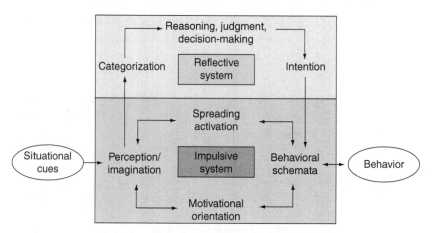

Figure 3.1 The Reflective-Impulsive Model (source: Strack and Deutsch 2004).

involved, and outputs are almost instantly available. The reflective system may not always be engaged, especially when arousal is low (e.g., during routine behavior) or high (e.g., when performing under pressure).

Automatic associations in the impulsive system and intentions from the reflective system may or may not be in accord. Friese *et al.* (2011) use the metaphor of a person riding a horse to illustrate how outputs from the two systems can diverge or converge: the horse (the impulsive/automatic process) may go in the direction intended by the rider (reflective/controlled process) or it may bolt and run in a completely different direction from the one chosen by the rider.

The *MODE* model (Motivation and Opportunity as Determinants; Fazio 1990) is an influential account of how attitudes can influence behavior. According to this model attitudes represent the extent to which the individual has learnt to associate a positive or negative evaluation with an attitude object (e.g., doping). These associations are assumed to be relatively stable and – in that sense – dispositional constructs. The MODE model (Fazio and Olson 2003) views an automatically activated attitude as the starting point from which attitude-relevant behavior can flow spontaneously, unimpeded by more conscious processes although an attitude's downstream consequences, its influence on overt judgments and behavior, are moderated by motivation and opportunity. According to the MODE model automatically activated attitudes are more likely to govern behavior when the time or capacity for deliberation is limited, whereas when people are motivated to deliberate and have the opportunity to do so it is more likely that they will engage in rational evaluations of an issue (e.g., whether or not to take an illegal substance) and take behavioral decisions in line with the outcome of their deliberations.

The *Associative-Propositional in Evaluation* Model (APE) (see Figure 3.2) goes beyond these two earlier models (RIM and MODE) as it focuses on the dynamics of associative (type 1) and propositional (type 2) processes of

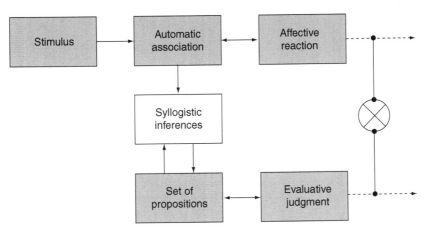

Figure 3.2 The Associative-Propositional in Evaluation Model (source: Gawronski and Bodenhausen 2006).

evaluation and attitude change (Gawronski and Bodenhausen 2006). The authors of the model assumed that associative processing is often characterized by automatic affective reactions; they emphasized that such automatic affective reactions – implicit attitudes in their terminology – were independent of truth values, i.e., associative evaluations can be activated irrespective of whether an individual considers them to be appropriate or inappropriate. In contrast the propositional process is based on evaluative judgments (explicit attitudes) which are the outcome of syllogistic inferences involving all propositional information that is considered relevant to the judgment in hand. This propositional process is generally concerned with the validation of evaluations and beliefs (i.e., it is dependent on truth values in the above-mentioned sense). The APE model posits that individuals base their evaluative judgment on their automatic affective reactions. It is proposed that affirmation of validity is the default mode of propositional processing and that the "perceived validity of a proposition depends on the consistency of this proposition with other propositions that are momentarily considered to be relevant for the respective judgment" (Gawronksi and Bodenhausen 2006: 694). The authors suggest that implicit and explicit attitude change should be understood as a function of the underlying associative and propositional processes. In the case of associative evaluations (type 1 thinking) these processes include changes in activation patterns. Evaluative judgments on the other hand (type 2 thinking) can be changed by adjusting associative evaluations, changing the set of propositions considered relevant to the judgment and altering the validity of some of these propositions to achieve propositional consistency.

In summary, these dual process approaches offer theoretical accounts of *how* type 1 and type 2 thinking are related; second, all dual process models propose that type 1 and type 2 thinking are linked in the *temporal dimension*. Correlations between type 1 (automatic) and type 2 (controlled) cognition, and – for example – between spontaneous and reasoned doping-related decisions and behavior should therefore be analysed with regard to the underlying *process*.

Response time-based testing of type 1 cognition: a necessary excursion on terminology

One can easily gain access to outputs from – in RIM terminology – the reflective system by asking people about their thoughts and feelings directly. However, impulsive processes cannot be inferred from participants' answers to a research questionnaire. In general terms this is because meaningful verbal responses to some extent are necessarily linked with reasoned thinking (i.e., a type 2 process). Developing empirical methods that can effectively dissociate type 2 and type 1 processes has long been one of the greatest challenges in social-cognitive research. The inaccessibility of the outputs of the impulsive system by using questionnaires prompted researchers to use reaction time-based tests to investigate type 1 processes.

One of these tests, the Implicit Association Test[1] (IAT; Greenwald *et al.* 1998), has already attracted some attention in doping research (Brand *et al.*

2011, 2014a, 2014b; Lotz and Hagemann 2007; Petróczi *et al.* 2008, 2010, 2011). An IAT is typically presented on a computer, in the form of a lexical sorting task in which two concepts (one target concept and one evaluative concept) are mapped to the same computer key. The sorting task is easier for respondents when the two concepts sharing the same response key are closely associated than when they are not. An athlete with a negative attitude to doping will respond more quickly when the words "steroids" and "bad" are mapped to the same key than when "steroids" and "good" are mapped to the same key. IAT scores are usually calculated using the difference between response times for related and unrelated word pairs (Greenwald *et al.* 2003). Low IAT scores, e.g., negative scores, indicate closer associations between doping and the negative attribute (i.e., a more negative attitude to doping) than between doping and the positive attribute (i.e., a more positive attitude to doping). Absolute scores are assumed to reflect associative and thus attitude strength.

One might argue that the IAT has been handicapped by being labeled as an "implicit" test. There is a wealth of literature on resulting misunderstandings and their origins (De Houwer and Moors 2010; Fiedler *et al.* 2006). These are outlined in the following section, together with terminology in which we believe addresses some of the misunderstandings affecting the IAT and alternative response time-based tests used in social-cognition research.

In this terminology (see De Houwer and Moors 2010: 177ff.) a "measure" is the outcome of applying a measurement procedure to an individual. A measure is "implicit" if the underlying process contains features of automaticity (e.g., it is unintentional, uncontrolled, unconscious, and efficient; Bargh 1994). These four features of automaticity do not always co-occur, so it is important to specify which features of automaticity characterize the processes underlying the IAT task. To date there has been relatively little empirical research on this and results have not been conclusive (De Houwer *et al.* 2009). It is worth noting that propositional (type 2 processes) interpretations of IAT effects (De Houwer 2006; Hughes *et al.* 2011) remain a viable alternative to accounts couched in terms of type 1 processes. But at present it seems unreasonable and premature to generally reject the assumption the IAT taps type 1 processes.

The case for classifying the IAT as an "indirect" test is much more clear-cut. In the IAT participants do not have to self-assess their attitude as they would in a direct test, for example in a doping attitude questionnaire. Instead participants' attitudes are inferred from behavior, in this instance differences in response latencies to target and control pairs on the IAT.

Taken in sum, tests are classified as "direct" or "indirect" on the basis of the procedure involved. Response time-based tests tend to reduce the opportunity participants have to engage in effortful type 2 processing. We will therefore refer to IAT effects (the outcomes of the IAT procedure) as indicators of attitude – not implicit attitudes – derived from an indirect attitude test (the IAT) that is intended to tap type 1 human thinking processes (see also Chapter 7).

Empirical findings on type 1 processes in doping research

To date few social-cognition studies have used recognized type 1 tasks to investigate doping-related type 1 processes and with the exception of a study by Schirlin *et al.* (2009) all have used variants of the IAT. The first study of type 1 processes in the context of doping was published by Lotz and Hagemann (2007); they used a standard IAT task with "doping" as the target and "tea blends" as the comparison concept, together with "positive" and "negative" as evaluative attributes (i.e., doping or tea blends paired with positive or negative attributes). In essence they showed that track and field athletes – a group of athletes prone to doping according to the authors – had a more lenient attitude to doping than table tennis players, who were assumed to be less prone to doping. Shortly after this Petróczi *et al.* (2008) reported that participants who declared that they would consider using doping had a more lenient attitude to doping according to a doping/nutritional supplements–good/bad standard IAT. These authors showed that the results of questionnaire-based direct attitude test (e.g., the Performance Enhancement Attitude Scale, PEAS; Petróczi and Aidman 2009) was partially dissociated from the results of an indirect attitude test, thereby suggesting that indirect tests had the potential to capture undeclared attitudes. Later, Brand *et al.* (2011) evaluated the psychometric properties of the two published doping IATs available at that time. They found that both procedures had substantial error rates and were subject to adaptive learning and concluded that both were suboptimal.

From a historical perspective the most important contribution of these seminal IAT studies was to show that reaction time-based attitude tests were an interesting alternative or complement to questionnaire-based direct testing which had been the standard method for examining attitudes until that point. These studies were an important starting point for later research in this area, making it possible to now investigate how indirect tests of attitude to doping could contribute to our understanding of doping behavior.

Two new lines of research have emerged in the past few years. The first line of research focuses on the relationship between athletes' answers to direct questions about doping or behavior and the results of indirect attitude tests (Petróczi *et al.* 2010, 2011). The second line of research was concerned with development of the IAT method and provided clear evidence that doping behavior and type 1 cognition are indeed connected (Brand 2014a, 2014b).

Petróczi *et al.* (2010) compared the attitudes of "doped" and "clean" athletes to doping using an indirect attitude test, the Brief IAT (BIAT), with a doping–bad/good–[supplements] format (the bracketed concept is the one that remains non-focal in the BIAT). Their most important finding related to six athletes who had biochemical traces of banned substances in their hair samples and denied doping in a questionnaire assessment. These athletes responded even more rapidly to the *good-doping* pairs than the four "doped" athletes who had admitted doping. The same authors analysed their findings in more detail in a subsequent article ("In Which Measure Do We Trust?"; Petróczi *et al.*

2011). Direct measures of attitude (e.g., PEAS score) aligned well with admitted use of banned substances, but biochemical test results were more closely aligned with indirect measures of attitude (e.g., BIAT results). The effects were very small and variance was large, so these relationships were not statistically significant. In summary, Petróczi *et al.* (2010, 2011) proposed that direct and indirect measures of attitude were dissociable and, hence, that strong rejection of doping in the PEAS combined with a (B)IAT result indicating a rather lenient attitude to doping might be indicative of unacknowledged doping.

The overarching goal of the work by Brand *et al.* (2014a) was to develop and test a doping BIAT which could be used internationally in research i.e., irrespective of the test taker's first language. In a preliminary validation study they showed that bodybuilders had more lenient attitudes to doping (use of performance-enhancing substances is widespread in bodybuilding) than handball players in a doping–dislike/like–[health food] task in which the test stimuli were pictures and emoticons. They found evidence to support and extend Petróczi *et al.*'s (2011) hypothesis that the dissociation between direct and indirect measures of doping attitudes may be indicative of athletes' unacknowledged doping behavior. Brand *et al.* (2014a) reported significant positive correlation between directly and indirectly measured attitudes to "doping" in bodybuilders but not handball players. This suggests that the dissociation between direct and indirect measures of attitude might only serve as an indicator of doping behavior in sports in which illegitimate use of doping substances is socially banned and/or prohibited.

A second study (Brand *et al.* 2014b) demonstrated the predictive validity of the pictorial doping BIAT for factual doping behavior. In a large sample of 61 bodybuilders the authors showed that BIAT score helped to identify the 26 bodybuilders whose urine samples contained biochemical traces of doping substances. This study was the first, and to date the only study, to have provided robust empirical evidence for the correlation between a psychological measure of attitude to doping and biochemical evidence of doping behavior.

So far only one study has investigated doping-related type 1 cognition using an alternative to the IAT family. Schirlin *et al.* (2009) used an emotional Stroop task in which participants had to respond as quickly as possible to the colors in which words related to doping or control words were presented on a computer screen. The response latencies for doping words were significantly longer (26 ms on average) than for control words. This emotional Stroop effect can be interpreted as an indication of the difficulty the test taker has in actively, deliberately disengaging his or her attention from a personally salient stimulus. Schirlin *et al.* (2009) showed that adolescents with low self-esteem (they were not athletes) exhibited an attentional bias toward doping-related words, thus demonstrating that an emotional Stroop task can be used to detect an apparently impulsive (type 1) interest in doping.

Conclusions

Dual process theories of cognition assume that there are two types of thinking: one is fast, automatic, and effortless (type 1) and the other is comparatively slow, reasoned, and controlled (type 2). There is undisputable evidence from general social-cognition research that type 1 processes play an important role in human decision-making and behavior (e.g., Hofmann *et al.* 2009). The RIM, MODE, and APE models offer different accounts of the relationship between type 1 and type 2 processes. Doping research has only recently begun to make use of reaction time-based paradigms based on these theories. Most of these studies have used the IAT or a variant on the IAT.

The IAT is based on a distinction between explicit and implicit memory (Greenwald and Banaji 1995). There is very good evidence from several behavioral domains that it can be used to predict behavior (Greenwald *et al.* 2009) and so the IAT has become an instrument for measuring socially sensitive attitudes in social psychological research (De Houwer *et al.* 2009). In one of the earliest and most frequently cited publications on the IAT its developers wrote that "the implicit association method may reveal attitudes and other automatic associations even for subjects who prefer not to express those attitudes" (Greenwald *et al.* 1998: 1465). This statement is capable of being misunderstood, as the IAT was never designed to serve as a "lie detector." It is rather the possibility to learn about an individual's spontaneous associations with an attitude object giving the IAT intuitive appeal as a means of addressing the central problem in social science doping research, which is that athletes will not always give report of their spontaneous thoughts about doping. In the language of dual process theories when responding to a questionnaire athletes may start to deliberate and give what they believe to be the socially desirable response (e.g., Gucciardi *et al.* 2010).[2] There are good reasons to believe that the IAT helps to address the problem of strategic answering in doping research; but it must be emphasized that even IAT tests can be faked, especially when participants are given information about how this can be done (e.g., Kim 2003).

Most researchers accept that IAT scores reflect type 1 processes (Nosek *et al.* 2007). One advantage of using this test is its relative robustness, compared to alternatives such as the emotional Stroop test (Mathews and MacLeod 1985) or the affective priming task (Fazio *et al.* 1995). Also, the IAT is comparatively easy to handle. It has superior internal consistency and test-retest reliability, and better predictive validity than, for example, the two tests mentioned as alternatives (Greenwald *et al.* 2009). On the other hand, these alternatives can more unambiguously be related to type 1 processes. We consider that at present the IAT is the most promising approach of measuring type 1 processes related to doping behavior.

Some of the extant doping-related findings can be interpreted in the light of dual process theories of cognition. The APE model and the RIM provide good accounts of the finding that the dissociation between indirect and direct measures of attitude was indicative of unacknowledged doping among athletes practicing sports in which doping is illegitimate and socially unacceptable (e.g., handball), but may be less useful in the context of sports in which doping is socially accepted (e.g., bodybuilding) (Brand *et al.* 2014a). This may be attributed to a difference between handball players and bodybuilders in the perceived necessity of deliberatively adjusting answers to direct questions about attitude to doping. However, it is very important to recognize that athletes can reflect on (type 2 process) and choose to reject a positive automatic affective evaluation of doping (type 1 process) as a basis for decisions about behavior; this is more likely when the automatic affective evaluation is inconsistent with other personal beliefs (e.g., that doping remains a socially and legally sanctioned behavior) than when it is not (e.g., "doping" is culturally accepted in one's sport or peer group).

We conclude with one main recommendation based on our analysis of the current state of research on doping-related cognition. Future research should address the *complex interaction* between type 1 and type 2 thinking processes (e.g., attitudes) and doping behavior, rather than continuing to debate *the existence of* correlations between doping behavior and the two types of thinking.

Notes

1 It is important to note that the IAT is a class of tests; several variants have been developed, for example the Single Category IAT (Karpinski and Steinman 2006), the Recoding Free IAT (Rothermund *et al.* 2009), and the Brief IAT (BIAT; Sriram and Greenwald 2009). One of these variants, the BIAT, has already been used in doping research.

2 The data from many empirical studies using questionnaires to measure attitude to doping are subject to floor effects (e.g., when athletes are asked to indicate their attitude to statements such as "Doping is an unavoidable part of competitive sport" on a Likert scale ranging from e.g., 1 = "strongly disagree" to 5 = "strongly agree" responses are often clustered at the bottom of the scale).

References

Bargh, J. A. (1994). The four horsemen of automaticity: Awareness, intention, efficiency, and control in social cognition. In R. S. Wyer Jr. and T. K. Srull (eds.), *Handbook of social cognition*, Volume 1. (1–4). Hillsdale, NJ and UK: Lawrence Erlbaum Associates.

Brand, R., Heck, P., and Ziegler, M. (2014a). Illegal performance enhancing drugs and doping in sport: A picture-based brief implicit association test for measuring athletes' attitudes. *Substance Abuse Treatment, Prevention, and Policy, 9*, 7.

Brand, R., Melzer, M., and Hagemann, N. (2011).Towards an implicit association test (IAT) for measuring doping attitudes in sports. Data-based recommendations developed from two recently published tests. *Psychology of Sport and Exercise, 12* (*3*), 250–256.

Brand, R., Wolff, W., and Thieme, D. (2014b). Using response-time latencies to measure athletes' doping attitudes. The brief implicit attitude test identifies substance abuse in bodybuilders. *Substance Abuse Treatment, Prevention, and Policy, 9*, 36.

De Houwer, J. (2006). Using the implicit association test does not rule out an impact of conscious propositional knowledge on evaluative conditioning. *Learning Motivation, 37*, 176–187.

De Houwer, J. and Moors, A. (2010). Implicit measures: Similarities and differences. In B. Gawronski and B. K. Payne (eds.), *Handbook of implicit social cognition: Measurement, theory, and applications* (176–196). New York: Guilford Press.

De Houwer, J., Teige-Mocigemba, S., Spruyt, A., and Moors, A. (2009). Implicit measures: A normative analysis and review. *Psychological Bulletin, 135*, 347–368.

Evans, J. S. (2008). Dual-processing accounts of reasoning, judgment, and social cognition. *Annual Review of Psychology, 59*, 255–278.

Evans, J. S. and Stanovich, K. E. (2013). Dual-process theories of higher cognition: advancing the debate. *Perspectives on Psychological Science, 8*, 223–241.

Fazio, R. A. (1990). Multiple processes by which attitudes guide behavior: The MODE model as an integrative framework. In M. P. Zanna (ed.), *Advances in experimental social psychology* (75–110). New York: Academic Press.

Fazio, R. H. and Olson, M. A. (2003). Implicit measures in social cognition research: Their meaning and use. *Annual Review of Psychology, 54*, 297–327.

Fazio, R. H., Jackson, J. R., Dunton, B. C., and Williams, C. J. (1995). Variability in automatic activation as an unobtrusive measure of racial attitudes: A bona fide pipeline? *Journal of Personality and Social Psychology, 69*, 1013–1027.

Fiedler, K., Messner, C., and Bluemke, M. (2006). Unresolved problems with the "I", the "A", and the "T": A logical and psychometric critique of the Implicit Association Test (IAT). *European Review of Social Psychology, 17*, 74–147.

Friese, M., Hofmann, W., and Wiers, R. W. (2011). On taming horses and strengthening riders: Recent developments in research on interventions to improve self-control in health behaviors. *Self and Identity, 10*, 336–351.

Gawronski, B. and Bodenhausen, G. V. (2006). Associative and propositional processes in evaluation: An integrative review of implicit and explicit attitude change. *Psychological Bulletin, 132*, 692–731.

Greenwald, A. G. and Banaji, M. R. (1995). Implicit social cognition: Attitudes, self-esteem, and stereotypes. *Psychological Review, 102*, 4–27.

Greenwald, A. G., McGhee, D. E., and Schwartz, J. L. K. (1998). Measuring individual differences in implicit cognition: The implicit association test. *Journal of Personality and Social Psychology, 74*, 1464–1480.

Greenwald, A. G., Nosek, B. A., and Banaji, M. R. (2003). Understanding and using the implicit association test: I. An improved scoring algorithm. *Journal of Personality and Social Psychology, 85*, 197–216.

Greenwald, A. G., Poehlman, T. A., Uhlmann, E. L., and Banaji, M. R. (2009). Understanding and Using the Implicit Association Test: III. Meta-Analysis of Predictive Validity. *Journal of Personality and Social Psychology, 97*, 17–41.

Gucciardi, D. F, Jalleh, G., and Donovan, R. J. (2010). Does social desirability influence the relationship between doping attitudes and doping susceptibility in athletes? *Psychology of Sport and Exercise, 11*, 479–486.

Hofmann, W., Friese, M., and Strack, F. (2009). Impulse and self-control from a dual-systems perspective. *Perspectives on Psychological Science, 4*, 162–176.

Hughes, S., Barnes-Holmes, D., and De Houwer, J. (2011). The dominance of associative theorizing in implicit attitude research: Propositional and behavioral alternatives. *Psychological Records, 61*, 465–496.

Kahneman, D. (2003). A perspective on judgement and choice. Mapping bounded rationality. *American Psychologist, 58*, 697–720.

Karpinski, A. and Steinman, R. B. (2006). The Single Category Implicit Association Test as a measure of implicit social cognition. *Journal of Personality and Social Psychology, 91*, 16–32.

Kim, D. Y. (2003). Voluntary controllability of the implicit association test (IAT). *Social Psychology Quarterly, 66*, 83–96.

Kruglanski, A. W., Erb, H. P., Pierro, A., Mannetti, L., and Chun, W. Y. (2006). On parametric continuities in the world of binary either ors. *Psychological Inquiry, 17*, 153–165.

Lotz, S. and Hagemann, N. (2007). Using the Implicit Association Test to measure athletes' attitude toward doping. *Journal of Sport and Exercise Psychology, 29 (Suppl.)*, 183–184.

Mathews, A. and MacLeod, C. M. (1985). Selective processing of threat cues in anxiety states. *Behaviour Research and Therapy, 23*, 563–569.

Nosek, B. A., Greenwald, A. G., and Banaji, M. R. (2007). The Implicit Association Test at age 7: A methodological and conceptual review. In J. A. Bargh (ed.), *Automatic processes in social thinking and behavior* (265–292). New York: Psychology Press.

Ntoumanis, N., Ng, J. Y., Barkoukis, V., and Backhouse, S. H. (2014). Personal and psychosocial predictors of doping use in physical activity settings: A meta-analysis. *Sports Medicine, 44 (11)*, 1603–1624.

Petróczi, A. and Aidman, E. V. (2009). Measuring explicit attitude toward doping: Review of the psychometric properties of the Performance Enhancement Attitude Scale. *Psychology of Sport and Exercise, 10*, 390–396.

Petróczi, A., Aidman, E. V., and Nepusz, T. (2008). Capturing doping attitudes by self-report declarations and implicit assessment: A methodology study. *Substance Abuse Treatment Prevention and Policy, 3 (9)*.

Petróczi, A., Aidman, E. V., Hussain, I., Deshmukh, N., Nepusz, T., Uvacsek, M., Tóth, M., Barker, J., and Naughton, D. P. (2010). Virtue or pretense? Looking behind self-declared innocence in doping. *PLoS One, 5 (5)*: e10457.

Petróczi, A., Uvacsek, M., Nepusz, T., Deshmukh, N., Shah, I., Aidman, E. V., Barker, J., Tóth, M., and Naughton, D. P. (2011). Incongruence in doping related attitudes, beliefs and opinions in the context of discordant behavioural data: in which measure do we trust? *PLoS One, 6 (4)*: e18804.

Rothermund, K., Teige-Mocigemba, S., Gast, A., and Wentura, D. (2009). Minimizing the influence of recoding in the Implicit Association Test: The Recoding-Free Implicit Association Test (IAT-RF). *Quarterly Journal of Experimental Psychology, 62*, 84–98.

Schirlin, O., Rey, G., Jouvent, R., Dubal, S., Komano, O., Perez-Diaz, F., and Soussignan, R. (2009). Attentional bias for doping words and its relation with physical self-esteem in young adolescents. *Psychology of Sport and Exercise, 10*, 615–620.

Sriram, N. and Greenwald, A. G. (2009). The Brief Implicit Association Test. *Experimental Psychology, 56*, 283–294.

Strack, F. and Deutsch, R. (2004). Reflective and impulsive determinants of social behavior. *Personality and Social Psychology Review, 8*, 220–247.

4 Social-cognitive predictors of doping use

An integrative approach

Lambros Lazuras

> Every psychological event depends upon the state of the person and at the same time on the environment, although their relative importance is different in different cases.
>
> (Kurt Lewin 1935)

From the preceding chapters it is clear that doping use is a multifaceted phenomenon that requires different levels of explanation, and a sound understanding of underlying psychosocial processes. These processes range from implicit social cognition, such as automatic attitude activation and action tendencies, to deliberate, purposeful action involving a consideration of expected costs and benefits, social norms, and perceived behavioral control (e.g., Brand *et al.* 2011; Ntoumanis *et al.* 2014; Petróczi and Aidman 2008). Integrative models of behavior (e.g., Fishbein and Cappella 2006) attempt to organize these different sources of influence into a coherent theoretical and explanatory framework. Such models may accordingly help research scientists, policymakers, and practitioners better understand when certain behaviors are likely to be enacted, and, most importantly, what types of interventions are suitable to prevent the onset – or decrease the likelihood – of undesirable and risky behaviors. This chapter provides an overview of integrative models for behavioral prediction and discusses relevant research in the context of doping use. Recommendations for future research in this area, as well as implications for policy-making and anti-doping campaign development, are also addressed.

Why is an integrative approach important?

As evidenced in the opening quote from Kurt Lewin (1935) human behavior does not stem from personal beliefs and traits alone, but it is rather explained through an understanding of the dynamic links between intra-personal characteristics, like beliefs and traits, and contextual features and influences. This principle is reflected in general integrative models of behavioral prediction, and is also embedded in domain-specific integrative models of doping use, such as

Petróczi and Aidman's (2008) life-cycle model of performance enhancement. But before turning to the discussion of these models, it is worth mentioning the importance of the "integrative" approach. And it is better to do so with an illustrative (and imaginary) example.

Consider Tom, a 23-year-old athlete competing in the professional football league. Tom has contemplated the use of prohibited substances with hopes of increasing endurance and markedly improving his performance. He has a firm intention to start using these substances, while at the same time acknowledging that their use can be life-threatening. But as in Goldman's dilemma (Connor and Mazanov 2009), Tom decides to pursue immediate glory and overlook potential health consequences placed somewhere in the future. He makes the necessary contacts and within a short time frame he starts using prohibited performance enhancement substances.

A simple reading of this case may lead someone to conclude that Tom's decision to engage in doping practices stems from a personal need to succeed in sports at all costs. Such an interpretation will heavily emphasize individual, intra-personal characteristics as the driving forces of the decision to engage in doping behavior. The tendency to think of doping in these terms is depicted in popular stories and related films. For example, the motion picture *A Body To Die For: The Aaron Henry Story*, starring Ben Affleck, describes the life of a teenage football player who resorted to steroids to increase muscularity and improve athletic performance, and totally neglected symptoms of ill health, aggressive behavior, and a deterioration of social relationships caused by continuous steroid use. Perhaps emphasizing intra-personal characteristics is an easy way for authorities to label athletes who engage in doping behaviors as "bad apples" (i.e., athletes with inherent traits and inclination to commit undesirable acts) rather than viewing doping behaviors as a complex interaction of environmental and interpersonal factors. It is easy to see an athlete as totally responsible for a doping incident and overlook the external forces that facilitated or led to that decision.

However, such a viewpoint neglects the broader environmental and contextual influences that might have played a role in shaping the decision to engage in doping behavior, and, thus, fails to capture the dynamism of human behavior suggested by Kurt Lewin some 80 years ago. As it is stated in different parts of this book, doping permeates all levels of sports and is evident across age groups and competence levels. These different contexts can have a profound and unique effect on an athlete's mindset about doping behavior. Interpreting doping incidents as the result of character flaws and personal weakness leads us to a moral model of doping that says nothing about the situations wherein doping occurs; thus leading us to a fundamental attribution error, and giving us an incomplete view of the problem in question. Therefore, for a better and more complete understanding of the psychological processes underlying doping use, it is important to understand the interaction between intra-personal traits and social/contextual features, and how the resultant dynamic relationships drive action-initiation. In this direction, integrative models of behavioral prediction (e.g., Fishbein 2009; Hagger and Chatzisarantis 2009) provide a helpful explanatory framework, and their application can be particularly useful in the context of doping prevention in sports.

Integrative models of behavioral prediction: deepening and broadening the Theory of Planned Behavior

In the first chapter, Kirby and colleagues eloquently described the role of attitudes in predicting doping use in sports, and also the importance of the Theory of Planned Behavior (TPB; Ajzen 1991) in explaining attitude–behavior relationships in this context. A recent meta-analysis showed that the TPB has guided most of the published studies on the social-cognitive correlates of doping use (Ntoumanis et al. 2014). However, this meta-analysis also presented studies that attempted to move beyond the standard TPB by adding new variables, and/or considering parallel processes to the ones described by the original model. For instance, Lazuras et al. (2010) extended the concept of social norms within the TPB framework and included descriptive norms (i.e., beliefs about what other athletes do), as well as the concept of situational temptation (i.e., the perceived temptation to engage in doping under certain conditions of normative influence), in an attempt to broaden the normative processes underlying doping use, and accordingly show a novel potential path to action through the norms-situational temptation link. This approach fits well with Perugini and Bagozzi's (2001) contentions about deepening and broadening existing theories. They argued that theories are broadened when new variables are added in parallel to other established predictors in a model. In this respect, Ajzen's TPB can be seen as a broadened Theory of Reasoned Action (Ajzen and Fishbein 1977) because the TPB added perceived behavioral control as a parallel predictor of behavior along attitudes and social norms. Accordingly, Lazuras et al. (2010) "broadened" the TPB by incorporating descriptive norms as a parallel variable to subjective norms in predicting doping intentions among adult elite-level athletes. Furthermore, Perugini and Bagozzi (2001) asserted that "deepening" an existing theory occurs when new variables are introduced in a model to explain how pre-existing predictor variables link with intentions and behavior. In this respect, Lazuras et al. (2010) incorporated situational temptation as a variable that explained the processes linking norms to doping intentions. Integrating new variables to the TPB has been a research tradition over the last 15 years, with several review articles and meta-analyses presenting related findings and explaining the theoretical underpinning of the reported integrations (Armitage and Conner 2001; Barkoukis et al. 2010; Hagger 2009; McEachan et al. 2011).

The "broadening and deepening" approach integrates new concepts and variables within an existing theoretical framework, but does not necessarily provide a new way of looking at underlying dynamic processes after Lewin. The main limitation being that the "broadening and deepening" is bound by the main postulates of the target model, and thus fails to provide a dynamism of intrapersonal and contextual/environmental influences as prerequisites of behavioral prediction. Rather, the interactions between interpersonal, contextual forces, and intra-personal characteristics is narrowly explained through the premises of a non-dynamic model where additional variables actually serve as remedies for weak relationships between cognitive/affective variables (Flay *et al.* 2009). To further justify this argument, consider that the incorporation of social influences in the original TPB stemmed from the need to better understand intra-personal processes (i.e., attitude–behavior relationships), rather than understanding contextual influences on behavior and their interactions with personal characteristics and traits. Furthermore, the TPB has been well known for its parsimony. A constant search for new variables added on top of the standard TPB conceptualization may eventually harm the theory's parsimony and make it impractical (Ajzen 2011; Fishbein and Ajzen 2010).

Fishbein (2000, 2009) attempted to retain the TPB's parsimony, while acknowledging the role of external sources of influence and their relationship with TPB's main components. Accordingly, he developed the "integrative model" of behavioral prediction (Fishbein 2009; Fishbein and Cappella 2006) in order to account for the effects of "distal" predictors, such as demographic variables, personality traits, and other individual differences, on intentions and behavior. The model was based on the mediation hypothesis of the TPB, whereby the effects of any variable falling outside the original TPB conceptualization on behavior should be mediated by TPB components (attitudes, social norms, perceived behavioral control, and intentions), also referred to as "proximal" predictors (Fishbein 2000; Fishbein and Yzer 2003). This integrative model is presented in Figure 4.1.

So far, the applications of the integrative model are mostly concerned with the design of health promotion campaigns and interventions to promote safe sex practices and cancer screening (Fishbein 2009; Fishbein and Yzer 2003; Smith-McLallen and Fishbein 2008). Nevertheless, there are certain limitations in the integrative approach suggested by Fishbein (2000, 2009). First, the way the model is presented does not account for the interaction between contextual features and intra-personal characteristics. Rather, the integrative model considers media exposure as a general (and vaguely described) distal predictor of attitudes, social norms, and self-efficacy beliefs. Environmental constraints are presented as external variables that may influence the effects of intentions on behavior, but are only seen as deterrents of behavioral inaction and not as fundamental sources of influence in the decision-making process. Thus, the model does not account for the principle of "adaptive co-regulation," which purports that behaviors are largely shaped by contextual influences and that (social) cognition is socially situated (e.g., Semin and Smith 2013). Furthermore, the integrative model (Fishbein 2000, 2009) does not specify the causal paths from distal to proximal variables. Thus, while the integrative model assumes that variables external to the TBP components may influence intention-formation and behavior, the ways this effect may occur are not detailed, and any set of external variables can potentially have an effect on all the core components of the TPB. Thus, it is hard to specify more detailed, theory-driven causal mechanisms and pathways

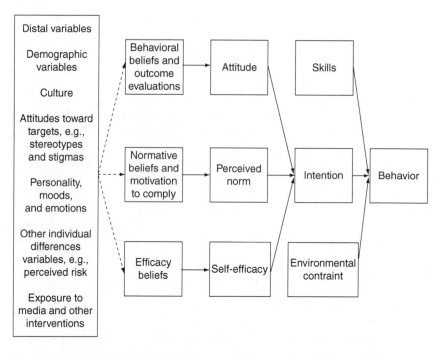

Figure 4.1 The Integrative Model (source: adapted by Fishbein and Yzer 2003).

between distal and proximal predictors a priori using this model. A couple of recent empirical studies on doping use have tried to overcome this issue by specifying how distal, background variables predicted doping-related social-cognitive beliefs and intentions.

In one of these studies, Barkoukis *et al.* (2013) made an explicit reference to, and adapted, the integrative model in the context of doping. More specifically, they assessed the effects of distal variables on attitudes, social norms, self-efficacy beliefs, and intentions to use prohibited performance enhancement substances among adult elite athletes in Greece. The distal variables included individual differences in motivational and moral characteristics (i.e., achievement motivation, self-determination, and sportspersonship), and their effects were assumed to be mediated by social-cognitive beliefs. Using regression-based multiple mediation modeling, Barkoukis *et al.* (2013) found that attitudes and self-efficacy beliefs mediated the effects of achievement motivation and sportspersonship on doping intentions. This finding was in line with the predictions of Fishbein's (2000) integrative model about the mediating properties of social-cognitive beliefs when external/background variables, such as individual differences, are taken into account. It is noteworthy that in their integration, Barkoukis *et al.* (2013) did not arbitrarily add random indices of individual differences as antecedents of social-cognitive beliefs. Rather, their approach rested on the theoretical integration of major theoretical framework in motivational psychology, such as Deci and Ryan's (2008) self-determination theory and achievement goal theory (Elliot and McGregor 2001). Barkoukis *et al.* (2013) extended previous work on the associations between self-determination dimensions and sportspersonship orientations (Donahue *et al.* 2006), and hypothesized that this motivational model of performance enhancement would explain more variance in substance use intentions by considering behavior-related social cognitions. This approach was in line with both Perugini and Baggozi (2001) and Fishbein and Ajzen's (2010) contentions about the use of theory-driven criteria in developing integrative models of behavioral prediction.

Another study utilized the Trans-contextual Model (TCM; Hagger *et al.* 2003) to assess the effects of motivation on social-cognitive variables related to anti-doping (abstinence from using banned performance enhancement substances) in a sample of young Australian sub-elite-level athletes (Chan *et al.* 2015). The TCM integrates three different theoretical perspectives, namely self-determination theory (Deci and Ryan 2008), the hierarchical model of motivation (Vallerand 2007), and the TPB (Ajzen 1991), and emphasizes the distinction between autonomous motivation (self-driven) and controlled motivation (externally driven). The main proposition of the TCM is that motivation in one context can shape motivation and related beliefs (attitudes, social norms, and PBC) and intentions toward performing that behavior in another context. Thus, motivation to take part in exercise in the school context (e.g., physical activity classes) influences the motivational impetus for exercise participation outside the school context, such as leisure-time physical activity (Barkoukis *et al.* 2010). This process specifies the causal paths of motivation between contexts, and addresses their link to social-cognitive variables and intentions. For instance, if autonomous motivation predicts physical activity participation in a primary context (e.g., school), then autonomous motivation will relate to more positive attitudes, social norms, PBC, and intentions to engage in physical activity in a secondary context (i.e., leisure time; Hagger *et al.* 2003).

Chan *et al.* (2015) hypothesized that athletes with higher autonomous motivation would be more likely to pre-emptively avoid doping substances, because doping is against the principles of sports, and represents a means to an end that is more relevant to contingent self-worth than autonomous motivation. Accordingly, controlled motivation for sports participation would have no effect in autonomous, proactive tendencies to avoid doping in sports. The model of the study is presented in Figure 4.2. The findings showed that autonomous motivation predicted both autonomous and controlled motivation to avoid doping. Furthermore, autonomous motivation to avoid doping predicted more positive attitudes, social norms, and PBC for doping avoidance, which, in turn predicted doping-avoidance intentions. Controlled motivation to avoid doping predicted intentions through its effect on subjective norms. First of all, these findings show that one type of motivation in a primary context (autonomous motivation for sports participation) can predict both similar and different types of motivation in a secondary context (autonomous and controlled motivation for doping

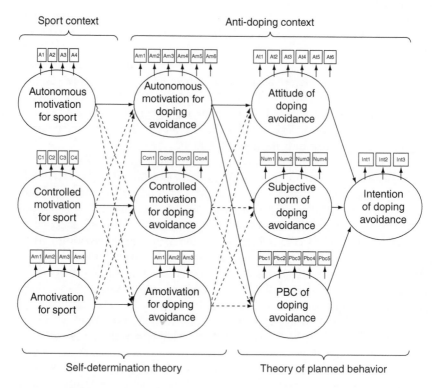

Figure 4.2 The Trans-contextual Model of anti-doping (source: adapted by Chan *et al.* 2014).

avoidance). In turn, these two types of motivation in the secondary context have differential effect on anti-doping-related social cognitions and intentions. Second, and more relevant to the scope of this chapter, Chan *et al.* (2015) showed that a general integrative model for behavioral prediction (TCM) can be successfully applied to the study of doping use, and, more specifically, to the study of doping avoidance – a topic that is largely underrepresented in the existing literature.

Overall, the studies by Barkoukis *et al.* (2013) and Chan *et al.* (2015) suggest that doping intentions and related social-cognitive variables can be, at least partly, understood within broader theoretical frameworks that take into account contextual influences and individual differences in such variables as motivation and moral tendencies (e.g., sportspersonship). Both models supported the "mediation hypothesis" embedded in Fishbein's (2000, 2009) integrative model, as well as the main premises of the TPB about the hierarchical positioning of social-cognitive variables and behavioral intentions. Our understanding of the social-cognitive correlates of doping use can be further enhanced by a look into theoretical models that have derived from different theoretical premises and adopted an ecological perspective of action-initiation. One such model is the Theory of Triadic Influence, which is thoroughly discussed in the following section.

Integrative models of behavioral prediction: an ecological perspective

The Theory of Triadic Influence (TTI; Flay *et al.* 2009) provides a comprehensive and integrative theoretical framework of the antecedents of social-cognitive predictors of health-related behaviors. Like the TPB and related models, the TTI provides a framework to explain and predict intentional behaviors and acknowledges that the effects of external variables on intentions and behavior can be mediated by attitudes, social norms, and self-efficacy. However, the TTI differs from the planned behavior perspective in two important and fundamental ways. First, the TTI is derived from different theoretical premises that use an ecological framework to understand action-initiation. In this respect, family, as well as genetic and heritable components (e.g., phenotype), individual differences, and institutions (e.g., laws and regulations) dynamically interact and produce human behavior. Thus, in sharp contrast to theories that fixate on cognitive/affective variable interactions, the TTI offers a broader perspective that focuses on the importance of background factors. Second, and perhaps more importantly, unlike other integrative models, the TTI organizes these background factors in three distinct categories, and specifies the causal paths that lead to cognitive/affective variables, intention formation, and action-initiation (Flay *et al.* 2009).

As shown in Figure 4.3, the TTI distinguishes between different groups of predictor variables organized hierarchically along three different levels of causation. Ultimate levels of causation include remote and generic influences on behavior, such as biological factors (e.g., testosterone levels), personality characteristics (e.g., neuroticism, extraversion), or social/environmental features (e.g., legal framework, parenting practices, schooling). Distal levels of causation represent influences that are more close to the behavior in question, they can be seen as predisposing influences, but still belong to the group of more general characteristics and beliefs. For instance, self-worth, self-determination, and moral values can all relate to a given behavior (e.g., doping use), however they are not behavior specific. Proximal levels of causation incorporate the group of predictor variables that are said to be more closely situated to decisions and action-initiation, and include cognitive and affective variables, such as attitudes, social norms and self-efficacy beliefs, and intentions. For a behavior to be established, however, feedback is important (e.g., social reinforcement, physiological and psychological experience). Thus, the TTI assumes that cognitive/affective variables are proximal to "trial" behavior, which, in turn, predicts if the behavior in question will re-occur or not (Flay *et al.* 2009). Furthermore, the theory suggests that these levels of causation reflect variables situated in three different streams: the personal stream, the social, and the environmental stream. As shown in Figure 4.3, all the streams include ultimate and predisposing/distal influences, as well as cognitive/affective proximal predictors of behavior initiation.

So, in an illustrative example in the context of doping behavior, the TTI would assume that doping-specific cognitive/affective variables, such as attitudes, norms, and self-efficacy beliefs, stem from more distal and ultimate causes. These causes could range from personality traits (personal stream/ultimate causes), parenting practices (social stream/ultimate causes), and anti-doping policies (e.g., environmental stream/ultimate causes), to achievement motivation and self-determination (personal stream/distal causes), the behavior of role models (social stream/distal causes), and mass media depictions of doping use (environmental stream/distal causes). So far, no study in the field of doping use has addressed the entire nexus of relationships and interactions between levels of causation and streams as suggested by the TTI. Nonetheless, a recent study made explicit reference to the TTI premises and tested specific causal paths from distal to proximal influences on doping intentions. Stemming from the work of Barkoukis et al. (2013) who used an integrative model of doping intentions in adult athletes, Lazuras et al. (forthcoming) used the TTI to specify causal paths between motivation and moral values (sportspersonship) and doping-specific cognitive/affective variables in youth competitive sports. They found that achievement goals, an aspect of motivation and self-competence, predicted doping intentions through self-efficacy beliefs, which is in line with the causal links depicted in the personal stream of the TTI. Accordingly, moral values reflected in sportspersonship orientations predicted doping intentions through outcome expectancy beliefs (attitudes and anticipated regret), which is also congruent with the TTI predictions in the environmental stream. Nevertheless, the study by Lazuras et al. used a cross-sectional design and this limits any conclusions about causality effects, the directionality of the reported associations, and the temporal relationships between the hypothesized distal and proximal influences on doping intentions.

The TTI can be a particularly useful model in the study of the psychological antecedents of doping use for the following reasons. First, it allows a comprehensive understanding of the interplay between ultimate causes of behavior (e.g., legal sanctions and policies against doping use), predisposing/distal influences (e.g., team-level characteristics), and proximal predictors, such as attitudes, social norms, and self-efficacy beliefs. Second, the model may account for the effects of first use (e.g., trial behavior as shown in Figure 4.3) on future use of doping substances. Mapping such feedback loops is important for policymaking and interventions designed to capture the beliefs and experiences of athletes at the early stages of experimentation and use of doping substances and methods. Finally, the TTI can show how training regimes, coaching, and team/motivation climate may act as predisposing influences that, over time, enforce pro-doping beliefs and intentions. This means that a longitudinal design can chart the pathways from broader features of coaching and training to more specific cognitive/affective processes underlying doping use. Thus, although TTI was primarily developed to explain health-related behaviors and guide preventive health policy,

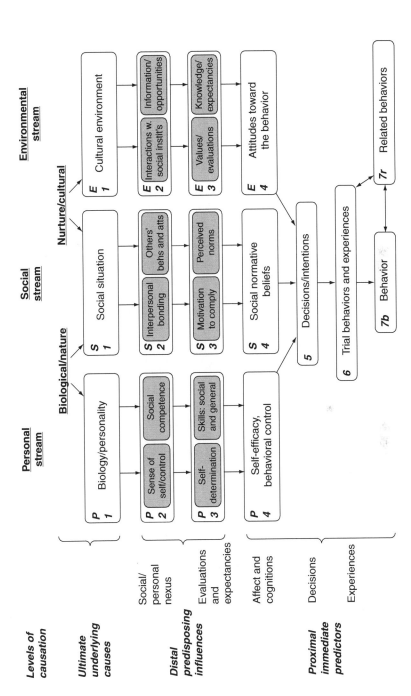

Figure 4.3 The Theory of Triadic Influence (source: adapted from Flay et al. 2009).

the model seems also pertinent to the study and policymaking in the context of doping use. A very similar way of thinking about doping use is also presented in Petróczi and Aidman's (2008) model that was specifically developed to explain doping use in sports. Doping-specific integrative models are discussed in more detail in the following section.

Domain-specific integrative models

Domain-specific integrative models are the ones that were developed to explain doping use and accordingly inform anti-doping policy. Unlike the TTI (Flay *et al.* 2009) and the integrative model (Fishbein 2009) that were either generic models of behavioral prediction, or were developed to explain health-related behaviors, the models discussed in this section came out of the need to better understand the social psychological processes underlying doping use in sports. As such, their main premises rest not only on theoretical foundations about human behavior in general, but also take into account the particularities of competitive sports, such as the existence and influence of legal performance enhancement methods (e.g., use of nutritional supplements), and the cultural beliefs and expectations about sports in present days. Petróczi and Aidman's (2008) Life-cycle Model (LCM) represents an illustrative example of domain-specific (i.e., doping-related) integrative models. The model rests on the assumption that the expectations and methods in competitive sport have changed radically over the last century, leading to a more "mechanistic" view of the (athlete's) body and relying on the pursuit of improving performance. The model accounts for the interplay between intra-personal characteristics (traits), situational factors, and systemic factors that interact and shape athletes' decisions to engage in doping, throughout the life cycle of performance enhancement – thus, the model's name.

Petróczi and Aidman's (2008) core argument is that doping use is intentional, self-regulated, and goal-directed, and not accidental, as other forms of substance use (e.g., alcohol or tobacco use). Accordingly, the use of chemically assisted performance enhancement can be seen as a continuum ranging from legal methods, such as the consumption of dietary/nutritional supplements (e.g., proteins, amino acids, and vitamins) to the use of illegal substances, such as testosterone and other hormone-derived and prohibited drugs. Petróczi and Aidman's model, therefore, was primarily developed to explain drug use in competitive athletes who are acquainted with the functional use of performance enhancement substances. Yet, they argue that their model could also apply to other contexts where the "pill-taking" norm prevails as a performance enhancement method. For instance, the LCM could apply in the case of amateur bodybuilders or leisure-time exercisers who are motivated to use drugs not to improve their athletic performance but to enhance their appearance. Thus, the LCM can be usefully extended to doping prevention policies outside the typical competitive sports contexts where most anti-doping action takes place.

What are the main features of the LCM that make the model so applicable to doping use? Petróczi and Aidman distinguish between three groups of risk or "vulnerability" factors: personality traits, systemic, and situational. Trait factors may range from self-esteem to cognitive ability, integrity, and beliefs about the efficacy of doping. Systemic factors include features of the athletic "system," such as motivational climate and performance enhancement culture in the team, as well as attributes of existing anti-doping policies and doping control mechanisms. Environmental or situational factors, on the other hand, encompass access to and availability of doping and other performance enhancement methods, interactions with peers and fellow athletes, and the salience of role models. It is noteworthy that personality variables are considered more stable than systemic ones, and that the relationships between personality and systemic factors is influenced by the more fluid situational/environmental factors.

Most importantly, the LCM describes the decision to engage in doping as the outcome of six distinct phases: choice, goal commitment, execution, goal attainment feedback, goal evaluation and adjustment, and the decision to exit the performance enhancement cycle. Athletes are assumed to progress through these phases sequentially, and transition between the phases is facilitated by the interplay between achievement goals, reflection on goals and outcomes, and situational factors, such as family or team/sports personnel support. At the final phase, athletes decide whether they will repeat the performance enhancement cycle, modify it to improve the outcomes, or totally abandon their performance enhancement goals. Petróczi and Aidman (2008) recognized that the model is too complex to be evaluated empirically, but the distinct phases of the LCM can be assessed by individual studies. Nevertheless, the LCM does not provide a comprehensive and detailed account of the anticipated relationships between risk/vulnerability and doping intentions or use in each stage, and, so far, no study has explicitly assessed the assumptions of the LCM. That said, unlike the more general integrative models of behavioral prediction, the LCM takes into account the specific context wherein doping is more likely to occur.

The Sports Drug Control Model (SDCM; Donovan *et al.* 2002) represents another domain-specific integrative model of doping use that, unlike Petróczi and Aidman's (2008) LCM, has been subject to empirical investigation. The SDCM has its origins in social cognition models, research on fear appeals, and normative approaches (Donovan *et al.* 2002). Thus, just like most of the models discussed above, the SDCM views doping use as a goal-directed behavior, and, thus, emphasizes the role of attitudes and intentions in the drug use process. Nevertheless, unlike other approaches the SDCM takes a slightly different angle and considers incentives and deterrents for doping use, and the role of both personality traits and reference groups' influence (see Figure 4.4). Doping attitudes in the SDCM are said to be influenced by an appraisal of threats (e.g., detection in a doping control, health side effects); incentives (e.g., anticipated benefits of doping use); reference group opinions (e.g., their approval/disapproval of doping use); moral agency (e.g., beliefs about the legitimacy of doping use); perceived legitimacy of anti-doping policies and laws; and personality traits, such as self-esteem and optimism. Attitudes predict doping intentions, which are influenced by the availability and affordability of doping. These processes are said to take place

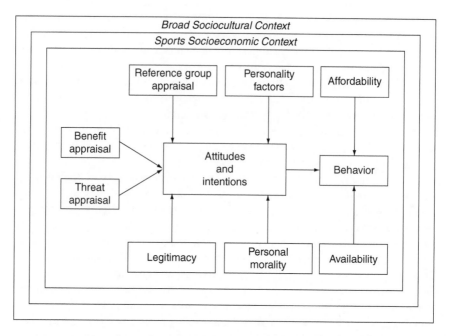

Figure 4.4 The Sport Drug Control Model (source: adapted from Gucciardi *et al.* 2011).

within two broader interacting contexts, the sports socioeconomic context and the broader sociocultural context (Gucciardi *et al.* 2011).

Gucciardi *et al.* (2011) assessed the SDCM in a sample of elite athletes in Australia. They found that, in accordance with the model's predictions, benefit and threat appraisals, and morality significantly predicted doping attitudes. Unlike the SDCM's tenets, however, personality factors (e.g., self-esteem), referent group opinions, and beliefs about the legitimacy of existing doping control methods and policies did not predict doping-related attitudes. In turn, attitudes predicted an indirect measure of doping intentionality (referred to as doping susceptibility). A more recent study with Australian athletes, however, found that attitudes toward doping were predicted by morality, reference group opinions, and personality factors, but not by appraisals of threats, benefits, and the legitimacy of anti-doping policies (Jalleh *et al.* 2014). Collectively, these two studies suggest that SDCM is a useful approach toward understanding how doping attitudes are formed, and how these attitudes relate to doping intentionality and actual doping use. Nevertheless, no study of the SDCM has yet studied the interaction between these person-centered beliefs or cognitive/affective variables with broader sociocultural or sports socioeconomic factors. Thus, although the SDCM identifies the importance of the broader contexts in which doping decisions are made, the existing evidence base has focused largely on the relationships between a narrow set of social-cognitive variables.

The future of integrative models of doping use

The preceding sections provided a detailed account of different integrative models that have been applied in the study of doping use. The majority of these models originate in more general models of behavioral prediction, such as the Theory of Planned Behavior (Ajzen 1991). The applications of the Theory of Triadic Influence and the integrative model (Barkoukis *et al.* 2013; Lazuras *et al.* forthcoming), as well as the Trans-contextual Model (Chan *et al.* 2015), the Sports Drug Control Model (Donovan *et al.* 2002), and the Life-cycle Model (Petróczi and Aidman 2008) explicitly addressed the dynamism suggested by the Lewinian perspective – the dynamic interplay between situations and personal attributes in behavioral performance. Accordingly, all of the models presented in this chapter heavily emphasized the role of decision-making, resting on the assumption that doping is goal-directed, intentional, and self-regulated behavior (Petróczi and Aidman 2008). Nonetheless, while providing important insights into the underlying processes, there is still room for improvement in the development of comprehensive, integrative models of doping use. Possible ways by which integrative models can be further improved are presented as follows.

First of all, most of the models have either implicitly or explicitly suggested that decisions occur in a specific context (e.g., socioeconomic and/or socio-cultural). Nevertheless, none of the empirical studies of these models have incorporated measures of these contextual influences, or ways of analysing the effects of contextual features on doping decisions. One way of overcoming this notable limitation is by directly measuring the aspects of the context that are directly pertinent to the model tested. For instance, if the sports socioeconomic context is relevant, then respective measures should be included. Another way of addressing contextual influences is through the analysis of nested or hierarchical models (Raudenbush 2004). For instance, if the model posits that individual athletes' doping decisions are partly shaped by team culture with respect to doping use, then a hierarchical modeling of team-level and athlete-level characteristics will be relevant to test this hypothesis.

Second, by heavily emphasizing the role of attitudes and intentions in doping use, most of the models discussed above do not leave room for alternative pathways to action, either through other risk factors that act in parallel to intentions, or through the integration of both reflective and controlled processes (see Chapter 3 for an example). For instance, Barkoukis *et al.* (2014) argued that situational temptation – a measure of the efficacy or temptation to engage in doping under specific circumstances – can predict doping initiation independently, or in parallel to one's explicit intentions. By assessing the direct effects of situational temptation on actual doping use, researchers can gain a better understanding of the most critical risk situations for doping use that may trigger behavior in a more automatic and spontaneous manner. It is important to note that this perspective does not neglect the goal-directed nature of doping use (e.g., Petróczi and Aidman 2008). Rather, it presents another way by which behavior can be enacted that does not necessarily require reflection on one's intentions. This view is similar to Ajzen's (2011) view of intentionality, whereby intentions and attitudes do not need to guide behavior through careful deliberation and reflection. Rather, these constructs may serve goal attainment in a more automatic manner.

Finally, the aforementioned models are meant to study doping use, but they actually tackle only one aspect of this problem: substance use. There is no evidence or study of integrative models that tackles alternative doping methods, such as blood doping, gene doping or more unobtrusive methods, such as the use of hypobaric chambers. Thus, the existing integrative models hold promise for a better understanding of doping use, but it remains to be tested if their predictions hold true in other doping methods than using pills and injections.

Conclusions

This chapter showed that the scientific understanding of the psychological factors that relate to doping use in sports is increasingly evolving. Contemporary empirical studies and theoretical positions have moved away from a narrow focus on single processes (e.g., attitude–behavior relationships), and try to draw a different picture by utilizing more ecological perspectives, allocating greater attention to background variables, such as motivation, moral tendencies, legal sanctions, and situational and environmental features. The move toward this direction is important and needed for two main reasons. First, an integrative approach can eloquently describe the dynamic interactions between different levels of risk (e.g., Barkoukis *et al.* 2013) and protective factors for doping use (Chan *et al.* 2015; Gucciardi *et al.* 2011). Second, equally important is the linkage between scientific knowledge and prevention practice and policymaking. Intervention designers and policymakers can greatly benefit from an integrative, holistic understanding of doping use. This will allow them to identify not only single target variables (e.g., attitude change), but rather whole processes (e.g., how motivation training can change attitudes toward doping), and risk-conducive settings (e.g., teams with maladaptive performance enhancement norms), and accordingly expand the range, reach, and impact of preventive interventions. Furthermore, integrative models can inform policymakers by showing how policy change or implementation impacts on doping decisions at different levels of sports, from youth and sub-elite to adult and elite-level athletes. As a concluding remark, doping use does not occur in a vacuum. Athletes are exposed to a wide range of influences in different contexts, and with different timing. These contexts can have a profound effect on action-initiation. Integrative models of doping use are needed to guide us through the doping mindset and shows us ways to more effectively prevent doping use in the future (Barkoukis *et al.* 2013; Petróczi 2014).

References

Ajzen, I. (1991). The theory of planned behavior. *Organizational Behavior and Human Decision Processes, 50,* 179–211.

Ajzen, I. (2011). The theory of planned behavior: Reactions and reflections. *Psychology and Health, 26,* 1113–1127.

Ajzen, I. and Fishbein, M. (1977). Attitude-behavior relations: A theoretical analysis and review of empirical research. *Psychological Bulletin, 84* (*5*), 888–918.

Armitage, C. J. and Conner, M. (2001). Efficacy of the theory of planned behavior: A meta-analytic review. *British Journal of Social Psychology, 40,* 471–499.

Barkoukis, V., Hagger, M. S., Lambropoulos, G., and Tsorbatzoudis, H. (2010). Extending the trans-contextual model in physical education and leisure-time contexts: Examining the role of basic psychological need satisfaction. *British Journal of Educational Psychology, 80* (*4*), 647–670.

Barkoukis, V., Lazuras, L., and Tsorbatzoudis, H. (2014). Beliefs about the causes of success in sports and susceptibility for doping use in adolescent athletes. *Journal of Sports Sciences, 32,* 212–219.

Barkoukis, V., Lazuras, L., Tsorbatzoudis, H., and Rodafinos, A. (2013). Motivational and social cognitive predictors of doping intentions in elite sports: An integrated approach. *Scandinavian Journal of Medicine and Science in Sports, 23,* e330–e340.

Brand, R., Melzer, M., and Hagemann, N. (2011). Towards an implicit association test (IAT) for measuring doping attitudes in sports: Data-based recommendations developed from two recently published tests. *Psychology of Sport and Exercise, 12* (*3*), 250–256.

Chan, D. K. C., Dimmock, J. A., Donovan, R. J., Hardcastle, S., Lentillon-Kaestner, V., and Hagger, M. S. (2015). Self-determined motivation in sport predicts anti-doping motivation and intention: A perspective from the trans-contextual model. *Journal of Science and Medicine in Sport, 18* (*3*), 315–322.

Connor, J. M. and Mazanov, J. (2009). Would you dope? A general population test of the Goldman dilemma. *British Journal of Sports Medicine, 43* (*11*), 871–872.

Deci, E. L. and Ryan, R. M. (2008). Self-determination theory: A macrotheory of human motivation, development, and health. *Canadian Psychology/Psychologie Canadienne, 49* (*3*), 182.

Donahue, E. G., Miquelon, P., Valois, P., Goulet, C., Buist, A., and Vallerand, R. J. (2006). A motivational model of performance-enhancing substance use in elite athletes. *Journal of Sport and Exercise Psychology, 28,* 511–520.

Donovan, R. J., Egger, G., Kapernick, V., and Mendoza, J. (2002). A conceptual framework for achieving performance enhancing drug compliance in sport. *Sports Medicine, 32* (*4*), 269–284.

Elliot, A. J. and McGregor, H. A. (2001). A 2×2 achievement goal framework. *Journal of Personality and Social Psychology, 80* (*3*), 501–519.

Fishbein, M. (2000). The role of theory in HIV prevention. *AIDS care, 12* (*3*), 273–278.

Fishbein, M. (2009). An integrative model for behavioral prediction and its application to health promotion. In R. J. DiClemente, R. A. Crosby, and M. C. Kegler (eds.), *Emerging theories in health promotion practice and research* (215–234). New York: John Wiley & Sons.

Fishbein, M. and Ajzen, I. (2010). *Predicting and changing behavior: The reasoned action approach.* New York: Psychology Press.

Fishbein, M. and Cappella, J. N. (2006). The role of theory in developing effective health communications. *Journal of Communication, 56 (s1)*, s1–s17.

Fishbein, M. and Yzer, M. C. (2003). Using theory to design effective health behavior interventions. *Communication Theory, 13 (2)*, 164–183.

Flay, B. R., Snyder, F. J., and Petraitis, J. (2009). The theory of triadic influence. In R. J. DiClemente, R. A. Crosby, and M. C. Kegler (eds.), *Emerging theories in health promotion practice and research* (215–234). New York: John Wiley & Sons.

Gucciardi, D. F., Jalleh, G., and Donovan, R. J. (2011). An examination of the Sport Drug Control Model with elite Australian athletes. *Journal of Science and Medicine in Sport, 14 (6)*, 469–476.

Hagger, M. S. (2009). Theoretical integration in health psychology: Unifying ideas and complimentary explanations. *British Journal of Health Psychology, 14*, 189–194.

Hagger, M. S. and Chatzisarantis, N. L. (2009). Integrating the theory of planned behaviour and self-determination theory in health behaviour: A meta-analysis. *British Journal of Health Psychology, 14 (2)*, 275–302.

Hagger, M. S., Chatzisarantis, N. L., Culverhouse, T., and Biddle, S. J. (2003). The processes by which perceived autonomy support in physical education promotes leisure-time physical activity intentions and behavior: A trans-contextual model. *Journal of Educational Psychology, 95 (4)*, 784.

Jalleh, G., Donovan, R. J., and Jobling, I. (2014). Predicting attitude towards performance enhancing substance use: A comprehensive test of the Sport Drug Control Model with elite Australian athletes. *Journal of Science and Medicine in Sport, 17*, 574–579.

Lazuras, L., Barkoukis, V., and Tsorbatzoudis, H. (forthcoming). Towards an integrative model of doping intentions: An empirical study with adolescent athletes. *Journal of Sport and Exercise Psychology*.

Lazuras, L., Barkoukis, V., Rodafinos, A., and Tsorbatzoudis, H. (2010). Predictors of doping intentions in elite-level athletes: A social cognition approach. *Journal of Sport and Exercise Psychology, 32*, 694–710.

Lewin, K. (1935). *A dynamic theory of personality*. New York: McGraw-Hill.

McEachan, R. R. C., Conner, M., Taylor, N. J., and Lawton, R. J. (2011). Prospective prediction of health-related behaviours with the theory of planned behaviour: A meta-analysis. *Health Psychology Review, 5 (2)*, 97–144.

Ntoumanis, N., Ng, J. Y., Barkoukis, V., and Backhouse, S. (2014). Personal and psychosocial predictors of doping use in physical activity settings: A meta-analysis. *Sports Medicine, 44 (11)*, 1603–1624.

Perugini, M. and Bagozzi, R. P. (2001). The role of desires and anticipated emotions in goal-directed behaviours: Broadening and deepening the theory of planned behaviour. *British Journal of Social Psychology, 40 (1)*, 79–98.

Petróczi, A. (2014). The doping mindset – Part I: Implications of the Functional Use Theory on mental representations of doping. *Performance Enhancement and Health, 2*, 153–163.

Petróczi, A. and Aidman, E. (2008). Psychological drivers in doping: The life-cycle model of performance enhancement. *Substance Abuse Treatment, Prevention, and Policy, 3 (1)*, 7.

Raudenbush, S. W. (2004). *HLM 6: Hierarchical linear and nonlinear modeling*. Lincoln Wood, IL: Scientific Software International.

Semin, G. R. and Smith, E. R. (2013). Socially situated cognition in perspective. *Social Cognition, 31 (2)*, 125–146.

Smith-McLallen, A. and Fishbein, M. (2008). Predictors of intentions to perform six cancer-related behaviours: Roles for injunctive and descriptive norms. *Psychology, Health and Medicine, 13 (4)*, 389–401.

Vallerand, R. J. (2007). A hierarchical model of intrinsic and extrinsic motivation for sport and physical activity. In M. S. Hagger and N. L. D. Chatzisarantis (eds.), *Intrinsic motivation and self-determination in exercise and sport* (255–279). Champaign, IL: Human Kinetics.

Part II

Methodological considerations in doping research

5 When the "how" may at least matter as much as the "what"

The value of qualitative approaches in doping research

Fabio Lucidi, Luca Mallia, and Arnaldo Zelli

In recent years, the study of the socio-cognitive determinants and correlates of doping use has been the focus of much psychological and psychosocial inquiry. Much of this scientific focus has departed from the general consensus that doping use is an illicit behavior which is unhealthy and intentionally adopted to achieve a specific objective or goal. In the broad sport arena, the specific objectives may obviously also vary with the professional level one has reached in a particular sport. It is, for instance, of no surprise that doping studies conducted with high-level athletes have shown that performance enhancement represents one of the key objectives athletes seek to achieve by using doping substances. Doping studies conducted either with amateur and young athletes or with those who habitually practice physical exercise show, on the contrary, that doping use may serve aesthetic purposes or one's need to achieve or match an idealized, socially constructed, body image. The present chapter will briefly summarize results from the main quantitative approaches based on surveys and will discuss the qualitative approaches used so far in doping research, and will provide suggestions for mixed-method designs that can be implemented in future studies.

Quantitative approaches in doping research

Aside from the nature of the specific goals guiding people's doping use, the scientific inquiry has generally utilized well-developed theoretical frameworks to study individuals' conscious and deliberate intentions to use doping substances and their possible determinants. Over the course of the last decade or so, this top-down approach has generated a series of studies that specifically utilized social-cognitive models to account for people's intentions to use doping substances (e.g., Lucidi *et al.* 2004) and that, over time, have established clear assessment protocols and structured and fully standardized self-report instruments to validly address people's intentions to use doping substances and their social-cognitive determinants. Many of these quantitative studies are described in other chapters of this book. Overall, they have been carried out according to several theoretical approaches, such as the "Theory of Planned Behavior" (TPB hereafter; Ajzen 1991), the "Achievement Goal Theory" (Nicholls 1989) and the "Social-Cognitive Theory" (Bandura 1986). In line with much of these theoretical frameworks' hypotheses or assumptions, the results of these studies highlighted the importance or contribution on doping use yielded by attitudes and social norms (e.g., Goulet *et al.* 2010; Lazuras *et al.* 2010; Allahverdipour *et al.* 2012; Gucciardi *et al.* 2011; Wiefferink *et al.* 2008), self-regulatory efficacy (e.g., Lucidi *et al.* 2008b; Zelli *et al.* 2010; Lucidi *et al.* 2013), moral disengagement (e.g., Lucidi *et al.* 2004, 2008b, 2013; see also Kavussanu's chapter in this volume), sportspersonship (e.g., Donahue *et al.* 2006; Barkoukis *et al.* 2011) and Task and Ego orientations (e.g., Lucidi *et al.* 2013).

In sum, as it also has been well highlighted by Petróczi and Aidman (2008) and strongly emphasized by a recent meta-analysis of doping literature funded by WADA (Ntoumanis *et al.* 2014), this quantitative survey-based research suggests that the choice of using doping substances is regulated by a complex system of dynamic relations linking motivations, cognitions, and moral convictions or evaluations. The complexity of these dynamic relations acquires further meaning if one considers the possibility that these relations might be embedded, generate, and develop within a system of specific social and interpersonal contexts and situations (see also Zelli and colleagues' chapter in this volume). The understanding of this complexity might not be well served by instead adopting a dichotomous perspective by which athletes are pushed from no-substance use directly to prohibited substance intake (Hauw 2013).

Limitations and flaws of survey-based research on doping

This research may, however, be somewhat problematic. Broadly speaking, quantitative research can be considered a "closed" scientific system, since it tests hypotheses (e.g., even by means of experiments, rather rarely utilized in doping research) or it explores a specific field (e.g., a sample survey on students' attitudes toward doping) by collecting structured data referring to variables with values that are determined a priori via operational definitions of the constructs that are studied. In this sense, researchers' evaluative processes are developed according to a top-down approach by which previous theories and knowledge inform specific assessment algorithms, which are then used to develop questionnaire items that, in turn, are "imposed" onto research samples of athletes (French and Hankins 2003). If we accept this general framework and the seemingly well-grounded notion that doping is a contextualized behavior (Hauw 2013; Hauw and Bilard 2012), a research approach that heavily relies on structured and fully standardized assessment protocols may undermine the complex system of events, situations, circumstances, and individual characteristics accounting for the relations linking doping attitude formation to explicit doping use. In this sense, research on athletes' doping attitudes and beliefs may too heavily have relied on quantitative investigations (e.g., Brand *et al.* 2011; Lotz and Hagemann 2007; Petróczi and Aidman 2008) that may have forged scientific causal explanations that are reductionist in nature and that, in turn, easily confirm dominant theories (e.g., Clark 1997; Juarrero 1999; Varela 1989).

Qualitative approaches to doping research

A qualitative approach to doping research may represent a valid means to resolve the limitations of a purely quantitative approach. It also may yield significant insights into the belief systems underpinning athletes' motivation and intentions to take banned performance-enhancing substances.

A qualitative approach in doping research is grounded in – and explicitly assigns meaning to – athletes' actual experiences. It scientifically focuses on phenomena or assesses hypotheses on the basis of "unstructured" data, without the constraint of having to operationally define what is being studied. That is, qualitative researchers use data collection techniques (e.g., open interviews and unstructured observations) that do not entirely define the variables and their values a priori, and this methodological choice may lead qualitative researchers to new information and knowledge. In this sense, qualitative research can be considered an "open" scientific system. An athlete-driven, bottom-up, inductive, and "open" approach can be extremely useful in increasing the comprehensiveness and breadth of the conceptualization and operationalization of psychological constructs implicated in doping use (Hagger and Chatzisarantis 2011; Lucidi *et al.* 2008a), particularly in the context of banned performance-enhancing substances (Mazanov *et al.* 2011). A key element of a qualitative approach is, then, the possibility of integrating factual events, experiences, and circumstances characterizing a specific behavior (e.g., doping use) to the peculiar meanings and representations individuals may personally assign or ascribe to those events, experiences, and circumstances (Kirshner and Whitson 1997).

A variety of qualitative methods: the ethnographic approach

In the existing doping research, there indeed exist studies that have embraced a qualitative approach and attempted to integrate a variety of methodologies. Some studies proposed ethnographic views of case studies, conducted with the aim of getting information in "the field" including participant observation, field notes, interviews, and surveys. This kind of approach is particularly useful in doping research since it helps in addressing specific cultural dimensions that can hardly be captured by the traditional assessments of both individualistic-collectivistic differences. More generally, ethnographic researchers set their data collection in order to obtain a more personal and in-depth portrait of the informants, while trying, at the same time, to control for personal bias on the data being collected. Illustratively, Monaghan (2002), for instance, provided a clear ethnographic account of and indirect support to a scientific topic in traditional doping research, namely, that of "moral disengagement." Briefly, traditional research has inquired and assessed through surveys and questionnaires the personal justifications that athlete and non-athlete users may adopt for moving away from the moral implications of an illicit behavior such as doping use. Monaghan's ethnographic study moved beyond this level and explored the social meanings that bodybuilders assigned to their "risk" doping practices, showing that the justifications that bodybuilders may adopt primarily stem from and are sustained by their drug subculture and self-identity negotiations they daily experience. This contribution could of course be appreciated only through an ethnographic research protocol. Similarly, the ethnographic study by Bailey (2013) – through in-depth interviews – contributed to the understanding of the role and the exchanges among different "actors" of the doping use arena and showed that bodybuilders may tend to rely on their own first-hand experiences with doping-related medical and pharmacological issues or their trusted bodybuilder friends, rather than on specialists or official warnings about the "dangers" of consuming certain products.

Focus groups and open interviews

Other qualitative research instead adopted other methodologies primarily utilizing an array of methods ranging from focus groups to individual open interviews in order to describe the narratives of athletes who have admitted using doping substances or who had confessed concerns and worries about the possibility of "falling" into doping use. This type of qualitative doping research has been summarized in a very recent review (Sagoe *et al.* 2014), which overall focused on steroid use and on key doping variables such as users' onset age, their main personality characteristics, as well as the motives and circumstances that contributed to their doping use. This review overall suggests that most of the participants of the 44 studies being reviewed reported to have begun using steroids in young adulthood (i.e., before the age of 30). Interview data also suggested that many participants had concerns and worries about their body image (see also Fudala *et al.* 2003; Pope *et al.* 1993) even prior to the onset of steroid use. Open interview accounts reveal that androgenic anabolic steroid (AAS) users experience psychological difficulties with self-esteem and with their sense of efficacy in dealing with or resolving body image issues and personal dissatisfaction with respect to physical capacities (e.g., Kusserow 1990; Maycock and Howat 2005, 2007; Petrocelli *et al.* 2008; Walker and Joubert 2011), anxiety or depression (e.g., Rashid 2000; Hegazy and Sanda 2013; Khorrami and Franklin 2002).

Finally, qualitative doping data also show that users significantly attribute their onset use of doping substances to the "pressure" that media, peers, coaches, trainers, or physicians and – more generally – existing norms in sport contexts have evoked or elicited (e.g., Copeland *et al.* 2000; Hegazy and Sanda 2013; Khorrami and Franklin 2002; Maycock and Howat 2005, 2007; Petrocelli *et al.* 2008; Rashid 2000). Psychosocial processes that support doping use in bodybuilders have been recently studied by Boardley and Grix (2014) utilizing Social Cognitive Theory of moral thought and action (Bandura 1991). Semi-structured interviews of bodybuilders who admitted to being doping users were content-analyzed and inductively coded, using Bandura's definitions for the eight mechanisms of moral disengagement. Only six mechanisms were cited in the interviews, namely moral justification, euphemistic labeling, advantageous comparison, displacement of responsibility, diffusion of responsibility, and distortion of consequences.

Sagoe and colleagues' review (2014) addressed qualitative studies that, for the most part, were concerned with bodybuilders, weightlifters, and the like. This focus is not surprising, as the review was addressing AAS use. Its findings are, however, consistent with those of qualitative studies focusing on other sport disciplines, at different professional levels. For instance, Lentillon-Kaestner and Carstairs (2010) conducted semi-structured interviews with young cyclists who were hoping to find a professional team and with cyclists who recently had become professional. The young cyclists believed that doping at the professional level in cycling was acceptable; they were open to using doping substances themselves, if that were to be the key to continuing their cycling career, but eventually only after joining the professional level. The more experienced cyclists, who doped or used to dope, transmitted the culture of doping to the young cyclists, teaching them doping methods and suggesting which substances to use. Chan and colleagues (2015) instead conducted thematic content analysis on focus-group interviews with 57 athletes and identified ten themes that were then classified into three higher-order themes including personal attitudes (i.e., reputation and getting caught, health effects, and financial incentives and rewards), social influence (perceived social pressure from coaches, parents, medical staff and sport scientists), and control beliefs (i.e., insufficiency of doping testing, resource availability, sport level and type). In a recent qualitative study, Erickson *et al.* (2014) looked at the complex interplay between protective and risk factors and emphasized that self-regulation, strong moral stance, and resilience may serve as personal protective factors against doping use in sport. Family, school, and community attachments resulted instead in being situational sources of protection.

Several other qualitative studies addressed motives underlying the decision to begin using doping substances. The most frequently cited motives for initiating AAS use were enhancing appearance (e.g., Bardick *et al.* 2006; Bilard *et al.* 2011; Copeland *et al.* 2000; Pappa and Kennedy 2012) or enhancing muscles (Nøkleby and Skårderud 2013; Schwingel *et al.* 2012; Tallon 2007; Walker and Joubert 2011), physiological recovery or injury prevention (Malone *et al.* 1995) and for sporting or competitive activities (Skårberg and Engstrom 2007; Vassallo and Olrich 2010). As suggested by Hauw (2013), the motives underlying the development of unethical actions such us doping consumption cannot be correctly understood if they are not situated: (1) in relation to the other constituents of human activity with which they interact; (2) over long timescales; and (3) by considering the points of view of the actors. Consistent with these aims, Hauw analysed the sporting life courses of 17 athletes who had positive doping controls or who admitted to having used banned substances, and took into account both the productive dimensions of action (what is done) and the developmental dimensions (what it generates for the actor). Following this approach, four different prototypical situations associated with doping use were described. The first situation occurs typically to high-level athletes who isolate themselves to hide the consumption of prohibited substances. In this case, the actions were closely related to the search of ways to reach high performance, protect against injury, or maintain a specific level of training. The second situation occurs within a set of coordinated actions common to a group of athletes and hierarchically managed. In this situation, athletes take substances together as an established group, i.e., a team. The types of substances, dosages, and consumption periods are all defined in the team. In the third situation, the action of prohibited substance use occurs in social situations dissociated from sport, for instance during vacations, whereas the fourth typical situation is identified in relation to the unintentional use of banned substances.

The value of qualitative data as a guide for interventions

Education programs need to be designed and include factors in order to move beyond the individual and his or her choices. Anti-doping activities in sport have shifted from secondary prevention (intervening after athletes have used) to educational strategies focusing on primary prevention through the promotion of abstinence. There is the need for empirical evidence guiding anti-doping initiatives. In this sense, qualitative research could be of great help. Mazanov and colleagues (2011) derived a heuristic guide to educational initiatives by re-analysing a series of interviews with athletes, coaches, sports managers, physiotherapists, and sports nutritionists. These scholars' findings showed that the efficacy of primary prevention of doping may be enhanced by timing it around periods of career instability, during which athletes' vulnerability to doping may increase as a function of obtaining or, rather, losing sponsorship. Lentillon-Kaestner's (2013) interviews with high-level cyclists highlighted a possible recent decrease in the subculture of doping and doping use in high-level cycling. There also has been an increase in individual cyclists' choice to use performance-enhancing substances and a change in cyclists' attitudes toward doping use. However, actual anti-doping measures also produce unexpected effects, including a decrease in medical supervision, an increase in health risks, and the development of a black market to obtain doping substances. These results provide a basis for targeting education interventions to promote abstinence. According to Mazanov *et al.* (2011), there are two options to mitigate the need to time prevention activity around career instability by lessening the effect of sponsorship on athlete doping. The first is liberalizing access to legitimate performance-enhancing technologies (e.g., training techniques or nutritional supplements). The second is to delay access to financial sponsorship (beyond living expenses) until retirement, with monetary gains (e.g., prize money) deposited into an account where penalties are debited if the athlete is caught doping.

Summarizing

In sum, qualitative studies seem to indicate that factors such as being male and under 30 years, using legal supplements, knowing friend(s) who dope, having a positive attitude toward doping, perceiving doping to be socially supported, being morally disengaged, perceiving a scarce personal efficacy to refrain from doping, having a low body image, lacking autonomous motivation in exercise or sport, and having an ego goal orientation may facilitate doping intentions and behaviors. In this sense, qualitative research seems to be generally consistent with the findings and the conclusions that are available from quantitative research framed within social-cognitive approaches, such as, for instance, the Theory of Planned Behavior. At the same time, qualitative research also seems to offer additional insights that may well complement the existing quantitative research addressing the social-cognitive processes regulating doping use in sport (Chan *et al.* 2015) and contribute to the development of anti-doping initiatives.

Mixed-method designs in doping research

This chapter in some way departed from highlighting some possible limitations of quantitative research and standardized questionnaires in the study of doping use to then qualify the value of qualitative research. Nonetheless, it seems important to also point out that the latter type of research is not immune to limitations or possible weaknesses. The advantage of framing qualitative research within a set of specific and definite situations that give high value to the subjective experiences of research participants may have the drawback of limiting findings' generalization. There also are limitations concerning the specific research methods and techniques. For instances, qualitative studies that are based on retrospective interviews or on information collected from champions' accounts and confessions tend to emphasize extrinsic reasons for doping, thus perhaps discounting personal responsibility and protecting one's overall self-esteem. Moreover, the "true story" might be modified to limit the risks of future sanctions (e.g., Brissonneau and Bui-Xuan 2006; Monaghan 2002). Furthermore, the motives for using prohibited substances seem to be of concern only to a minority of athletes, namely those who are at a high level and those who have tested positive in doping controls. The motives offered by these athletes, such as enhancing performance, increasing financial gain, and making a sporting name for oneself, are associated with common social representations and influenced by social desirability.

According to Petróczi (2014), doping behavior research would benefit from closing the gap between qualitative and quantitative research. Doping researchers should in particular promote pluralism, embrace multiple frameworks (i.e., qualitative and quantitative), and accept situational embeddedness. Along these lines, doping investigations should also embrace and consider mixed-method research design to overcome the epistemological and methodological differences between the two distinct paradigms and to create positive synergies between them. The so-called mixed methods stand as a fruitful perspective for addressing both the limitations derived from a quantitative approach and those derived from a qualitative approach. This perspective provides a broader picture of the phenomenon being studied and/or valuable corroborations to research findings. In the mixed-method research, any feature of quantitative and qualitative research (e.g., objectives, data type, instruments, data analysis) can be combined at any stage of the mixed research design. In the methodological social science literature, the idea of combining different methods within the same study can be traced back to Campbell and Fiske's (1959) article on convergent and discriminant validation by the multitrait–multimethod matrix. However, according to Johnson and colleagues (2007), the specific idea of blending qualitative and quantitative methods, while studying the same phenomenon, first appeared in Denzin's (1978) book titled *The research act: a theoretical introduction to research methods*. The practice of combining qualitative and quantitative methods has changed a great deal over the years and numerous mixed-method research designs have been proposed.

With the goal of integrating the existing classifications, Leech and Onwuegbuzie (2009), for instance, suggested a three-dimensional typology of mixed-method research designs. The first dimension is the level of mixing, which distinguishes between fully mixed methods and partially mixed methods. Fully mixed methods combine quantitative and qualitative techniques within or across one or more stages of the research process (i.e., research objectives, type of data and operations, type of analysis, and type of inferences). For example, in the same study there might be the presence of both qualitative objectives (e.g., free exploration) and quantitative objectives (e.g., prediction), data collection using qualitative instruments (e.g., open interviews) and quantitative instruments (e.g., closed answers to a questionnaire), as well as qualitative analysis (e.g., coding) and quantitative analysis (e.g., inferential statistics). Partially mixed methods, on the other hand, do not mix quantitative and qualitative components within or across stages: each component is performed separately and it is mixed only when the results are discussed and interpreted. The second dimension of the proposed mixed-method research typology is "time orientation," since the quantitative and qualitative methods can either be concurrent (i.e., applied at the same time) or sequential (i.e., taking place one after the other). The third and last dimension is concerned with an emphasis on approaches, which establishes whether qualitative methods and quantitative methods have the same importance or if there is a prevalence of one over the other.

In mixed-methods research, a specific definition of the various components of a research process, such as sampling, data collection, data analysis, and type of inferences, has been proposed. Mixed-methods sampling (Teddlie and Yu 2007), for instance, involves the combination of quantitative sampling – in which the probability of the inclusion of a population's case is known – with qualitative techniques, such as purposive sampling – in which the units are selected according to the specific aim of the study rather than according to a statistical criterion. Likewise, mixed methods of data collection may involve the gathering of qualitative information, such as textual data from interviews or unstructured observational data, as well as quantitative information, such as the closed answers to a set of questionnaire items.

Along the same lines, according to Teddlie and Tashakkori (2009), the main types of mixed-method data analysis techniques can be defined as follows:

- Parallel mixed data analysis. In this case, there are separate analyses of qualitative and quantitative data, and these analyses are then combined into meta-inferences.
- Conversion mixed data analysis. This technique is concerned with the possibility of converting qualitative data into quantitative data or vice versa. The "quantifying" of qualitative data usually refers to the process of coding interview data and then converting these codes into numbers, whereas the "qualitizing" of quantitative data generally refers to the elaboration of typologies on the basis of numerical data by means of cluster analysis or other statistical techniques.
- Sequential mixed data analysis. This technique takes place when the qualitative and quantitative parts of a study occur at different moments. For example, in qualitative to quantitative analysis, a typology of subjects is generated from the qualitative data and those distinct groups are then compared using the quantitative data. In quantitative to qualitative analysis, instead, subjects who have high scores on a test (quantitative analysis) can be successively interviewed, and the more detailed qualitative data can then be analyzed to search for factors linked to their high test scores. In iterative sequential mixed analysis, the data comes from studies that have more than two phases and there is the possibility of various combinations of qualitative and quantitative stages of analysis.
- Multilevel data analysis. When studying settings with a hierarchical structure, such as athletes who are grouped into teams, qualitative and quantitative techniques can be used at different levels. For instance, a qualitative method could be adopted to analyze team documentation and manager interviews (team level) and a quantitative method could be used to analyze athletes' answers to a closed questionnaire analysis (athlete level).
- Fully integrated data analysis. In this case, qualitative and quantitative analysis of data is combined in an interactive, interrelated, and iterative process.
- Application of analytical techniques from one tradition to another. An example of this technique is the use of matrices derived from quantitative methods into the context of qualitative research.

Finally, with regards to inferences in mixed-methods research, Morgan (2007) describes the qualitative interpretation as inductive and subjective, whereas quantitative interpretations are described as deductive and objective. The author proposes a pragmatic approach that is based on abduction, a form of reasoning that moves back and forth between induction and deduction and intersubjectivity, in a process of communication and shared meaning.

Conclusion

To the best of our knowledge, mixed-method approaches are not yet common or utilized in research focusing on the psychosocial variables associated with doping intentions and behaviors. Nonetheless, the features and characteristics that briefly have been outlined in this chapter suggest that mixed-method approaches might be particularly conducive to the study of the myriad of situations, circumstances, and contradictions possibly characterizing one's experience with doping use. Doping use is, at the same time, a clear violation of sport ethics or rules and a possible outcome of well-accepted norms within sport groups; it is an immoral or reprehensible behavior and, yet, users find ways to accept or justify its moral implications; it clearly damages one's health and, yet, physicians may support it; it seems an oxymoron to "reasoning" and "mindfulness" and, yet, it also is conceived as the result of "reasoned" actions.

References

Ajzen, I. (1991). The theory of planned behavior. *Organizational Behavior And Human Decision Processes*, *50*, 179–211.

Allahverdipour, H., Jalilian, F., and Shaghaghi, A. (2012). Vulnerability and the intention to anabolic steroids use among Iranian gym users: An application of the theory of planned behavior. *Substance Use and Misuse*, *47*, 309–31.

Bailey, B. J. (2013). Ethnopharmacology and male bodybuilders' lived experience with consuming sports nutrition supplements in Canada. *Sport in Society*, *16* (*9*), 1105–1119.

Bandura, A. (1986). *Social foundations of thoughts and action: A social cognitive theory.* Englewood Cliffs, NJ: Prentice-Hall.

Bandura, A. (1991). Social cognitive theory of moral thought and action. In W. M. Kurtines and J. L. Gewirtz (eds.), *Handbook of moral behavior and development: Theory research and applications* (71–129). Hillsdale, NJ: Lawrence Erlbaum Associates.

Bardick, A. D., Bernes, K. B., and Nixon, G. (2006). In pursuit of physical perfection: Weight lifting and steroid use in men. *Journal of Excellence*, *11*, 135–145.

Barkoukis, V., Lazuras, L., Tsorbatzoudis, H., and Rodafinos, A. (2011). Motivational and sportspersonship profiles of elite athletes in relation to doping behavior. *Psychology of Sport and Exercise*, *12*, 205–212. doi: 10.1016/j.psychsport.2010.10.003.

Bilard, J., Ninot, G., and Hauw, D. (2011). Motives for illicit use of doping substances among athletes calling a national antidoping phone-help service: An exploratory study. *Substance Use and Misuse*, *46*, 359–367.

Boardley, I. D. and Grix, J. (2014). Doping in bodybuilders: A qualitative investigation of facilitative psychosocial processes. *Qualitative Research in Sport, Exercise and Health*, *6* (*3*), 422–439.

Brand, R., Melzer, M., and Hagemann, N. (2011). Towards an implicit association test (IAT) for measuring doping attitudes in sports. Data-based recommendations developed from two recently published tests. *Psychology and Sport Exercise*, *12*, 250–256.

Brissonneau, C. and Bui-Xuan, K. (2006). Analyse psychologique etsociologique du dopage. Rationalisation du discours, du mode de vie et de l'entraînement sportif [Psychological and sociological analysis of doping. Rationalization, lifestyle and sport training]. *Sciences et techniques des activities physiques et sportives* (STAPS), *70*, 57–73.

Campbell, D. T. and Fiske, D. W. (1959). Convergent and discriminant validation by the multitrait-multimethod matrix. *Psychological Bulletin*, *56*, 81–105.

Chan, D. K. C., Hardcastle, S., Dimmock, J. A., Lentillon-Kaestner, V., Donovan, R. J., Burgin, M., and Hagger, M. S. (2015). Modal salient belief and social cognitive variables of anti-doping behaviors in sport: Examining an extended model of the theory of planned behavior. *Psychology of Sport and Exercise*, 16 (*P2*), 164–174. doi: 10.1016/j. psychsport.2014.03.002.

Clark, A. (1997). *Being there. Putting the brain, body and the world together again.* Cambridge, MA: MIT Press.

Copeland, J., Peters, R., and Dillon, P. (2000). Anabolic-androgenic steroid use disorders among a sample of Australian competitive and recreational users. *Drug and Alcohol Dependence*, *60*, 91–96.

Denzin, N. K. (1978). *The research act: A theoretical introduction to sociological methods.* New York: McGraw-Hill.

Donahue, E. G., Miquelon, P., Valois, P., Goulet, C., Buist, A., and Vallerand, R. J. (2006). A motivational model of performance-enhancing substance use in elite athletes. *Journal of Sport and Exercise Psychology*, *28*, 511–520.

Erickson, K., McKenna, J., and Backhouse, S. H. (2014). A qualitative analysis of the factors that protect athletes against doping in sport. *Psychology of Sport and Exercise.* doi: 10.1016/j.psychsport.2014.03.007.

French, D. P. and Hankins, M. (2003). The expectancy-value muddle in the theory of planned behaviour and some proposed solutions. *British Journal of Health Psychology*, *8*, 37–55.

Fudala, P. J., Weinrieb, R. M., Calarco, J. S., Kampman, K. M., and Boardman, C. (2003). An evaluation of anabolic-androgenic steroid abusers over a period of 1 year: Seven case studies. *Annals of Clinical Psychiatry*, *15*, 121–130.

Goulet, C., Valois, P., Buist, A., and Cote, M. (2010). Predictors of the use of performance enhancing substances by young athletes. *Clinical Journal of Sport Medicine*, *20*, 243–248. doi: 10.1097/JSM.0b013e3181e0b935.

Gucciardi, D., Jalleh, G., and Donovan, R. (2011). An examination of the Sport Drug Control Model with elite Australian athletes. *Journal of Science and Medicine in Sport*, *14*, 469–476. doi:10.1016/j.jsams.2011.03.009.

Hagger, M. S. and Chatzisarantis, N. L. D. (2011). Never the twain shall meet? Quantitative psychological researchers' perspectives on qualitative research. *Qualitative Research in Sport, Exercise and Health*, 16 (*3*), 266–277.

Hauw, D. (2013). How unethical actions can be learned: The analysis of the sporting life courses of doping athletes. *International Journal of Lifelong Education*, 32 (*1*), 14–25.

Hauw, D. and Bilard, J. (2012). Situated activity analysis of elite track and field athletes' use of prohibited performance-enhancing substances. *Journal of Substance Use*, 17 (*2*), 183–197.

Hegazy, B. and Sanda, C. (2013). A 28-year-old man with depression, PTSD, and anabolic-androgenic steroid and amphetamine use. *Psychiatric Annals*, *43*, 408–411.

Johnson, R. B., Onwuegbuzie, A. J., and Turner, L. (2007). Toward a definition of mixed methods research. *Journal of Mixed Methods Research*, 1 (*2*), 112–133.

Juarrero, A. (1999). *Dynamics in action. Intentional behavior as a complex system.* Cambridge, MA: MIT Press.

Khorrami, S. and Franklin, J. (2002). The influence of competition and lack of emotional expression in perpetuating steroid abuse and dependence in male weightlifters. *International Journal of Men's Health*, *1*, 119–133.

Kirshner, D. and Whitson, J. A. (1997). *Situated cognition. Social, semiotic and psychological perspectives.* Mahwah, NJ: Lawrence Erlbaum Associates.

Kusserow, R. P. (1990). *Adolescents and steroids: A user perspective.* Washington, DC: Office of Inspector General.

Lazuras, L., Barkoukis, V., Rodafinos, A., and Tzorbatzoudis, H. (2010). Predictors of doping intentions in elite-level athletes: A social cognition approach. *Journal of Sport and Exercise Psychology, 32* (5), 694–710.

Leech, N. L. and Onwuegbuzie, A. J. (2009). A typology of mixed methods research designs. *Quality and Quantity, 43*, 265–275.

Lentillon-Kaestner, V. (2013). The development of doping use in high-level cycling: From team-organized doping to advances in the fight against doping. *Scandinavian Journal of Medicine and Science in Sports, 23*, 189–197.

Lentillon-Kaestner, V. and Carstairs, C. (2010). Doping use among young elite cyclists: A qualitative psychosociological approach. *Scandinavian Journal of Medicine and Science in Sports, 20*, 336–345.

Lotz, S. and Hagemann, N. (2007). Using the implicit association test to measure athletes' attitude toward doping. *Journal of Sport and Exercise Psychology, 29*, S183–S184.

Lucidi, F., Alivernini, F., and Pedon, A. (2008a). *Metodologia della ricerca qualitativa* [Methodology of qualitative research]. Bologna, Italy: Mulino Editore.

Lucidi, F., Mallia, L., and Zelli, A. (2013). The contribution of moral disengagement to adolescents' use of doping substances. *International Journal of Sport Psychology, 44*, 331–350. doi: 10.7352/IJSP 2013.00.000.

Lucidi, F., Grano, C., Leone, L., Lombardo, C., and Pesce, C. (2004). Determinants of the intention to use doping substances: An empirical contribution in a sample of Italian adolescents. *Journal of Sport Psychology, 35* (2), 133–148.

Lucidi, F., Zelli, A., Mallia, L., Grano, C., Russo. P. M., and Violani, C. (2008b). The social-cognitive mechanisms regulating adolescents' use of doping substances. *Journal of Sport Sciences, 26* (5), 447–456. doi: 10.1080/02640410701579370.

Malone, D. A. Jr., Dimeff, R. J., Lombardo, J. A., and Sample, R. B. (1995). Psychiatric effects and psychoactive substance use in anabolic-androgenic steroid users. *Clinical Journal of Sport Medicine, 5*, 25–31.

Maycock, B. and Howat, P. (2005). Overcoming the barriers to initiating illegal anabolic steroid use. *Drugs Education, Prevention and Policy, 14*, 317–325.

Maycock, B. and Howat, P. (2007). Social capital: Implications from an investigation of illegal anabolic steroid networks. *Health Education Research, 22*, 854–863.

Mazanov, J., Huybers, T., and Connor, J. (2011). Qualitative evidence of a primary intervention point for elite athlete doping. *Journal of Science and Medicine in Sport, 14* (2), 106–110.

Monaghan, L. F. (2002). Vocabularies of motive for illicit steroid use among bodybuilders. *Social Science and Medicine, 55*, 695–708.

Morgan, D. L. (2007). Paradigms lost and pragmatism regained: Methodological implications of combining qualitative and quantitative methods. *Journal of Mixed Methods Research, 1*, 48–76.

Nicholls, J. G. (1989). *The competitive ethos and democratic education.* Cambridge, MA: Harvard University Press.

Nøkleby, H. and Skårderud, F. (2013). Body practices among male drug abusers. Meanings of workout and use of doping agents in a drug treatment setting. *International Journal of Mental Health and Addiction, 11*, 490–502.

Ntoumanis, N., Ng, J. Y., Barkoukis, V., and Backhouse, S. (2014). Personal and psychosocial predictors of doping use in physical activity settings: A meta-analysis. *Sports Medicine, 44* (11), 1603–1624.

Pappa, E. and Kennedy, E. (2012). "It was my thought ... he made it a reality": Normalization and responsibility in athletes' accounts of performance enhancing drug use. *International Review for the Sociology of Sport*, *48*, 277–294.

Petrocelli, M., Oberweis, T., and Petrocelli, J. (2008). Getting huge, getting ripped: A qualitative exploration of recreational steroid use. *Journal of Drug Issues*, *38*, 1187–1206.

Petróczi, A. (2014). The doping mindset – Part I: Implications of the Functional Use Theory on mental representations of doping. *Performance Enhancing and Health* (forthcoming) doi: 10.1016/j.peh.2014.06.001.

Petróczi, A. and Aidman, E. (2008). Psychological drivers in doping: The life-cycle model of performance enhancement. *Substance Abuse Treatment, Prevention, and Policy*, *3* (*7*). doi: 10.1186/1747-597X-3-7.

Pope, H. G. Jr., Katz, D. L., and Hudson, J. I. (1993). Anorexia nervosa and "reverse anorexia" among 108 male bodybuilders. *Comprehensive Psychiatry*, *34*, 406–409.

Rashid, W. (2000). Testosterone abuse and affective disorders. *Journal of Substance Abuse Treatment*, *18*, 179–184.

Sagoe, D., Schou, S. A., and Pallesen, S. (2014). The aetiology and trajectory of anabolic androgenic steroid use initiation: A systematic review and synthesis of qualitative research. *Substance Abuse Treatment, Prevention, and Policy*, *9*, 27.

Schwingel, P. A., Cotrim, H. P., dos Santos, C. R. Jr., Salles, B. C. R., de Almeida, C. E. R., and Zoppi, C. C. (2012). Non-medical anabolic-androgenic steroid consumption and hepatitis B and C virus infection in regular strength training practitioners. *Journal of Pharmacy and Pharmacology*, *6*, 1598–1605.

Skårberg, K. and Engstrom, I. (2007). Troubled social background of male anabolic-androgenic steroid abusers in treatment. *Substance Abuse Treatment, Prevention, and Policy*, *2*, 20.

Tallon, V. (2007). *An exploratory investigation of anabolic-androgenic steroid use in Lanarkshire*. Paisley: University of Paisley. Available at www.ibrarian.net/navon/paper/An_Exploratory_Investigation_Of.pdf?paperid=10804537.

Teddlie, C. and Tashakkori, A. (2009). *Foundations of mixed methods research: Integrating quantitative and qualitative approaches in the social and behavioral sciences*. London: SAGE.

Teddlie, C. and Yu, F. (2007). Mixed methods sampling: A typology with examples. *Journal of Mixed Methods Research*, 1 (*1*), 77–100.

Varela, F. J. (1989). *Cognitive science. A cartography of current ideas*. Cambridge, MA: MIT Press.

Vassallo, M. J. and Olrich, T. W. (2010). Confidence by injection: Male users of anabolic steroids speak of increases in perceived confidence through anabolic steroid use. *International Journal of Sport and Exercise Psychology*, *8*, 70–80.

Walker, D. M. and Joubert, H. E. (2011). Attitudes of injecting male anabolic androgenic steroid users to media influence, health messages and gender constructs. *Drugs and Alcohol Today*, *11*, 56–70.

Wiefferink, C. H., Detmar, S. B., Coumans, B., Vogels, T., and Paulussen, T. G. (2008). Social psychological determinants of the use of performance-enhancing drugs by gym users. *Health Education Research*, *23*, 70–80. doi: 10.1093/her/cym004.

Zelli, A., Mallia, L., and Lucidi, F. (2010). The contribution of interpersonal appraisals to a social-cognitive analysis of adolescents' doping use. *Psychology of Sport and Exercise*, *11*, 304–311. doi: 10.1016/j.psychsport.2010.02.008.

6 Substantive and methodological considerations of social desirability for doping in sport

Daniel F. Gucciardi, Geoffrey Jalleh, and Robert J. Donovan

Have you taken illicit drugs? Are you mentally tough? How often do you display aggressive acts toward your opponents in sport? Would you assist a stranger in need of help? These questions and many others like them are central to several academic disciplines within the social sciences. Asking people to respond truthfully to these questions, however, is a complex endeavor given the propensity for some people to excessively overestimate desirable attributes or actions and underestimate or deny undesirable qualities or behaviors on self-report scales (Paulhus 2002). Referred to as socially desirable responding (SDR), this response distortion has the potential to contaminate the accuracy of peoples' self-reports and therefore the validity of empirical findings. In this chapter, we will provide an overview of the literature on SDR as it pertains to the social science of use of banned performance-enhancing substances or methods in sport, otherwise referred to as doping.

Substantive considerations of SDR

Several definitions of social desirability or SDR have appeared over the years (for reviews, see Holden and Passey 2009; Paulhus 2002; Uziel 2010). Although there does not appear to be a universally agreed upon definition of this concept, common themes suggest that SDR is best described as a conscious or unconscious attempt to distort responses by overestimating positive or underestimating negative qualities or behaviors. A key point is that SDR can be either a deliberate *or* unintentional act to present oneself in the best possible light for others (Paulhus 2002). The former is concerned with a conscious effort to distort responses in order to present oneself in a desirable manner to others (i.e., impression management), whereas the latter is an unconscious tendency to view oneself in a positive light through biased responses toward socially desirable qualities or behaviors that are considered true by the individual (i.e., self-deception enhancement). In either case, the process results in individuals to some degree distorting their responses to convey a desirable impression on others and therefore influencing their attitudes, beliefs, or behavior (Kuncel and Tellegen 2009).

The issue of whether SDR is best conceptualized as trait (substance) or error (style) variance has been the subject of considerable debate for over 40 years (e.g., Block 1965; Edwards 1967). On the one hand, the observed covariation between SDR scales and personality traits such as neuroticism, agreeableness, and conscientiousness (e.g., Ones *et al.* 1996; Paulhus 1991) supports an interpretation that SDR represents a substantively meaningful trait (see also Smith and Ellingson 2002). To truly understand valid variance that belongs to the scales of substantive interest, scholars have proposed that it is necessary to remove SDR from measures of (un)desirable traits or behaviors (McCrae and Costa 1983). The dilemma, however, is to accurately delineate what a person's score on an inherently (un)desirable trait or behavior means if the items designed to capture the construct are free from any desirability component (cf. Paunonen and LeBel 2012). Doping is an inherently undesirable behavior and is therefore a prime example of this challenge because self-reports dominate methodological approaches in this research area (Ntoumanis *et al.* 2014). Nevertheless, without estimating and controlling for SDR, speculations will remain as to whether individuals' true level of the trait or behavior, their tendency to distort responses toward the desirable pole, or some combination of both accounts for respondents' high or low scores on an (un)desirable construct (Paunonen and LeBel 2012).

Conceptualized as a style rather than a substantive trait, SDR is thought to comprise a source of artificial variance (i.e., systematic bias or error variance) and covariance (i.e., common method) attributable to social desirability and not the intended construct, and therefore threatens construct validity (e.g., factor structure) and interpretations of relations among two or more variables (Chan 2009). If SDR does affect criterion-related validities, it could do so in two primary ways. First, it could moderate the relations among predictor and outcome variables, such that different criterion-related validities would be observed for groups of differing levels of SDR (e.g., low, moderate, high). In other words, high levels of SDR results in a loss of meaningful information or a large degree of error variance. However, this expectation has been questioned in personality assessments (Hough *et al.* 1990) and applicant testing settings (Ones *et al.* 1993; see also McGrath *et al.* 2010). Second, SDR could serve as a suppressor variable, such that it inflates the association between two or more variables. In other words, SDR shifts one's "true" response on the predictor variable toward the desirable end. Meta-analytic data in which zero-order and SDR-partialed correlations between personality and job performance are compared does not support a suppressor explanation (Li and Bagger 2006; Ones *et al.* 1996). It is important to note that the limited support for these interpretations regarding criterion-related validities might be a result of the validity of the SDR scales rather than the effect itself (Uziel 2010). Alternatively, it may be that everyone in a sample engaged in SDR to a similar degree (Rosse *et al.* 1998).

Both the content and context of the survey can influence the likelihood of SDR (Chan 2009; McFarland and Ryan 2000; Paunonen and LeBel 2012). For example, topics which are sensitive (e.g., criminal offences, drug use) or have a high degree of perceived social appeal (e.g., mental toughness, altruism) are likely to be more susceptible to SDR than issues in which there is an absence of any clear sensitivity (e.g., use of nutritional supplements) or desirable social norms (e.g., extraversion versus neuroticism). There might also be an elevated degree of SDR in those contexts where respondents can be identified or the consequences of the assessment are important or valued (e.g., job application, talent identification tests). Finally, if people possess a high amount of a desirable attribute or regularly engage in a desirable behavior (i.e., true level is high), then there should be little need for them to engage in SDR to present themselves in the best possible light for others. Simply put, contamination of self-reports from SDR may not always be a major concern with some people, contexts, or topics (Chan 2009; Paunonen and LeBel 2012; Peidmont *et al.* 2000).

Methodological considerations of SDR

As science is largely concerned with evidence, one requires data demonstrating that self-reports depart from reality to support any allegation that responses are biased or distorted in some way (Paulhus 2002). Unsurprisingly, scholars have devoted considerable effort toward developing and evaluating ways to assess or detect and, if necessary, control for such distortions in self-reports (Nederhof 1985; Paulhus 1991; see also Tourangeau and Yan 2007; Krumpal 2013). In this section, we review both proactive and *post hoc* approaches to minimizing, detecting, and controlling for SDR, and provide examples pertinent to the study of doping in sport. Interested readers are referred to other chapters of this book for detailed overviews of techniques not discussed here including the randomized response technique and implicit measurements.

Proactive approaches to minimizing SDR

Techniques employed during scale development

The social desirability of items (or item desirability) is often a primary focus during scale development. Typically, the aim is to develop items with SDR in mind, such that one identifies and eliminates potentially problematic items during scale construction. Perceived desirability of each item can be obtained by directly asking participants (e.g., Kuncel and Tellegen 2009; Randall and Fernandes 1991) or indirectly by correlating items with a presumed measure of SDR (e.g., Kam 2013). A number of psychometric scales have been developed to assess SDR and published in peer-reviewed outlets. The most commonly employed questionnaires include the Marlowe-Crowne Social Desirability Scale (M-CSDS; Crowne and Marlowe 1960; see also Reynolds 1982; Strahan and Gerbasi 1972), Balanced Inventory of Desirable Responding (BIDR; Paulhus 1991), and Social Desirability Scale-17 (SDS-17; Stöber 2001). Both the M-CSDS and SDS-17 are unidimensional and capture behaviors that are socially approved or desirable yet infrequent, as well as socially disapproved or undesirable but frequent. In contrast, the BIDR measures the dualistic model of SDR (Paulhus 1991, 2002), including items to capture impression management (i.e., conscious deception to make a favorable impression on others) or self-deceptive enhancement (i.e., unconscious deception to protect self-esteem).

Despite the intuitive appeal, the elimination of items that capture a target concept can result in a reduction in the validity of the scale (Johnson 2004). To alleviate this concern, researchers might focus their attention on developing items that maximize content validity and minimize SDR through careful attention to the content of items during their development (Chan 2009; Holden 2010). For example, it is important to minimize value-laden content (e.g., "Doping is a trivial issue in my sport") as it can lead to responses based on both the content and tone of the statement. The content validity index (Lynn 1986) represents one approach that researchers might find useful in making an informed judgment on the representativeness and clarity of items using assessments from expert raters (see also Polit and Beck 2006). Nevertheless, some attributes or behaviors are inherently desirable (e.g., mental toughness, altruism) or undesirable (e.g., neuroticism, doping) and therefore it is important to recognize that it might be difficult to minimize SDR through scale development processes for these topics (Paunonen and LeBel 2012).

Techniques employed during scale completion

Rational techniques are designed to minimize the extent to which individuals respond to items in a desirable fashion through measures that are built into the scale itself (Paulhus 1991). Researchers can employ forced-choice items, which require respondents to choose between two alternatives with an equal degree of un/desirableness, or single statements that are neutral in social desirability (Nederhof 1985; see also Converse *et al.* 2010). However, a limitation of these techniques is that the researcher's judgment of social desirability may differ from those of participants and therefore SDR may still have an influence on their responses. Demand reduction techniques such as maximizing anonymity and confidentiality, and reminding participants that honest responses are important to obtain useful feedback, are considered effective for minimizing SDR (Chan 2009; Paulhus and Vazire 2007). However, the evidence regarding the usefulness of anonymity for SDR is equivocal (e.g., Holden *et al.* 1999; Lautenschlager and Flaherty 1990), and there are situations in which the desire to distort one's responses would be expected to be exceptionally high regardless of such reminders (e.g., job or school related assessments, illegal activities; Paunonen and LeBel 2012). It is important that this feature of the survey administration process is tested as it pertains to doping research; for example, athletes could be randomized to complete a survey package with or without the traditional instructional set (i.e., honesty, confidentiality, anonymity). Nevertheless, there is evidence that people are more likely to report socially undesirable behaviors or activities when the survey is self-administered rather than interviewer-administered (Tourangeau and Yan 2007).

Another methodological approach that can be applied during the testing phase is to compare individuals who complete a survey package as per normal (i.e., honest responses) with people who have a strong incentive or motivation to convey a desirable impression on others (e.g., applicants versus non-applicants), or have been instructed to "fake good" on the test (i.e., report the most desirable impression). For example, doping scholars might randomize athletes to complete a survey in a desirable condition (e.g., scholarship application for institute of sport) or as per normal. There is ample evidence that instructions to fake good in experimental settings change mean scores in predictable directions, with social desirability scales particularly susceptible to response distortion under faking conditions (Viswesvaran and Ones 1999). Such changes in scale scores can have dramatic effects on test validity (e.g., Holden 2007; Jackson *et al.* 2000). Nevertheless, although people can consciously distort their responses on self-reports to make a favorable impression on others in experimental settings (Ones *et al.* 1996), it does not necessarily mean they do it to the same degree (or at all) in real-world settings (Hough *et al.* 1990).

The bogus pipeline technique is designed to maximize motivation to provide accurate self-reports of socially sensitive behaviors by informing participants that dishonest responses can be detected by an objective device such as a polygraph (Jones and Sigall 1971). Participants are typically connected to equipment and led to believe that the machines assess the truthfulness of peoples' verbal statements through objective psycho-physiological indicators that cannot be consciously manipulated by the respondent. For example, doping scholars could integrate heart rate measures as part of the data collection process, and inform athletes that their pulse (relative to baseline) provides an indication as to whether or not they are telling the truth in their survey responses. One variant of this technique is to check public records (e.g., voting activity; Hanmer *et al.* 2014). Although requiring specialized equipment in most instances (e.g., polygraph, galvanic skin response), this technique has been shown to reduce SDR and encourage honest responses in an attempt to avoid being detected as a liar (Roese and Jamieson 1993).

Specialized equipment can also offer more objective methods of detecting SDR than self-report scales. Eye-tracking equipment, for example, has been used to gain insight into the response processes during conditions in which individuals are instructed to respond honestly or fake good (van Hooft and Born 2012). Using a repeated-measures design, van Hooft and Born (2012) found that response latencies are 0.25 seconds faster when responding in a socially desirable manner when compared to answering honestly ($d=0.23$). Furthermore, eye-tracking data revealed that SDR involved approximately one eye fixation less per scale item, greater attention to extreme response options, and more immediate movement to the extreme response option after having read the scale item when compared with the honest condition. These findings suggest that SDR involved a less cognitively complex process of information retrieval when compared with honest responses, such that there was little emphasis on the retrieval of accurate information relating to self-referenced information but rather a focus on the instructional set and desirability of the item (van Hooft and Born 2012).

Post hoc approaches to detecting and controlling SDR

A number of approaches have been proposed to estimate or control for the effects of SDR on construct and criterion-related validities (Chan 2009; Paunonen and LeBel 2012; Ziegler and Buehner 2009; for a review, see Podsakoff *et al.* 2012). Perhaps the most common approach is to administer a scale presumed to capture SDR alongside tools that target the constructs of substantive focus; people who report high SDR scores are assumed to have distorted their responses to the primary constructs of interest. Typically, researchers statistically test this assumption by ascertaining if SDR moderated or suppressed criterion-related validities. Despite its intuitive appeal, it is ineffective to use self-report measures of SDR to statistically control or correct for SDR bias (Li and Bagger 2006; Ones *et al.* 1996) because they typically remove valid variance (Paulhus and Vazire 2007), particularly when such scales do not adequately capture SDR (Uziel 2010; see also Paunonen and LeBel 2012). Given that SDR scales have meaningful correlations with personality traits such as neuroticism, agreeableness, and conscientiousness (Ones *et al.* 1996; Paulhus 1991), it is difficult to conclude that extreme scores on SDR scales represent response bias rather than extreme personalities (Ziegler and Buehner 2009).

When conceptualized as spurious measurement error or systematic variance that is caused by a person's perception of situational demands or characteristics (Schmidt *et al.* 2003), statistical techniques commensurate with common method variance can be applied to model the effects of SDR (Ziegler and Buehner 2009). Common method variance is typically represented as a latent variable within a structural equation modeling framework whereby all items or scales distorted by SDR load on their respective trait variable and a latent variable representing common method (for a review, see Podsakoff *et al.* 2012). Nevertheless, although method variance could be due to SDR (Ziegler and Buehner 2009), one cannot rule out other explanations such as response sets or styles (e.g., Wetzel *et al.* 2013) or acquiescence (e.g., Rammstedt and Kemper 2011). The use of marker variables has been recommended as a method by which to provide insight into the nature of the latent variable (Podsakoff *et al.* 2012). In the case of social desirability, correlating a scale presumed to capture SDR with the latent variable does not necessarily mean this response bias was modeled; rather, it could well mean that some higher-order personality construct was extracted given the substantive overlap evidence in previous research (Ones *et al.* 1996; Paulhus 1991). An alternative approach might be the use of bogus items, which are designed on the surface to appear similar to real tasks or behaviors but are actually fake or non-existent (e.g., Dwight and Donovan 2003); thus, no respondent should report engaging in such fictitious behaviors. An example of a bogus item for athletes might be "How often do you utilize mesotechnic stretching during a warm-up activity?" Bogus items are embedded within the survey and subsequently used as a proxy for SDR. Researchers might also consider the integration of statistical and experimental methodologies. For example, Ziegler and Buehner (2009) demonstrated the usefulness of an approach whereby two groups completed measurements at two time points, with one group instructed to provide honest assessments for both ratings (control group) and the other group asked to "fake good" at the second assessment (experimental group). Common method variance was modeled at both time points within a latent variable framework and allowed for the separation of trait and SDR variances, alongside the reversal of the effects of SDR on means and covariance structure.

Monte Carlo simulations have also been used to examine the effects of SDR (e.g., Berry and Sackett 2009; Komar *et al.* 2008; Paunonen and LeBel 2012). Rather than estimating or manipulating variables using real participants, Monte Carlo simulations enable researchers to sample means from a given population distribution that represents people's scores on constructs of interest, and assess the performance of the model by varying specific features (e.g., sample size, effect sizes, covariance matrices) that may have bearing on the interpretation of substantive outcomes (Paxton *et al.* 2001). For example, Paunonen and LeBel (2012) varied the amount of SDR to trait scores of a bipolar personality inventory (e.g., honesty-dishonesty) and examined the effects on three levels of criterion-related validity (ρ_{XY}=0.20, 0.40, and 0.60) in three different sample sizes (n=90, 180, and 270). They found that there was little influence of SDR on criterion-related validity, even when some respondents' test scores were highly distorted due to response bias. Consistent with meta-analytic data (Hough *et al.* 1990; McGrath *et al.* 2010; Ones *et al.* 1993; Ones *et al.* 1996), they also found little evidence to support a moderation or suppressor effect of SDR.

SDR and doping in sport: current status and future directions

Contamination of self-reports from SDR may not always be a major concern with some samples or topics (Chan 2009; Peidmont *et al.* 2000). However, doping is a sensitive issue and therefore represents a behavior that individuals might be highly motivated to intentionally minimize or deny when asked about their involvement in this activity. Thus, the presence of SDR may pose a threat to the validity of findings in which individuals are asked to self-report key variables of interest (e.g., attitudes to doping, engagement in doping). A recent meta-analysis of doping research revealed that scholars have relied primarily on self-report data (Ntoumanis *et al.* 2014). Despite the potential threats of this response bias to the validity of empirical findings, there have been few attempts to delineate an understanding of the effects of SDR for research on doping in sport. As depicted in Table 6.1, we located only seven published studies in which the influence of SDR for self-reports of doping-related variables has been considered.

Our review of the doping literature with regard to SDR revealed two noteworthy considerations. First, researchers have relied on *post hoc* approaches to detect and control for SDR in cross-sectional designs, exclusively by the use of presumed SDR scales. This approach is not ideal (Li and Bagger 2006; Ones *et al.* 1996) because there is an assumption that they validly capture the SDR construct (Uziel 2010). Particularly when SDR scales correlate with substantive variables, correcting for this construct typically removes valid variance (Paulhus and Vazire 2007). Clearly, there is a need for researchers to utilize alternative methodological (e.g., faking paradigm) and statistical techniques (e.g., Monte Carlo simulations) to enhance our understanding of SDR as it pertains to doping research.

Second, there is conflicting evidence in the available literature. With the exception of one null finding (Gucciardi *et al.* 2010), SDR has been shown to be inversely associated with doping-related variables (e.g., attitudes, intentions, susceptibility) in adolescent (Barkoukis *et al.* 2014) and adult Greek athletes (Barkoukis *et al.* 2011; Lazuras *et al.* 2010), college athletes (Petróczi 2007; Petróczi and Nepusz 2011) and competitive athletes (Whitaker *et al.* 2013). These findings suggest that SDR shares some conceptual overlap with substantively important variables. Yet the evidence regarding the influence of SDR on criterion-related validities is equivocal. Controlling for SDR did not significantly alter the association between doping intentions and variables such as attitudes, subjective norms, and perceived behavioral control (Barkoukis *et al.* 2014; Lazuras *et al.* 2010), thereby providing null results with regard to a suppressor effect interpretation. However, SDR has been shown to moderate the relation between attitudes to doping and doping susceptibility (Gucciardi *et al.* 2010). Similarly, strong and significant relations among study variables (e.g., attitudes, internal deterrence factors) were observed for athletes high in SDR, but these associations were low and non-significant in a low SDR group (Petróczi and Nepusz 2011). There is also evidence to suggest that the inclusion of SDR in structural equation modeling can enhance the variance explained and model-data fit (Petróczi and Nepusz 2011). Such inconsistencies in evidence could be clarified through designs that provide insight into cause and effect, that is, the manipulation of features related to the content and context of the study. One could compare theoretical sequences under varying conditions where SDR may be minimized or maximized; for example, anonymous surveys excluding all personal information versus assessments in which participants provide such information or responses that increase the likelihood that their data could be identified (e.g., birthdate, linked code for multiple assessment points) (e.g., Smith and Ellingson 2002).

Validation studies are considered the gold standard for assessing whether or not responses depart from reality because they compare self-reports with the "true" value from external sources such as medical or administrative records (Krumpal 2013). Though not directly targeting SDR, one study to date has revealed an interesting methodological finding. In a sample of competitive athletes, evidence of doping behavior from a bioanalysis of hair samples was denied in athletes' self-reported data; moreover, self-reported doping behavior was not reflected in bioanalysis of hair samples (Petróczi *et al.* 2011). Alternatively, researchers might sample athletes who have and have not been convicted of an anti-doping rule violation from formal records (e.g., Australian Sports Anti-Doping Authority), and ascertain if self-reports converge with these

Table 6.1 Overview of doping research which has focused on or included a measure of SDR[1]

Reference	Sample	Design	Measure of SDR	Analyses and results
Barkoukis et al. (2011)	1,040 Greek elite adult athletes ($M_{age} = 22.97$; $SD = 6.39$; 62.6% males)	Cross-sectional survey	10-item version of the Marlowe-Crowne Social Desirability Scale (Strahan and Gerbasi 1972)	• SDR included as a covariate in ANOVA to examine differences in past doping use and intentions according to motivation and achievement goals • SDR had a significant effect on past use and intentions both when groups were formed on self-determined motivation and achievement goals • SDR inversely related to doping intentions ($r = -0.16$, $p < 0.001$)
Barkoukis et al. (2014)	309 Greek elite adolescent athletes ($M_{age} = 16.64$; $SD = 1.15$; 57.6% males)	Cross-sectional survey	10-item version of the Marlowe-Crowne Social Desirability Scale (Strahan and Gerbasi 1972)	• Variance reduction rate (VRR; see Chen and Spector 1991) used to control for SDR in regression (VRR = [zero-order correlation]^2 − [partial correlation]^2)/[zero-order correlation]^2) • SDR associated with susceptibility for doping use ($r = -0.25$, $p < 0.001$) • Correlations between study variables (attitudes, subjective norms, descriptive norms, deception) and doping susceptibility did not change significantly after controlling for SDR
Gucciardi et al. (2010)	224 Australian elite athletes ($M_{age} = 22.68$; $SD = 6.70$; 61.2% males)	Cross-sectional survey	16-item Social Desirability Scale-17 (Stöber 2001)	• SDR unrelated to attitudes to doping ($r = -0.13$, $p = 0.06$) or doping susceptibility ($r = 0.10$, $p = 0.13$) • Indirect effect of attitudes toward doping to doping susceptibility via SDR ($\beta = 0.05$, 95% CI = 0.01 to 0.11, $p = 0.017$) within a structural equation modeling (SEM) framework • Moderation analyses indicated that the strength of the relation between attitudes to doping and doping susceptibility was influenced by SDR (intact for low, less for medium and high SDR)
Lazuras et al. (2010)	750 Greek elite adult athletes ($M_{age} = 25$; $SD = 5.89$; 63.9% males)	Cross-sectional survey	10-item version of the Marlowe-Crowne Social Desirability Scale (Strahan and Gerbasi 1972)	• VRR employed to examine the influence of SDR • SDR associated with susceptibility for doping intentions ($r = -0.16$, $p < 0.001$) and situational temptations ($r = -0.27$, $p < 0.001$) • Correlations between study variables (past doping behavior, attitudes, subjective norms, descriptive norms, perceived behavioral control, situational temptation) and doping intentions did not change significantly after controlling for SDR

Study	Sample	Design	Measure	Findings
Petróczi (2007)	199 college athletes ($M_{age}=20.1; SD=1.9$; 71.6% males)	Cross-sectional survey	33-item Marlowe-Crowne Social Desirability Scale (Crowne and Marlowe 1960)	• SDR associated with attitudes to doping ($r=-0.22, p<0.001$)
Petróczi and Nepusz (2011)	278 male college athletes ($M_{age}=20.2; SD=2.15$)	Cross-sectional survey	33-item Marlowe-Crowne Social Desirability Scale (Crowne and Marlowe 1960)	• SDR associated with doping attitudes ($r=-0.22, p<0.001$), internal deterrence factors such as moral values and health concerns ($r=0.14, p<.05$), and opinion regarding legalizing doping for top athletes ($r=-0.18, p<0.01$) or all athletes ($r=-0.14, p<0.05$) • Stronger associations between SDR and the study variables for the high SDR group, but non-significant relations for the low SDR group (sample split using cluster analysis) • SEM without SDR was a poor fit with the data and contained a large degree of unexplained variance; the addition of SDR enhanced variance explained and model-data fit
Whitaker et al. (2013)	729 competitive athletes ($M_{age}=28.8; SD=10.1$; 63% males)	Cross-sectional survey	20-item impression management subscale of the Balanced Inventory of Desirable Responding (Paulhus 1991)	• SDR associated with willingness to dope ($r=-0.19, p<0.001$), PES[2] user favorability[3] ($r=-0.08, p<0.05$), PES user similarity[4] ($r=-0.10, p<0.05$), nonuser similarity ($r=-0.08, p<0.001$), subjective norms attitudes to doping ($r=-0.15, p<0.001$), and positive outcome expectancies associated with the use of PES ($r=-0.13, p<0.001$)

Notes
1 SDR = socially desirable responding.
2 PES = performance enhancing substances.
3 Favorability refers to perceptions of how favorable individuals perceived PES user/nonuser to be.
4 Similarity refers to perceptions of whether or not characteristics perceived to describe a PES user/nonuser also described them.

records. There is evidence that the likelihood of SDR is low when the accuracy of item responses is verifiable (Becker and Colquitt 1992). Nevertheless, there is an implicit assumption in this approach that formal records are reliable estimates of the target behavior and this assumption might not hold with doping in sport. Indeed, a recent probability and cost analysis of worldwide data on positive doping tests from 93 sports revealed that the likelihood of catching a doping athlete is only 2.9 percent (Hermann and Henneberg 2013).

Conclusion

In this chapter, we have reviewed the literature on SDR with regard to its conceptualization, and methods to assess or detect and, if necessary, control for such distortions in self-reports. Although much of the evidence supports an interpretation that SDR represents a substantively meaningful trait (e.g., Ones *et al.* 1996; Smith and Ellingson 2002), one cannot completely rule out its influence as a response bias for construct and criterion validity (e.g., Holden 2007; Viswesvaran and Ones 1999). A variety of proactive (e.g., bogus pipeline) and *post hoc* techniques (e.g., latent variable modeling) have been proposed to detect and control for SDR, yet researchers interested in the psychosocial aspects of doping have not yet capitalized on these methods. Technological (e.g., eye-tracking) and statistical advancements (e.g., Monte Carlo simulations) represent avenues for future research on the effects of SDR for self-reported doping attributes or behaviors. It is our hope that this chapter will provide the foundation upon which to stimulate future research in this important area.

References

Barkoukis, V., Lazuras, L., and Tsorbatzoudis, H. (2014). Beliefs about the causes of success in sports and susceptibility for doping use in adolescent athletes. *Journal of Sports Sciences*, *32*, 212–219. doi: 10.1080/02640414.2013.819521.

Barkoukis, V., Lazuras, L., Tsorbatzoudis, H., and Rodafinos, A. (2011). Motivational and sportspersonship profiles of elite athletes in relation to doping behavior. *Psychology of Sport and Exercise*, *12*, 205–212. doi: 10.1016/j.psychsport.2010.10.003.

Becker, T. E. and Colquitt, A. L. (1992). Potential versus actual faking of biodata form: An analysis along several dimensions of item type. *Personnel Psychology*, *45*, 389–406. doi: 10.1111/j.1744-6570.1992.tb00855.x.

Berry, C. M. and Sackett, P. R. (2009). Faking in personnel selection: Tradeoffs in performance versus fairness resulting from two cut-score strategies. *Personnel Psychology*, *62*, 833–863. doi:10.1111/j.1744-6570.2009.01159.x.

Block, J. (1965). *The challenge of response sets*. New York: Appleton-Century-Crofts.

Chan, D. (2009). So why ask me? Are self-report data really that bad? In C. E. Lance and R. J. Vandenberg (eds.), *Statistical and methodological myths and urban legends: Doctrine, verity and fable in the organizational and social sciences* (309–336). New York: Routledge.

Chen, P. Y. and Spector, P. E. (1991). Negative affectivity as the underlying cause of correlations between stressors and strains. *Journal of Applied Psychology*, *76*, 398–407. doi: 10.1037//0021-9010.76.3.398.

Converse, P. D., Pathak, J., Quist, J., Merbedone, M., Gotlib, T., and Kostic, E. (2010). Statement desirability ratings in forced-choice personality measure development: Implications for reducing score inflation and providing trait-level information. *Human Performance*, *23*, 323–342. doi: 10.1080/08959285.2010.501047.

Crowne, D. P. and Marlowe, D. (1960). A new scale of social desirability independent of psychopathology. *Journal of Consulting Psychology*, *24*, 349–354. doi: 10.1037/h0047358.

Dwight, S. A. and Donovan, J. J. (2003). Do warnings not to fake reduce faking? *Human Performance*, *16*, 1–23. doi: 10.1207/S15327043HUP1601_1.

Edwards, A. L. (1957). *The social desirability variable in personality assessment and research*. New York: Dryden.

Gucciardi, D. F., Jalleh, G., and Donovan, R. J. (2010). Does social desirability influence the relationship between doping attitudes and doping susceptibility in athletes? *Psychology of Sport and Exercise*, *11*, 479–486. doi:10.1016/j.psychsport.2010.06.002.

Hanmer, M. J., Banks, A. J., and White, I. K. (2014). Experiments to reduce the over-reporting of voting: A pipeline to the truth. *Political Analysis*, *22*, 130–141. doi: 10.1093/pan/mpt027.

Hermann, A. and Henneberg, M. (2013). *Anti-doping systems in sports are doomed to fail: A probability and cost analysis*. Unpublished manuscript, The University of Adelaide. Available at www.adelaide.edu.au/news/binary9861/Doping.pdf.

Holden, R. R. (2007). Socially desirable responding does moderate personality scale validity both in experimental and in nonexperimental contexts. *Canadian Journal of Behavioral Science/Revue canadienne des sciences du comportment*, *39*, 184–201. doi: 10.1037/cjbs2007015.

Holden, R. R. (2010). Social desirability. In I. B. Weiner and W. E. Craighead (eds.), *The Corsini Encyclopedia of Psychology* (4th edn, 1–2). Hoboken, NJ: Wiley. doi: 10.1002/9780470479216.corpsy0889.

Holden, R. R. and Passey, J. (2010). Social desirability. In M. R. Leary and R. H. Hoyle (eds.), *Handbook of individual differences in social behavior* (441–454). New York: Guilford Publications.

Holden, R. R., Magruder, C. D., Stein, S. J., Sitarenios, G., and Sheldon, S. (1999). The effects of anonymity on the Holden Psychological Screening Inventory. *Personality and Individual Differences*, *27*, 737–742. doi: 10.1016/S0191–8869(98)00274–8.

Hough, L. M., Eaton, N. K., Dunnette, M. D., Kamp, J. D., and McCloy, R. A. (1990). Criterion-related validities of personality constructs and the effect of response distortion on those validities. *Journal of Applied Psychology*, *75*, 581–595. doi:10.1037/0021–9010.75.5.581.

Jackson, D. N., Wroblewski, V. R., and Ashton, M. C. (2000). The impact of faking on employment tests: Does forced choice offer a solution? *Human Performance*, *13*, 371–388. doi: 10.1207/S15327043HUP1304_3.

Johnson, J. (2004). The impact of item characteristics on item and scale validity. *Multivariate Behavioral Research*, *39*, 273–302. doi:10.1207/s15327906mbr3902.

Jones, E. E. and Sigall, H. (1971). The bogus pipeline: A new paradigm for measuring affect and attitude. *Psychological Bulletin*, *76*, 349–364. doi: 10.1037/h0031617.

Kam, C. (2013). Probing item social desirability by correlating personality items with Balanced Inventory of Desirable Responding (BIDR): A validity examination. *Personality and Individual Differences*, *54*, 513–518. doi: 10.1016/j.paid.2012.10.017.

Komar, S., Brown, D. G., Komar, J. A., and Robie, C. (2008). Faking and the validity of conscientiousness: A Monte Carlo investigation. *Journal of Applied Psychology*, *93*, 140–154. doi:10.1037/0021–9010.93.1.140.

Krumpal, I. (2013). Determinants of social desirability bias in sensitive surveys: A literature review. *Quality and Quantity*, *4*, 2025–2047. doi: 10.1007/s11135–011–9640–9.

Kuncel, N. R. and Tellegen, A. (2009). A conceptual and empirical reexamination of the measurement of the social desirability of items: Implications for detecting desirable response style and scale development. *Personnel Psychology*, *62*, 201–228. doi: 10.111 1/j.1744–6570.2009.01136.x.

Lautenschlager, G. J. and Flaherty, V. L. (1990). Computer administration of questions: More desirable or more social desirability? *Journal of Applied Psychology*, *75*, 310–314. doi: 10.1037/0021–9010.75.3.310.

Lazuras, L., Barkoukis, V., Rodafinos, A., and Tsorbatzoudis, H. (2010). Predictors of doping intentions in elite-level athletes: A social cognition approach. *Journal of Sport and Exercise Psychology*, *32*, 694–710.

Li, A. and Bagger, J. (2006). Using the BIDR to distinguish the effects of impression management and self-deception on the criterion validity of personality measures: A meta-analysis. *International Journal of Selection and Assessment*, *14*, 131–141. doi: 10 .1111/j.1468–2389.2006.00339.x.

Lynn, M. R. (1986). Determination and quantification of content validity. *Nursing Research*, *35*, 382–385. doi: 10.1097/00006199–198611000–00017.

McCrae, R. R. and Costa, P. T., Jr. (1983). Social desirability scales: More substance than style. *Journal of Consulting and Clinical Psychology*, *51*, 882–888. doi: 10.1037/ 0022–006X.51.6.882.

McFarland, L. A. and Ryan, A. M. (2000). Variance in faking across noncognitive measures. *Journal of Applied Psychology*, *85*, 812–821. doi: 10.1037/0021–9010.85.5.812.

McGrath, R. E., Mitchell, M., Kim, B. H., and Hough, L. (2010). Evidence for response bias as a source of error variance in applied assessment. *Psychological Bulletin*, *136*, 450–470. doi: 10.1037/a0019216.

Nederhof, A. J. (1985). Methods of coping with social desirability bias: A review. *European Journal of Social Psychology*, *15*, 263–280. doi: 10.1002/ejsp. 2420150303.

Ntoumanis, N., Ng, J. Y., Barkoukis, V., and Backhouse, S. (2014). Personal and psychosocial predictors of doping use in physical activity settings: A meta-analysis. *Sports Medicine*, *44* (*11*), 1603–1624. doi: 10.1007/s40279–014–0240–4.

Ones, D. S., Viswesvaran, C., and Reiss, A. D. (1996). Role of social desirability in personality testing for personnel selection: The red herring. *Journal of Applied Psychology*, *81* (*6*), 660–679. doi:10.1037/0021–9010.81.6.660.

Ones, D. S., Viswesvaran, C., and Schmidt, F. L. (1993). Comprehensive meta-analysis of integrity test validities: Findings and implications for personnel selection and theories of job performance. *Journal of Applied Psychology*, *78*, 679–703. doi: 10.1037/0021–9010.78.4.679.

Paulhus, D. L. (1991). Measurement and control of response bias. In J. P. Robinson, P. R. Shaver, and L. S. Wrightsman (eds.), *Measures of personality and social psychological attitudes* (17–59). San Diego: Academic Press.

Paulhus, D. L. (2002). Socially desirable responding: The evolution of a construct. In H. I. Braun, D. N. Jackson, and D. E. Wiley (eds.), *The role of constructs in psychological and educational measurement* (49–69). Mahwah, NJ: Erlbaum.

Paulhus, D. L. and Vazire, S. (2007). The self-report method. In R. W. Robins, R. C. Fraley, and R. Krueger (eds.), *Handbook of research methods in personality psychology* (224–239). New York: Guilford Press.

Paunonen, S. V. and LeBel, E. P. (2012). Socially desirable responding and its elusive effects on the validity of personality assessments. *Journal of Personality and Social Psychology, 103*, 158–175. doi: 10.1037/a0028165.

Paxton, P., Curran, P. J., Bollen, K. A., Kirby, J., and Chen, F. N. (2001). Monte Carlo experiments: Design and implementation. *Structural Equation Modeling, 8*, 287–312. doi: 10.1207/S15328007SEM0802_7.

Peidmont, R. L., McCrae, R. R., Riemann, R., and Angleitner, A. (2000). On the invalidity of validity scales: Evidence from self-reports and observer ratings in volunteer samples. *Journal of Personality and Social Psychology, 78*, 582–593.

Petróczi, A. (2007). Attitudes and doping: A structural equation analysis of the relationship between athletes' attitudes, sport orientation and doping behavior. *Substance Abuse Treatment, Prevention, and Policy, 2 (34)* doi: 10.1186/1747–597X-2–34.

Petróczi, A. and Nepusz, T. (2011). Methodological considerations regarding response bias effect in substance use research: Is correlation between the measured variables sufficient? *Substance Abuse Treatment, Prevention, and Policy, 6 (1)*. doi: 10.1186/1747–597X-6–1.

Petróczi, A., Uvacsek, M., Nepusz, T., Deshmukh, N., Shah, I., Aidman, E., Barker, J., Tóth, M., and Naughton, D. P. (2011). Incongruence in doping related attitudes, beliefs and opinions in the context of discordant behavioral data: In which measures do we trust? *PLoS ONE 6*, e18804. doi:10.1371/journal.pone.0018804.

Podsakoff, P. M., MacKenzie, S. B., and Podsakoff, N. P. (2012). Sources of method bias in social science research and recommendations on how to control it. *Annual Review of Psychology, 63*, 539–569. doi: 10.1146/annurev-psych-120710–100452.

Polit, D. F. and Beck, C. T. (2006). The content validity index: Are you sure you know what's being reported? Critique and recommendations. *Research in Nursing and Health, 29*, 489–497. doi: 10.1002/nur.20147.

Rammstedt, B. and Kemper, C. J. (2011). Measurement equivalence of the Big Five: Shedding further light on potential causes of the educational bias. *Journal of Research in Personality, 45*, 121–125. doi: 10.1016/j.jrp. 2010.11.006.

Randall, D. M. and Fernandes, M. F. (1991). The social desirability response bias in ethics research. *Journal of Business Ethics, 10*, 805–817. doi: 10.1007/BF00383696.

Reynolds, W. M. (1982). Development of reliable and valid short forms of the Marlowe-Crowne social desirability scale. *Journal of Clinical Psychology, 38*, 119–125. doi: 10.1002/1097–4679(198201)38:1<119::AID-JCLP2270380118>3.0.CO;2-I.

Roese, N. J. and Jamieson, D. W. (1993). Twenty years of bogus pipeline research: A critical review and meta-analysis. *Psychological Bulletin, 114*, 363–375.

Rosse, J. G., Stecher, M. D., Miller, J. L., and Levin, R. A. (1998). The impact of response distortion on preemployment testing and hiring decisions. *Journal of Applied Psychology, 83*, 634–644. doi:10.1037/0021–9010.83.4.634.

Schmidt, F. L., Le, H., and Ilies, R. (2003). Beyond alpha: An empirical examination of the effects of different sources of measurement error on reliability estimates for measures of individual-differences constructs. *Psychological Methods, 8*, 206–224. doi: 10.1037/1082–989X.8.2.206.

Smith, D. B. and Ellingson, J. E. (2002). Substance versus style: A new look at social desirability in motivating contexts. *Journal of Applied Psychology, 87*, 211–219. doi: 10.1037//0021–9010.87.2.211.

Stöber, J. (2001). The Social Desirability Scale-17 (SDS-17): Convergent validity, discriminant validity, and relationship with age. *European Journal of Psychological Assessment, 17*, 222–232. doi: 10.1027//1015–5759.17.3.222.

Strahan, R. and Gerbasi, K. C. (1972). Short, homogeneous versions of the Marlowe-Crowne social desirability scale. *Journal of Clinical Psychology, 28*, 191–193.

Tourangeau, R. and Yan, T. (2007). Sensitive questions in surveys. *Psychological Bulletin, 133*, 859–883. doi: 10.1037/0033-2909.133.5.859.

Uziel, L. (2010). Rethinking social desirability scales: From impression management to interpersonally oriented self-control. *Perspective on Psychological Science, 5*, 243–262. doi: 10.1177/1745691610369465.

van Hooft, E. A. J. and Born, M. P. (2012). Intentional respond distortion on personality tests: Using eye-tracking to understand response processes when faking. *Journal of Applied Psychology, 97*, 301–316. doi: 10.1037/a0025711.

Viswesvaran, C. and Ones, D. S. (1999). Meta-analyses of fakability estimates: Implications for personality measurement. *Educational and Psychological Measurement, 59*, 197–210. doi: 10.1177/00131649921969802.

Wetzel, E., Carstensen, C. H., and Böhnke, J. R. (2013). Consistency of extreme response style and nonextreme response style across traits. *Journal of Research in Personality, 47*, 178–189. doi: 10.1016/j.jrp. 2012.10.010.

Whitaker, L., Long, J., Petróczi, A., and Backhouse, S. H. (2013). Using the prototype willingness model to predict doping in sport. *Scandinavian Journal of Medicine and Science in Sport, 24* (5), e398–e405. doi: 10.1111/sms.12148.

Ziegler, M. and Buehner, M. (2009). Modeling socially desirable responding and its effects. *Educational and Psychological Measurement, 69*, 548–565. doi: 10.1177/0013164408324469.

7 Indirect measures in doping behavior research

Andrea Petróczi

In quantitative psychological research, "data reproducibility is necessary but not sufficient for replicability, and replicability is necessary but not sufficient for generalizability" (Asendorpf *et al.* 2013: 110).[1] Reproducibility can be ensured by proper data treatment, analyses, and transparency. However, even with the best intention, replicability and generalizability are at jeopardy in cases where measurements are devised and tested in an ad hoc manner as part of the observation or intervention. Emerging social science research of doping is particularly prone to this problem. Research into doping behavior is characterized by studies that often encompass new methods and their applications within a single design. Purely methodological papers focusing on measurements of doping-related social cognitions are rare.

To move doping psychology research forward for the next decade, more attention must be paid to measurements of doping-related constructs by re-examining the existing methods and incorporating new methodologies. Specifically, and in line with the key focus of this chapter, there is a need to have a better understanding about (1) athletes' mental representations of doping before we attempt to develop methods for capturing the key elements of this important mental construct; (2) the nature and interpretation of the data obtained through projections; and (3) the conceptual alignment of response-time measures to explicit and implicit thought processing and behavior. The aim of this chapter is to provide a narrative overview of the *indirect measurements* and *measures*[2] already employed or having potential in researching the psychology behind doping.

Overview of indirect methods

Data in doping behavior research, by definition, must come from the information directly or indirectly provided by the athletes and the athlete entourage. Owing to the prevailing social norms surrounding doping, its sensitivity and potentially career-changing consequences, obtaining reliable, valid, and relevant information on doping prevalence, perceived norms, beliefs, preferences, and attitudes poses multiple methodological challenges on empirical investigations. Researchers in favor of incorporating indirect assessments and using innovative techniques typically justify this choice on counterbalancing social desirability bias (addressed in Chapter 6) and trying to capture thinking processes that cannot be easily faked (discussed in Chapter 3); or rationalize the choice on the fact that not all of a person's mind is introspectively and consciously accessible.

Taxonomy of indirect measures (Figure 7.1) can be formulated along two major dimensions: (1) the target concept (i.e., doping behavior or social cognition relating to doping behavior); and (2) the way the information is obtained on the target concept. The main role of social cognition in doping research is to develop an understanding of doping behavior through the exploration of the psychosocial factors that influence doping decisions and act as either a catalyst or deterrent of doping use. However, owing to the difficulty of obtaining reliable information on a sensitive behavior directly, social-cognitive variables such as attitudes or perceived norms are sometime used as proxy indicators for doping (Figure 7.1A). Attempts at using implicit measurements such as the autobiographical Implicit Association Test (aIAT; Agosta and Sartori 2013) or Timed

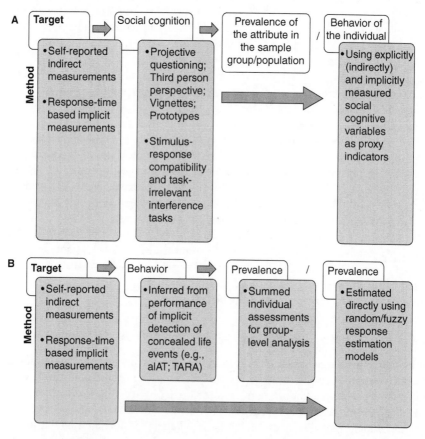

Figure 7.1 Taxonomy of indirect measures. (A) Target measure is a social cognitive variable; (B) Target measure is information on doping behavior and/or prevalence of doping.

Antagonistic Response Althiometer (TARA; Gregg 2007) to obtain information on concealed life events have been made (Figure 7.1B) but owing to the host of influencing factors on test performance (Vargo *et al.* 2014), forensic diagnostic use in a field setting is not recommended (Petróczi *et al.* 2015).

Having accurate assessment of the size of hidden, hard-to-count populations (i.e., people with attributes hidden from the public eye, such as drug users or doping users among athletes) is a challenging task. When the interest is not identifying doping user individuals but establishing prevalence for the athletic group or population (Figure 7.1B), Random/Fuzzy response models – discussed in Chapter 8 – can be used. These indirect estimation techniques have been specifically developed for group-level prevalence estimation and work by making the survey situation safe. In this set-up, although the answer is directly reported to the interviewer or self-reported by the respondent, the deliberately added "noise" makes relating the sensitive information to individuals impossible.

For this chapter, "*behavior*" is a specific life event (e.g., doping use) and represents information on a single individual with or without the target behavior, which then can be summed for the sample to obtain prevalence rates. "*Prevalence*" refers to the occurrence of the target behavior in the population and can either be derived as a sum of individuals with the behavior in the sample or calculated from knowledge-based information about others' target attribute and personal network size. Note that this definition excludes *perceived prevalence*, which is a subjective state that may derive from social projection of the self or heuristic thinking. "*Social cognition*" encapsulates attitudes, views, perceptions, beliefs, opinions, and motivations which can be explicitly expressed in surveys or interviews (covered in Chapter 5), indirectly assessed through hypothetical situations and/or as a third-person perspective; or inferred from performance on response-time based measurements (aka implicit tests). Although in the literature, *indirect* and *implicit* are often used interchangeably, in this chapter the term "*implicit*" is exclusively reserved for measures based on response time differences, whereas "*indirect*" is used as a broader term encompassing all measurement techniques where the attribute of the person or population is assessed via an intermediary variable (e.g., response time, third-person projection). Therefore an implicit measure is also an indirect measure but not all indirect measures are implicit.

Projective questioning

Although the answer is directly sought and explicitly reported, projective questioning counts as an indirect method because of the shift from the *self* to asking about *others* instead of the respondent. Interpretation of the results from projective questioning varies in the doping literature. Unfortunately, the ambiguity surrounding the terminology, definitions, and underlying assumptions often lead to some confusion as to what projective measures actually represent. The interpretation of projections is highly dependent upon how the projection is obtained, namely whether it is specific knowledge or perceptions; or it is an estimate for "most people" or for a specific group or a hypothetical "third person." Despite being underlined by different cognitive mechanisms, results from both the factual and specific information of the *known others* and the general perceptions of the *unknown others* (also referred to as social projection) are somewhat reflective of the respondent. Athletes who are doping users tend to know more doping users, compared to their "clean" counterparts. This feature is exploited in estimation methods that are based on social networks. Social projection is rooted in the *self* and manifests in thinking processes where people assume others to be similar to themselves (Robbins and Krueger 2005). On one hand, this allows people to make quick predictions about what others are like or how they are likely to behave but it also automatically fills the gap if factual information is required but not readily available in memory. As such, it has a tendency for biased perception of the prevalence of one's own behavior among others, driven by uniqueness bias (Goethals *et al.* 1991) or false consensus (Ross *et al.* 1977), which in turn results in subjective over- and underestimation. Being rooted in the *self* makes social projection an attractive – if somewhat elusive – candidate for being a proxy measure for doping behavior. Knowing doping users is also indicative of the person's own involvement in doping by either being a user or knowing and surrounded by users.

Projective questions (PQ) ask respondents to answer the question for "most people" or for a specific protagonist in hypothetical situations, which allows the respondent to detach him-/herself from the target behavior. Because respondents are not likely to have exact information on "most people" (unless it is a small and defined group to which the respondents belong), their responses may stem from the self. Projective techniques utilize this phenomenon when presenting deliberately ambiguous situations where respondents have to fill the gap in order to complete the task. In the absence of information, it is assumed that in this process a person uses his/her own (and thus egocentrically biased) views without being aware of doing so. Accordingly, PQ is likely to produce estimates with more accuracy in situations where the social distance is small (i.e., projection is made for people with similar traits or attributes) (Jones 2004).

PQ is not limited to behavior but it can also be employed for investigating a wide range of psychological constructs, such as attitudes, prototype characteristics, willingness, and social norms. One specific form of social projection manifests in prototype heuristics, which "share a common mechanism and a remarkably consistent pattern of cognitive illusions" (Kahneman 2003: 712). Prototypes, as cognitive representations of features that are shared as common attributes of an object or person among the members of the object or person group and distinctive from the non-members (i.e., typical doping user vs. nonuser) can be exploited as a feasible and effective tool for indirectly measuring attitudes toward doping via the perceived distinctive characteristics of doping users.

Whilst the deducted conclusion from most projected social constructs is relatively straightforward, measures of social norms are prone to misinterpretation.

Social norms have two components (Lapinski and Rimal 2005): (1) the per-ceived prevalence of the target behavior itself exerting informative influence (also referred to as *descriptive* norm); and (2) the perceived social judgment of this behavior serving as normative influence (also referred to as *injunctive* norm). Because of the first behavioral element, estimations of doping prevalence can be – and have been – erroneously interpreted as an indirectly obtained but objective estimate of the doping prevalence. Egocentric social projection assesses a dif-ferent mental construct than factual knowledge about the social network, thus social projection is not a bona fide measure of prevalence but an indirect assess-ment of the related social cognition.

Network scale-up

The Network Scale-Up Method (NSUM) is an elegantly simple, yet powerful, approach to acquire prevalence information on hard-to-reach or hard-to-find populations (Bernard *et al.* 2010). The method is rooted in the premise that peo-ple's social networks (i.e., the set of people they know) are, at the cumulative level, representative of the general population in which they "exist" (e.g., elite athletes belong to the population of competitive athletes). In this set-up, respond-ents are simply asked to report *exact data* on two segments of their social network: (1) the number of people in their environment; and (2) the number of people in their environment they *know* that carry the attribute of interest. One example is asking athletes to report the exact number of athletes they know and the number of athletes among these they know that use anabolic steroids). Then, the estimated prevalence rate is simply calculated by dividing the total number of people with the attribute by the cumulative number of people in personal net-works (Bernard *et al.* 2010). One variant, the Game of Contacts (Salganik *et al.* 2011), can be used for estimating the social visibility of groups with the target attribute.

Hypothetical situations

Presenting hypothetical situations to respondents and asking about their impres-sions and hypothetical decisions in the described situation has a long history in experimental psychology and sociology (Finch 1987). These hypothetical situ-ations (often called vignettes) describe everyday situations and are designed to evoke the target emotions and activate relevant social knowledge in participants who are required to make judgments on how the person in the vignette situation might feel, think, or should behave. The underlying assumption is that this demand would activate the self-concept and respondents make – consciously or unconsciously – inferences from their own thoughts or positions and project these onto the scenario described in the vignette, and thus indirectly revealing attitudes, values and perceived norms about the construct of interest (e.g., doping). Vignettes may also be combined with a third-person approach, remov-ing the respondents even one step further from the pressure of revealing their own thoughts directly – even if the decision or position to be revealed is purely hypothetical. The advantage of using hypothetical scenarios beyond protecting the respondents from directly revealing their views on sensitive topics is that the method enables controlled experiments to capture mental processes difficult or impossible to study via observations or classic experiments. The disadvantage is the ever-present caveat that making decisions in hypothetical situations is never the same as in real life. Stating that one would do something is not the same as actually doing it.

Implicit methods utilizing response-time differences

The inherent limitation of self-report methodology is the assumption that respondents are not only willing but also able to report their feelings, thoughts, motivations, beliefs, and explicitly express their preferences and attitudes. However, what is available to conscious self-examination is only a small fraction of people's thought processes. Although people may experience cognitive certainty of knowing their preferences and motives for their actions, this self-assured feeling is deceptive because mental experiences one is aware of are not equivalent to the mental processes that determined or influenced the behavioral choices (Nosek *et al.* 2011).

In contrast to explicit reports, implicit measurements do not make explicit connection between the test and the target construct. The key difference between implicit and the explicit measurements is that respondents are not asked to make evaluations directly (e.g., recording agreement with direct attitude statements or placing the target construct on a bipolar semantic-differential scale) but, rather, these "evaluations" are inferred from performance on an experimental, reaction-time based task.

A significant proportion of implicit measures utilizes dimensional overlap influence between the stimuli and response (S-R). The tests typically contrast one compatible S-R pair with one incompatible S-R pair and use the difference between the response times in each task to asses which of the two pairs is "more" or "less" compatible for, and thus implicitly preferred by, the individual (De Houwer 2001). Other tests in the implicit measurement family exploit task-irrelevant feature inferences (e.g., De Houwer 2003; Rinck and Becker 2007). These tests rely on the measurable interfering effect of the seemingly hidden relevant feature. Characteristically, the stimuli used in implicit measures of social cognition have valence (pleasant, unpleasant, desired, undesired, etc.). In fact, the test builds on this valence to measure, for example, implicit attitudes, preferences, or motivation (e.g., Greenwald *et al.* 1998). An exemption to this is the group of implicit tests, such as the autobiographical IAT (Agosta and Sartori 2013) and the Timed Antagonistic Response Alethiometer (Gregg 2007), which aim to capture memory of a specific life event.

Indirect methods in doping research

Network Scale-up

To date, only a limited number of studies used techniques that resemble NSUM to a varying degree. The first survey was conducted among Finnish Olympic athletes, which showed that whilst no athlete admitted doping, 37 percent of endurance athletes and 42.5 percent among those in power sports reported that they personally knew another athlete who engaged in doping (Alaranta *et al.* 2006). Nevertheless, without knowing the degree of overlap between the respondents' social circles, such figures put doping prevalence estimation anywhere up to 42.5 percent (with the top figure assuming that there is no overlap at all). From interviews with eight top-level athletes, Morente-Sánchez *et al.* (2013) reported that half of the athletes (three cyclists and one triathlete) knew a doping user. In the absence of information on the personal network size or sampling strategy, it is difficult to conclude anything else but doping may be more prevalent in cycling than in triathlon – providing that the participant selection was random. In a larger study, 6 percent of 706 English professional football players reported that they personally knew someone who used doping, compared to 45 percent having knowledge of a player using illicit drugs (Waddington *et al.* 2005). Again, personal network size was not reported but the majority (68 percent) of the players who knew someone using doping stated that such knowledge comes from their previous clubs (with 20 percent knowing someone in the current club and 12 percent knowing doping users in both previous and current clubs).

The underlying assumption of the NSUM, namely that people who use drugs tend to know more drug users and vice versa, was clearly evidenced in projected illicit drug use among elite athletes (Dunn *et al.* 2012). The proportion of athletes who knew another athlete or athletes using illicit drugs increased from 18.1 percent to 37.4 percent for lifetime users, but not current use, to 62.7 percent among self-admitted current users of illicit substances. Despite this, the NSUM estimation, which takes the number of friends known with the attribute and the personal network size, was used only once to date. This study used NSUM for validating prevalence figures obtained via two different indirect estimation models and showed that the number of cases definitely known for doping among friends is much less than the suspected number of cases, yielding NSUM prevalence estimates of 1.30 percent and 17.67 percent respectively (James *et al.* 2013).

Projections

Normative estimations

The first projected estimation for doping appeared in the media in 1992, reporting that 34 percent of US Olympic athletes thought that steroid use was up to 10 percent among their peers, while a further 43 percent put this figure higher than 10 percent (Pearson and Hansen 1992). Almost two decades later, a *Sports Illustrated* survey (2010) reported that a quarter of 71 professional golfers believed that Tiger Woods used HGH or other performance-enhancing drugs. Projective questioning has appeared in the scientific doping literature and following the same line of investigation has solely focused on normative beliefs.

With showing the interplay between the projected prevalence estimations and involvement (self-admitted doping behavior), the presence of the False Consensus Effect (FCE) was established (Petróczi *et al.* 2008b), and set a distinct path for researching projected prevalence estimation of doping. Typically, self-confessed doping users give a significantly higher estimate of general doping prevalence compared to those athletes who claimed abstinence (Morente-Sánchez *et al.* 2014; Petróczi *et al.* 2008b). Notably social projections for a non-sensitive behavior (e.g., use of nutritional supplements) are independent of the relevant behavior. Domain specificity in prevalence estimations (i.e., lack of cross-interference between illegal social drugs and doping) was established by Uvacsek *et al.* (2011) showing that self-admitted doping users who abstained from illegal drugs gave higher estimation for doping but not for illegal drugs, and vice versa. Projective questioning has also been used independently of doping behavior to establish perceived descriptive norms for doping use with or without comparison between sports, roles, and/or nations (e.g., Ćorluka *et al.* 2011; Dunn *et al.* 2012; Jalleh and Donovan 2008; Moston *et al.* 2014a, 2014b; Waddington *et al.* 2005).

In summary, a significant proportion of athletes perceive doping more widespread than one would expect from the official doping test statistics. The observed doping estimations (even those made by nonusers) were considerably higher than the 2 percent benchmark of the reported adverse analytical findings by WADA laboratories; and even higher among those who confessed doping use. It is yet to be ascertained whether this elevated perception of doping use is subconsciously used to justify own behavior or is, in fact, the initiator of doping use. The considerable discrepancy between the official figures and the consistently reported higher perceptions of doping prevalence underscore the urgent need for reliable information on how widespread doping is in competitive and recreational sport.

Third-person questioning

In the study of Huybers and Mazanov (2012), sets of vignettes regarding a doping decision situation with a gender-neutral athlete, whose characteristics were commensurate with the respondents' career stage and level, were used to indirectly assess the respondents' perceptions of facilitating and deterring factors of doping. Overall, the outcome of this study provided support for previous findings about the influence of the coach or senior peers and the desire for instant gains in performance as facilitator; and risk of failing the doping test, financial consequences, and severe health risks as deterrence.

With a few exceptions (Huybers and Mazanov 2012; Dodge *et al.* 2012), studies tend not to specify the hypothetical athlete's characteristics or circumstances, often not even having reference to gender, sport, club/team affiliation, or country, when using some form of third-person-questioning. Using the "me (us) vs. others" reference frame, the outcomes of these studies are more reflective of the in- and out-group bias in projection than indicative for what the respondent personally would do in the given choice situation. Other doping-focused studies asked participants to indicate what they think other athletes do or what other athletes would do in doping-related hypothetical situations that require a decision choice (as detailed later in this chapter).

Hypothetical scenarios

The Goldman dilemma

The most cited pair of doping vignettes is often referred to as the "Goldman dilemma," named after Bob Goldman, physician, who asked elite athletes in combat and power sports whether they would take a magic drug that could make them Olympic champion – but also kill them afterwards (Bamberger and Yaeger 1997). In fact, the question was prompted by an earlier informal poll among top-level runners by Gabe Mirkin in the 1970s (Mirkin and Hoffman 1978), suggesting that a considerable number of athletes (greater than 50 percent) would take the Faustian bargain.

As with projected estimations, the Goldman-type dilemma became an enticing scenario for doping research. Connor and colleagues repeated Goldman's "death for success" scenario in two independent studies. An overwhelming 210/212 rejection rate of such a bargain was noted among elite track and field athletes (Connor *et al.* 2013). Even with the grave consequence removed, only 12 percent of the athletes registered willingness, which still remains well below Goldman's estimations.

Other hypothetical scenarios in the literature diverge to some degree from Goldman's vignettes. Interestingly, the significant proportion of studies using projective questioning also included hypothetical scenarios in the battery of assessments. These typically asked directly about how the respondents would act or decide in the given situation (Morente-Sánchez *et al.* 2013; Petróczi *et al.* 2008b) while a small number of studies combined hypothetical scenarios with projection (Backhouse *et al.* 2013; Bloodworth *et al.* 2012; Huybers and Mazanov 2012; Petróczi *et al.* 2008b).

As part of a larger study, eight athletes were interviewed and only one indicated that he/she would use an undetectable drug that would significantly improve performance (Morente-Sánchez *et al.* 2013). The same vignette with a substance that is effective but undetectable was posed to emerging young athletes but also in combination with third-person projection for fellow competitors (Bloodworth *et al.* 2012). Congruently with the pattern expected from drug use projection, the low willingness (less than 10 percent without consequences and less than 1 percent if the drug shortens lifespan) of self-reported use increased radically for the perception of what others would do. Seventy-three percent of the athletes believed that at least some of the others would take the drug if there was no effect on health and more than 40 percent would still do so, even if it meant a reduction in their lifespan. Notably, the time invested in athletic career corresponded to the increased willingness, providing that there were no health consequences. Recovery from injuries and the economic pressures of elite sport emerged as potential pressure points in which doping use is more enticing than it would be otherwise. A significant minority expressed willingness to take a hypothetical performance-enhancing drug if it would guarantee success and was undetectable.

Choice scenarios

The first systematically created vignettes for doping choices appear in Huybers and Mazanov (2012) where the 64 pairs of scenarios were combined with third-person questioning. Choice attributes were based on an empirically derived list of cost and benefits from previous qualitative phase of the study and varied across the vignettes to ascertain how attributes are traded off. The results suggested that the choice about doping was based on rational assessments of gains and consequences (as opposed to being emotional or based on morals). From the methodological point of view, this work highlighted some important issues. The first is the nature of the dependent variable, whether it is consideration, willingness, or actual doping use, with the way doping is established being critical. The second is how to capture the dynamics and synergy between motivating and deterring factors, and whether athletes' thinking and decision-making process is linear or "spiral-like" with constant feedback loops or best captured as a loosely connected network of influencing factors. Finally, but perhaps most importantly for this chapter, is the value of systematically developed set of choice scenarios as a valid and relevant research tool for doping investigations.

One study used a doping vignette as contrast to cognitive performance enhancement with drugs and depicted two males (one in each scenario) who performed above expectation after having taken a performance enhancer before a sports competition, where the hypothetical athlete won, and prior to an exam, where the student received a better grade than expected (Dodge *et al.* 2012). The results showed that those who participated in sport viewed the athlete protagonist more as being a cheater compared to the student protagonist. However, because the vignettes contrasted a zero-sum game (sport) to a non-zero-sum game (exam), it remains unclear whether the drug and/or performance types or zero-sum game scenarios were compared.

Doping prototypes

To some degree, research dated more than two decades ago has already aimed to capture the anchoring process of the perception of doping users. Targeting anabolic steroids specifically, Schwerin and Corcoran (1996) found that the drug itself was seen differently by users and nonusers, each with respective congruence between views and actions. Thus athletes' views of doping substances could be used as an indirect method of assessing disposition toward doping. In more general terms, doping user and nonuser prototypes were explored among current or former competitive athletes (Whitaker *et al.* 2013). In this study, self-identification with doping user prototype characteristics correlated more strongly with explicit doping attitude and favorable view of doping user characteristics than with self-identification with nonusers or favorability of nonusers. The prototype measures also showed the same pattern for relationships with willingness to use doping, subjective norms, descriptive norms, and outcome expectancies, in order of decreasing strength, suggesting that prototype methodology can be employed as indirect measures of attitudes and, to a lesser degree, of other doping-related social cognition. Future research into how these prototype heuristics link to explicitly and implicitly retrieved attitudes and other social-cognitive measures would move the application of indirect methodologies to doping research forward.

Response-time based measurements in doping research

Utilizing stimulus-response compatibility to measure "implicit doping attitude"[3]

The early phase of incorporating implicit assessments into doping research was dominated by tests built on stimulus-response compatibility. First adaptations of the IAT concept (Greenwald *et al.* 1998) to doping mirrored the classic pleasant/unpleasant valenced target categorization with doping and nutritional supplements (Petróczi *et al.* 2008a), doping and tea blend with real word/not word target labels (Lotz and Hagemann 2007) and doping and tea blend with good/bad attributes (Brand *et al.* 2011; Lotz and Hagemann 2007). The results in these IAT studies showed preference for the target category set to contrast doping, which was interpreted as negative implicit attitude toward doping.

General preference for nutritional supplements over doping was also reported in two mixed-method studies using the Brief IAT concept coupled with explicit measures and hair analysis to corroborate self-reported behavior (Petróczi *et al.* 2011). The unique aspect was the combination of social science techniques with analytical chemistry which, for the first time in doping implicit cognition research, differentiated between doping user athletes based on admittance/denial. Whilst all groups of athletes exhibited negative implicit doping attitudes, the implicit preference for nutritional supplements was reduced in the group of athletes who used but denied doping. At the same time, their explicit responses took on values that indicated extreme negative view on all doping related cognitions, which resulted in increased dissociation between explicit and implicit measures for these athletes. This distinctive cognitive pattern, separating doping users according to whether they are admitting (under anonymity) their doping behavior or denying it, suggests that the "action–admission" congruency has a moderating effect on both explicit and implicit measures.

Using the brief IAT format, the malleability of implicit associations was tested in an information-based intervention study (James *et al.* 2010). The initial dominant association of functional foods with being healthy changed to perform-ance enhancing after reading an information pamphlet about the performance-enhancing effect of nitrate-rich foodstuffs. Uniquely, this test contrasted a single target-category (foodstuff) with two attributes that were not mutually exclusive (performance enhancing or health), nor did they form the bipolar ends of the same scale. This approach, in line with Petróczi's conceptualization of mental representation of performance enhancement and doping (2013a, 2013b), may capture more ecologically relevant associations than the classic attitude categor-ization with good/bad or pleasant/unpleasant affective tags.

In contrast to the lexical-processing tests, where respondents were invariably asked to categorize words based on their meaning, two recent studies used images as an implicit assessment of doping attitudes. The pictures presented in the Brief IAT framework were either associated with pharmacological perform-ance enhancements (e.g., pills and syringes) or healthy food items (a bowl of Greek salad and a bowl of granola, an apple and a medley of fruits and vege-tables), and paired with emoticons for "liking" and "disliking" (Brand *et al.* 2014a; Brand *et al.* 2014b). Because the test structure kept the health food cat-egory non-focal, the obtained implicit measurement was indicative of the degree of liking associated with pharmacological performance enhancements. The general outcomes were in line with previous assessments showing negative implicit attitude toward pharmacological performance enhancements across the sample but to a lesser degree among bodybuilders (as opposed to handball players). Discriminatory power for the pictorial BIAT was shown in a study with bodybuilders, where doping use was established via urinalyses (Brand *et al.* 2014b). However, owing to the high sensitivity-low specificity (i.e., obtaining relatively high percentage of false positives as a price for identifying true posit-ives), the test use should be limited to making comparisons at the group level.

In addition to the published full papers, several implicit measurements have been tested to capture various doping-related social-cognitive variables within affective, moral, functional, and self-referential frames (Petróczi 2013c). Instead of using affective attributes, other brief IAT variants for doping were also developed and tested. These included self-referential anchoring (*me/others*), implicit norms (*widespread/rare*), instrumental attitudes, or utility (*useful/ useless*), as well as two variants of doping autobiographical IATs (aIATs). Pre-liminary results from these applications showed that the self-referential doping BIAT contrasting target words with *me/not me* categories had better discrimina-tory power for doping use in settings where doping behavior categories were based on self-reports. Moral and instrumental attitudes alone, although each showed some difference in the expected direction at the aggregated level, did not produce significantly different implicit measures between self-admitted doping users and nonusers. Normative IATs showed that doping was implicitly associated with being rare, whereas nutritional supplements were associated with being prevalent, mirroring the explicit reports in the literature. Contrasting moral and functional frames (using BIAT and aIAT formats) has led to ambivalent outcomes at the individual level, suggesting that the moral dimension may not be the only relevant frame for doping cognition; and thus providing strong evidence for a framing effect on implicit measures. These results provide support to the previous observation (De Houwer 2003) that category labels have an influence on implicit measures and that anchoring doping to the *self* could increase discriminatory power. The latter is in line with the conclusion that personalized IAT predict behavior better than a standard IAT because it eliminates all reference to normative information from the attribute categories (Olson and Fazio 2004). Although further research and replication of the findings are required to make a definite conclusion and to develop a better understanding of the underlying cognitive mechanism, researchers should exercise caution when setting up implicit measures of doping cognition.

Exploiting task-irrelevant interference effect

Task-irrelevant interference was only exploited in one study using emotional Stroop task with doping and cheating words and showed that non-athletic adolescents exhibited some degree of attentional bias toward doping (Schirlin *et al.* 2009). Because the sample consisted of non-athletic individuals, the outcome of this study supports more the possibility that the implicit measurements tap into the person's environment than the assumption that response-time differences in performing the implicit tasks are measures of the intended intra-personal construct (e.g., attitude). However, the findings from this study should be interpreted with caution. The target stimuli set contained a mix of, presumably unfamiliar, words related to doping, most likely familiar words related to cheating, along with some ambiguous words. Furthermore, participants took part in a familiarization exercise to mitigate against unfamiliarity, which also could have functioned as priming. As a consequence, it remains unclear what exactly influenced the observed response-time difference.

Future directions

The more we know about doping behavior, the more we have come to realize that our knowledge is determined by the way we measured the relevant underlying psychological constructs. After 15 years of sustained effort, doping research has reached its saturation point with the currently existing measurements. The next decade will only be partly characterized by expanding the scope of subjects of our interest (i.e., moving beyond the elite athlete and incorporating different developmental ages and various stakeholders into the sampling protocol). The other important trend will be the expansion of the array of research tools utilized in data collection. Thus, it is expected that the number and variety of measures of doping-related social cognitions will be on the rise in the contemporary doping research armory. This will unequivocally benefit doping research, but also poses some danger. If ever, now there is a greater need for theorists and methodologists to be involved in experimental work to provide tools for applications in field settings.

As discussed in detail earlier in this chapter, caution about a clear differentiation between prevalence estimation using NSUM or similar methods and social projection using projective questioning or third-person method is warranted, because these "estimations" arise from distinctly different social knowledge structures. Research design with social projection should consider comparability and set to make research into in- and out-group bias feasible. Establishing the temporal sequence of *behavior–projection of own behavior* vs. *perceived high prevalence–behavior* will make a significant contribution to doping research and prevention.

Hypothetical questions and vignettes hold much underutilized potential for doping research. Future directions should include systematic vignette construction based on possible combinations of the key facilitating and deterring factors. Established potent vignettes can be further developed into game-like computerized tests resembling strategy games with simulated performance-related, financial, moral, and reputational gains and consequences; and in turn used as interactive educational tools to help athletes, particularly adolescents, to learn to develop alternative strategies for performance enhancement within the acceptable, thus less risky, limits.

Following Payne and Gawronski (2010), instead of asking how implicit measures can predict a behavior (e.g., doping) that is goal-oriented, effortful, and sustained (and thus primarily deliberative), researchers should consider what is in the behavior that might influence one's performance on implicit tests of doping-related social cognition. An athlete's thoughts about doping, including cognitive ambivalence, must have imprints on his/her mental representation of doping which in turn influences his/her performance on an implicit test recalling part of this mental mindset. One's mental representation of doping can be a collage of accumulated social knowledge, shaped by personal and vicarious experiences, formed in social context and stored in memory, which exerts influence on behavioral choices regarding doping. It is the recall situation that makes the manifestation of a *segment* of this information pool explicit or implicit. We may capture this temporal characteristic and refer to it as "*situated mental representation.*" From the methodological point of view, it is important to note that what *segment* manifests in explicit or implicit assessments is determined by the recall situation and it is temporary, thus should not be interpreted as if it would be a stable entity or the *whole* construct. In other words, we only learn about the part we measure, and what we learn is also influenced by the framework we impose on the measure in the assessment process. Researchers working with measures of doping-related social cognition must be aware of this limitation, which is particularly acute in research settings using implicit assessments.

It is clear that relying solely on explicit self-reports in explorative doping studies and anti-doping interventions can leave much variability unaccounted for. Equally, treating implicit measures as a panacea for obtaining information on people's "true" thoughts (i.e., as a lie detector) is a very deceptive view that locks researchers into a rigid frame when it comes to making sense of the implicit measures and the relationship between the implicit or explicit measures and the relevant behavior. In the next decade, implicit assessments of doping-related social cognition are likely to gain popularity in doping research. In order to fully utilize the potential of response-time methodology, doping research must move beyond straightforward application of established implicit measurements and focus on the mental processes that are captured with response-time methodology.

Finally, but perhaps most importantly, it must be noted that the indirect measures and proxy indicators for doping behavior are potent research tools to explore differences at group level but they are unsuitable for individual diagnostics. Forensic application of the indirect measures to identify dopers is inappropriate and thus is discouraged.

Acknowledgments

AP received funding for investigating the utility of indirect assessments of doping-related social cognitions and transition markers from the World Anti-Doping Agency (2008–2013). The assistance received from students and colleagues (Ricky James, Alex Kharadi, Árpád Kovács, Saira Khan, Jaime Morente-Sánchez, Aisling Naughton, Tamás Nepusz, Márta Ránky, Ihsan Sari, Attila Szabó, Martina Uvacsek, Julie Elisabeth Vargo, and Attila Velenczei) with aspects of data collection for the ongoing investigations is gratefully acknowledged.

Notes

1 Reproducibility is shown by independently re-analysing the same data set and coming to the same conclusion. Replicability refers to obtaining comparable results with a new data set which was sampled using a similar population, methodology, and conditions. Generalizability is only established if the phenomenon is evidenced independently of the original operationalizations of the involved constructs, situations, or populations.
2 *Measurement* refers to the assessment process, whereas *measures* are the outcomes (results) of the relevant measurements.
3 To remain congruent with the literature, outcomes of the SRC-based implicit tests are referred to as "implicit attitudes" but noted that it is debated whether the construct itself or the retrieval process is implicit; and what implicit tests actually measure.

References

Agosta, S. and Sartori, G. (2013). The autobiographical IAT: a review. *Frontiers in Psychology*, 4, 519.

Alaranta, A., Alaranta, H., Holmila, J., Palmu, P., Pietila, K., and Helenius, I. (2006). Self-reported attitudes of elite athletes towards doping: differences between type of sport. *International Journal of Sport Medicine*, 27, 842–846.

Asendorpf, J. B., Conner, M., De Fruyt, F., De Houwer, J., Denissen, J. J., Fiedler, K., Fiedler, S., Funder, D. C., Kliegl, R., Nosek, B. A., Perugini, M., Roberts, B. W., Schmitt, M., Vanaken, M. A. G., Weber H., and Wicherts, J. M. (2013). Recommendations for increasing replicability in psychology. *European Journal of Personality*, *27*, 108–119.

Backhouse, S. H., Whitaker, L., and Petróczi, A. (2013). Gateway to doping? Supplement use in the context of preferred competitive situations, doping attitude, beliefs, and norms. *Scandinavian Journal of Medicine and Science in Sports*, *23*, 244–252.

Bamberger, M. and Yaeger, D. (1997). Over the edge. *Sports Illustrated*, April 14, 1997.

Bernard, H. R., Hallett, T., Iovita, A., Johnsen, E. C., Lyerla, R., McCarthy, C., Mahy, M., Salganik, M. J., Saliuk, T., Scutelniciuc, O., Shelley, G. A., Sirinirund, P., Weir, S., and Stroup, D. F. (2010). Counting hard-to-count populations: the network scale-up method for public health. *Sexually Transmitted Infections*, *86*, ii11–ii15.

Bloodworth, A. J., Petróczi, A., Bailey, R., Pearce, G., and McNamee, M. J. (2012). Doping and supplementation: the attitudes of talented young athletes. *Scandinavian Journal of Medicine and Science in Sports*, *22*, 293–301.

Brand, R., Heck, P., and Ziegler, M. (2014a). Illegal performance enhancing drugs and doping in sport: a picture-based brief implicit association test for measuring athletes' attitudes. *Substance Abuse Treatment, Prevention, and Policy*, *9*, 7.

Brand, R., Melzer, M., and Hagemann, N. (2011). Towards an implicit association test (IAT) for measuring doping attitudes in sports. Data-based recommendations developed from two recently published tests. *Psychology of Sport and Exercise*, *12*, 250–256.

Brand, R., Wolff, W., and Thieme, D. (2014b). Using response-time latencies to measure athletes' doping attitudes. The brief implicit attitude test identifies substance abuse in bodybuilders. *Substance Abuse Treatment Prevention and Policy*, *9*, 36.

Connor, J., Woolf, J., and Mazanov, J. (2013). Would they dope? Revisiting the Goldman dilemma. *British Journal of Sports Medicine*, *47*, 697–700.

Ćorluka, M., Gabrilo, G., and Blažević, M. (2011). Doping factors, knowledge and attitudes among Bosnian and Herzegovinian football players [Dejavnikidopinga, znanje in odnos do dopinga med nogometaši Bosne in Hercegovine]. *KinesiologiaSlovenica*, *17*, 49–59.

De Houwer, J. (2001). A structural and process analysis of the Implicit Association Test. *Journal of Experimental Social Psychology*, *37*, 443–451.

De Houwer, J. (2003). The Extrinsic Affective Simon Task. *Experimental Psychology*, *50*, 77–85.

Dodge, T., Williams, K. J., Marzell, M., and Turrisi, R. (2012). Judging cheaters: is substance misuse viewed similarly in the athletic and academic domains? *Psychology of Addictive Behaviors*, *26*, 678–682.

Dunn, M., Thomas, J. O., Swift, W., and Burns, L. (2012). Elite athletes' estimates of the prevalence of illicit drug use: evidence for the false consensus effect. *Drug and Alcohol Review*, *31*, 27–32.

Finch, J. (1987). The vignette technique in survey research. *Sociology*, *21* (*1*), 105–114.

Goethals, G. R., Messick, D. M., and Allison, S. T. (1991). The uniqueness bias: studies of constructive social comparison. In J. Suls and T. A. Wills (eds.), *Social comparison: Contemporary theory and research* (149–176). Hillsdale, NJ and UK: Lawrence Erlbaum Associates.

Greenwald, A. G., McGhee, D. E., and Schwartz, J. L. (1998). Measuring individual differences in implicit cognition: the implicit association test. *Journal of Personality and Social Psychology*, *74*, 1464–1480.

Gregg, A. P. (2007). When voting reveals lying: the Timed Antagonistic Response Alethiometer. *Applied Cognitive Psychology, 21,* 631–647.

Huybers, T. and Mazanov, J. (2012). What would Kim do: a choice study of projected athlete doping considerations. *Journal of Sport Management, 26,* 322–334.

Jalleh, G. and Donovan, R. (2008). *Survey of Australian elite athletes' attitudes towards and beliefs about sport issues: May 2008 Survey.* Social Marketing Research Unit, School of Marketing, Curtin University, Perth, Australia.

James, R., Naughton, D. P., and Petróczi, A. (2010). Promoting functional foods as acceptable alternatives to doping: potential for information-based social marketing approach. *Journal of International Society for Sports Nutrition, 7,* 37.

James, R. A., Nepusz, T., Naughton, D. P., and Petróczi, A. (2013). A potential inflating effect in estimation models: Cautionary evidence from comparing performance enhancing drug and herbal hormonal supplement use estimates. *Psychology of Sport and Exercise, 14,* 84–96.

Jones, P. E. (2004). False consensus in social context: Differential projection and perceived social distance. *British Journal of Social Psychology, 43,* 417–429.

Kahneman, D. (2003). A perspective on judgment and choice: mapping bounded rationality. *American Psychologist, 58,* 697–720.

Lapinski, M. K. and Rimal, R. N. (2005). An explication of social norms. *Communication Theory, 15,* 127–147.

Lotz, S. and Hagemann, N. (2007). Using the Implicit Association Test to measure athletes' attitude toward doping. *Journal of Sport and Exercise Psychology, 29,* S183.

Mirkin, G. and Hoffman, M. (1978). *The Sportsmedicine Book.* Boston: Little, Brown & Co.

Morente-Sánchez, J., Femia-Marzo, P., and Zabala, M. (2014). Cross-cultural adaptation and validation of the Spanish version of the Performance Enhancement Attitude Scale (Petróczi, 2002). *Journal of Sports Science and Medicine, 13,* 430–438.

Morente-Sánchez, J., Leruite, M., Mateo-March, M., and Zabala, M. (2013). Attitudes towards doping in Spanish competitive female cyclists vs. triathletes. *Journal of Science and Cycling, 2,* 40–48.

Moston, S., Engelberg, E. T., and Skinner, J. (2014a). Perceived incidence of drug use in Australian sport: a survey of athletes and coaches. *Sport in Society.* doi: 10.1080/17430 437.2014.927867.

Moston, S., Engelberg, T., and Skinner, J. (2014b). Self-fulfilling prophecy and the future of doping. *Psychology of Sport and Exercise.* doi:10.1016/j.psychsport.2014.02.004.

Nosek, B. A., Hawkins, C. B., and Frazier, R. S. (2011). Implicit social cognition: from measures to mechanisms. *Trends in Cognitive Science, 15,* 152–159.

Olson, M. A. and Fazio, R. H. (2004). Reducing the influence of extra-personal associations on the implicit association test: Personalizing the IAT. *Journal of Personality and Social Psychology, 86,* 653–667.

Payne, B. K. and Gawronski, G. B. (2010). A history of implicit social cognition: where is it coming from? Where is it going? In B. Gawronski and K. Payne (eds.), *Handbook of implicit social cognition: measurement, theory, and applications* (1–8). New York: Guilford Press.

Pearson, B. and Hansen, B. (1992). Survey of U.S. Olympians. *USA Today,* February 5, 10C.

Petróczi, A. (2013a). The doping mindset – Part I: Implications of the functional use theory on mental representations of doping. *Performance Enhancement and Health, 2,* 153–163.

Petróczi, A. (2013b). The doping mindset – Part II: Potentials and pitfalls in capturing athletes' doping attitudes with response-time methodology, *Performance Enhancement and Health*, 2, 164–181.

Petróczi, A. (2013c). Getting inside the athletes' minds: potentials and pitfalls of self-reports and timed response measures in doping research. Keynote paper presented at the 5th International INHDR Conference, August 15–16, Aarhus, Denmark, 67.

Petróczi, A., Aidman, E. V., and Nepusz, T. (2008a). Capturing doping attitudes by self-report declarations and implicit assessment: a methodology study. *Substance Abuse, Treatment, Prevention and Policy*, 3, 9.

Petróczi, A., Mazanov, J., Nepusz, T., Backhouse, S., and Naughton, D. P. (2008b). Comfort in big numbers: False consensus in hypothetical performance enhancing situations. *Journal of Occupational Medicine and Toxicology*, 3, 19.

Petróczi, A., Uvacsek, M., Nepusz, T., Deshmukh, N., Shah, I., Aidman, E. V., Barker, J., Tóth, M., and Naughton, D. P. (2011). Incongruence in doping related attitudes, beliefs and opinions in the context of discordant behavioural data: in which measure do we trust? *PLoS One*, 6, 4.

Petróczi, A., Backhouse, S. H., Barkoukis, V., Brand, R., Elbe, A. M., Lazuras, L., and Lucidi, F. (2015). A call for policy guidance on psychometric testing in doping control in sport. *International Journal of Drug Policy*, doi:10.1016/j.drugpo.2015.04.022.

Robbins, J. M. and Krueger, J. I. (2005). Social Projection to ingroups and outgroups: a review and meta-analysis. *Personality and Social Psychology Review*, 9, 32–47.

Rinck, M. and Becker, E. S. (2007). Approach and avoidance in fear of spiders. *Journal of Behavior Therapy and Experimental Psychiatry*, 38, 105–120.

Ross, L., Greene, D., and House, P. (1977). The "false consensus effect": an egocentric bias in social perception and attribution processes. *Journal of Experimental Social Psychology*, 13, 279–301.

Salganik, M. J., Mello, M. B., Abdo, A. H., Bertoni, N., Fazito, D., and Bastos, F. I. (2011). The game of contacts: estimating the social visibility of groups. *Social Networks*, 33, 70–78.

Schirlin, O., Rey, G., Jouvent, R., Dubal, S., Komano, O., Perez-Diaz, F., and Soussignan, R. (2009). Attentional bias for doping words and its relation with physical self-esteem in young adolescents. *Psychology of Sport and Exercise*, 10, 615–620.

Schwerin, M. J. and Corcoran, K. J. (1996). Beliefs about steroids: user vs. non-user comparisons. *Drug and Alcohol Dependence*, 40, 221–225.

Sports Illustrated (2010). Ninth Annual PGA Tour Players Survey. May 3, 2010.

Uvacsek, M., Nepusz, T., Naughton, D. P., Mazanov, J., Ránky, M. Z., and Petróczi, A. (2011). Self-admitted behavior and perceived use of performance-enhancing vs psychoactive drugs among competitive athletes. *Scandinavian Journal of Medicine and Science in Sports*, 21, 224–234.

Vargo, E. J., Petróczi, A., Shah, I., and Naughton, D. P. (2014). It is not just memory: propositional thinking influences performance on the autobiographical Implicit Association Test. *Drug and Alcohol Dependency*. doi: 10.1016/j.drugalcdep. 2014.10.008.

Waddington, I., Malcolm, D., Roderick, M., and Naik, R. (2005). Drug use in English professional football. *British Journal of Sport Medicine*, 39, e18.

Whitaker, L., Long, J., Petróczi, A., and Backhouse, S. H. (2013). Using the prototype willingness model to predict doping in sport. *Scandinavian Journal of Medicine and Science in Sports*. doi: 10.1111/sms.12148.

8 Minimizing response bias

An application of the randomized response technique

Werner Pitsch

Until 2002, it was common knowledge in the scientific community as well as in the field of anti-doping that sport scientists had no means to reliably estimate the proportion of dopers among elite athletes. This was still questioned in 2010 by Lentillon-Kaestner and Ohl (2010). This conviction also implied a severe limitation to the believed possibility of testing theories on doping empirically as well as the estimation that the efficiency of anti-doping measures cannot be measured. In the recent past, the application of Randomized Response Techniques in doping research has allowed a more robust measurement of doping behaviors. This chapter will discuss the application of a Randomized Response method in the field of doping use and indicate how this method can generate reliable responses while maintaining confidentiality. As this chapter can only provide an outline of the development of this class of techniques, they will be described without reference to the mathematical background. Readers who are interested in applying these techniques by themselves should use the original literature, cited below or refer to literature reviews (e.g., see Lensvelt-Mulders *et al.* 2005; Lee 1993; Coutts and Jann 2011; Antonak and Livneh 1995) to become familiar with the mathematics behind these techniques.

The idea which drove the development of indirect questioning techniques is the well-known fact that individuals demonstrate a significant bias toward socially desirable answers as soon as sensitive questions are asked (see e.g., Lee 1993; Holbrook and Krosnik 2010, 2012). Approaches to deal with this bias include non-reactive or unobtrusive research (see Lee 2000), social desirability scales (e.g., Stöber 2001; Thompson and Phua 2005) and techniques which are designed to increase the respondents' confidence in the fact that they can safely confess socially unwanted behavior (e.g., Unmatched Count Technique or Item Count Technique, see Ahart and Sackett 2004; Coutts and Jann 2011; Tourangeau and Yan 2007; Randomized Count Technique, see Frenger *et al.* 2013; or Single Sample Count Technique, see James *et al.* 2013). Among the last techniques, the Randomized Response Technique was developed first and remains the most widely used, the most evaluated, and the most elaborated technique in the research on sensitive topics.

Theoretical background and development of Randomized Response Techniques

In the first Randomized Response Model, introduced by Warner in 1965, two different questions were used to ask if an interviewee belonged to a group X:

1   Are you a member of group X?
2   Are you not a member of group X?

Based on the result of a randomization device, the respondents were forced with a probability $p \neq 0.5$ to answer question 1 or question 2. As the result of the randomization remained unknown to the researcher, an answer "yes" could not be used to infer that the person under study had the embarrassing property X, but the difference in the rate of "yes" answers was used to estimate the prevalence of X in the population under study. Warner showed that his estimator Π_X was an unbiased, normally distributed estimator of the true proportion of X in the population. This model as well as the most important models, which were developed based on Warner's first RRT, are depicted in Figure 8.1. After Warner had introduced this technique, several refinements and new developments occurred. The developments which later also became effective in doping research in sport were:

• the unrelated question model;
• the forced answer model and;
• the cheater detection model.

These techniques will be briefly described in the following section.

The unrelated question model

The fact that all respondents in Warner's model had to answer the embarrassing question led to the suspicion that respondents might be more willing to answer truthfully if there were two different questions, one referring to the embarrassing property and one totally unrelated to it (Horvitz *et al.* 1967). Thus, in addition to the randomizing effect, neither a "yes" nor a "no" could unambiguously be related to the fact if the respondent had the sensitive property X or if he/she didn't have it. The theoretical framework for this model was developed by Greenberg *et al.* (1969).

When applying this model, a respondent is asked to use a randomization device (e.g., a coin or a dice) without reporting the outcome of the randomization to the researcher. Dependent on the outcome the respondent is asked to answer with a probability p the first or with the probability $(1-p)$ the second of the following questions:

Instruction: Please roll a dice.

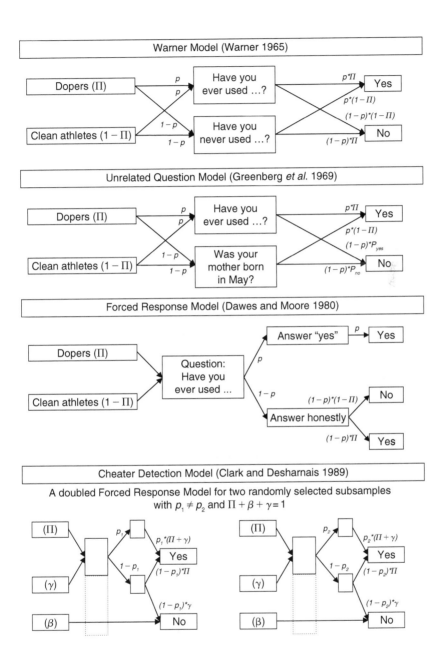

Figure 8.1 Comparison of different RRT models.

If the result is a 1, 2, 3, or a 4, please answer question 1; if the result is a 5 or a 6, please answer question 2.

1   Are you a member of group X?
2   Are you a member of group Y?

With X being the embarrassing property while Y is an unrelated, insensitive property (e.g., "Have you ever visited New York?", "Were you born in North Carolina?"). Greenberg *et al.* (1969) showed that the unrelated question technique can perform better than Warner's original model as long as the (unknown) prevalence of X, π_X is far smaller than 0.5, if several restrictions for *p* are met and if an unrelated property Y is chosen in such a way that π_X and π_Y are both either >0.5 or <0.5. They simulated the relative efficiency for the unrelated question model even for cases when the presence of the embarrassing property X is not totally truthfully reported.

   In later applications, unrelated question models were developed for known properties of the insensitive property Y (e.g., "Were you born in April?" Scheers 1992) as well as for properties with unknown prevalence (e.g., "Have you ever been to New York?" Tracy and Fox 1981).

The forced response model

The forced response model was first mentioned, although not formally developed, by Greenberg *et al.* (1969). Fidler und Kleinknecht (1977) report its first application. As a deviation from the unrelated question model, they instructed their respondents to answer "yes," "no," or to answer honestly, depending on the outcome of a randomization device. Without referring to these sources, Dawes and Moore (1980) suggested an "asymmetric" model. In this model, the randomization device is used to decide if the respondent is asked to answer the embarrassing question honestly or if he/she is forced to answer "yes," irrespective of if he/she has the property X or not (in cases where the absence of the property X would be the embarrassing answer, the forced response would be "no").

   An application of this model would be:

Instruction: Please roll a dice.
If the result is a 1 or a 2, please answer "yes" to the following question.
If the result is a 3, 4, 5, or a 6, please answer honestly.
Question: "Are you a member of group X?"

With this model, an answer "yes" also cannot be unambiguously linked to the presence of the embarrassing property X thus providing complete anonymity to the respondents having this attribute. Nevertheless, although the embarrassing property X is perfectly protected by this method, its perceived security is not as high as the security of "symmetric" forced response models (see Bourke 1984).

The cheater detection model

The fact that even in randomized response surveys, there is still a certain amount of jeopardizing interviewees was already discussed by Greenberg *et al.* (1977). Besides the many ideas to develop RRT models which led to an increased confidence of the respondents, Clark and Desharnais (1998) developed the first cheater detection model. In order to achieve this, the sample is split randomly into two subsamples. Each subsample gets a forced response-RRT-question with differing probabilities of the forced response. By using this technique, the increased number of degrees on freedom allows not only to calculate for the share of two groups in the population (π_X and $1 - \pi_X$) but to calculate for the share of the three groups:

- π_X – the rate of "honest yes" responders, indicating the lowest possible prevalence of the embarrassing property X;
- β – the rate of "honest no" responders, indicating the least possible rate of members of the population without the property X; and
- γ – indicating the share of "cheaters" who do not answer according to the RRT instructions.

In this context, it is important that "cheating" occurs if respondents having the property X answer "no" in cases when they are to answer "yes" either honestly or as a forced answer. Additionally, cheating can occur if respondents who do not have the property answer "no" although the randomization process has led to a result which would force them to answer "yes." Reluctance to obey the RRT instructions may be a result of misunderstanding the instructions, of misinterpreting the result of the randomization or of mistrust in the anonymity of the answer. Whatever the reasons may be, the method reveals no information about the "cheaters." In the first publication of the method, Clark and Desharnais (1998) therefore provided a χ^2-test of the hypothesis $\gamma > 0$ and suggested to abstain from using the results if this test would render a significant proportion of cheaters. In later applications, this practice was replaced by reporting the estimated rate of honest "yes" responses and the sum of this rate plus the rate of cheaters as lower respectively upper level of an interval, containing the true score of the prevalence of X in the population (e.g., Musch *et al.* 2001; Pitsch and Emrich 2012).

Use and application of RRT models in surveys

In order to use an RRT in a survey, there are several methodological decisions to take. They include:

1   the estimation if an RRT will outperform a direct question in terms of accuracy;
2   which RRT model to use;

3   the parameters controlling for the special RRT model that is used;
4   the randomization device; and
5   the sample size.

It is important to note that RRT methods are not generally superior to direct questioning. Typically, the RRT can lead to more reliable results due to the increased confidence of respondents but this comes at the costs of an increased variance and a need for larger samples. By and large, if the property under study is highly embarrassing, which is typically combined with a low prevalence, (according to Greenberg *et al.* 1969 between 5 percent and 25 percent), RRT questions are typically more efficient than direct questions. This is highly independent from the special RRT model which is to be used. Accordingly, the question which model should be used was mostly driven by methodological considerations and less by content-related decisions.

When selecting a special RRT model, several methodological and statistical issues have to be accounted for:

- Until now, there are no clear hints concerning the question of whether the unrelated question or the forced answer model is superior in terms of the trust of the respondents in the method. Methodologically, the forced answer model equals the unrelated question model with known prevalence of the innocuous property. These two models were also estimated to provide the best results in comparison to other RRTs (Lensvelt-Mulders *et al.* 2005).

- When deciding for or against cheater detection, it is important to keep in mind that the RRT does not guarantee honest answering. It is highly plausible that cheating due to social desirability also occurs in RRT surveys (e.g., Tracy and Fox 1981; van der Heijden *et al.* 2000). This is a strong argument in favor of cheater detection techniques but they are not by principle advantageous compared to the standard model. The most important issue is that they do not provide an estimate of the prevalence X, implying also the prevalence of the absence of X. In the plausible case of cheating, they partition the population into a share having property X, a share not having property X, and a third share with unknown status. Especially depending on the extent of this third group, the results may be totally useless in single cases.

- Generally, conducting an RRT study comes at the cost of increased sample sizes which are needed. This is even more severe for cheater detection models. Numerical simulations have shown that for the standard models, a response set of approximately 200 records lead to stable estimates, while simple cheater detection models are applicable starting with sample sizes of ~300–400, and for more sophisticated cheater detection models samples containing more than 1,500 records are needed. Therefore, the decision to use cheater detection models also largely depends on these practical limitations.

After a certain RRT model is selected, the parameters which control for the model in the field application have to be chosen. Typically, this refers to the probability to answer the innocuous question in unrelated question models or the forced yes and forced no probabilities in forced response settings. In general, this decision should balance out methodological issues and the need to provide the respondents a security guarantee. An example based on the unrelated question model (Greenberg *et al.* 1969) shall be used to describe this problem: the statistical power of the estimation increases with an increasing difference between the "yes" response to the non-sensitive question from 0.5. Logically, this would lead to selecting an innocuous property with a prevalence score either close to zero or close to 1, depending on the question if the answer "yes" or the answer "no" is embarrassing. This would nevertheless foil the logic of the RRT as the respondents would no longer perceive protected anonymity when confessing to having the embarrassing property. Therefore, probabilities must be chosen that give the respondents a strong feeling of protection while also satisfying the methodological demand.

The number of randomization devices which have been used in the past is immense (see e.g., Antonak and Livneh 1995). In RRT surveys which were conducted in face-to-face interviews, often dice, coins, card decks with colored cards, or boxes with marbles were used. In self-administered RRT surveys, the selection of a randomization device is even more difficult. With mailed questionnaires (e.g., Stem and Steinhorst 1984), spinners were used to ensure that the respondents had the randomization device at their convenience. Other randomizations used the respondent's birthday (Pitsch *et al.* 2007) or the birthday of a person known to the respondent (e.g., Dietz *et al.* 2013a, 2013b) in postal or web-based surveys.

When selecting a randomization device for a survey, it is important to regard the form of the interview (face-to-face, self-administered postal survey, web-based survey) as well as to ensure that the respondents trust the property of a random outcome. The study by Breuer and Hallmann (2013) as well as the RRT study by James *et al.* (2013) in elite sport and by Dietz *et al.* (2013b) in mass sport (see below) provide examples of the problems which can be caused by an inappropriate decision on the randomization.

Findings from empirical social research on the prevalence of doping in sport

The first researchers using an RRT on doping in sport were Plessner and Musch (2002). In an RRT survey with cheater detection on 467 competitive athletes, they reported a lifetime prevalence of at least 42 percent and at maximum 84 percent. Unfortunately, this study was only published as an abstract to a conference. Therefore, it remains unclear for which disciplines and for which level of athletic performance these figures hold. Nevertheless, this study inspired a series of RRT surveys on doping in sport.

Although this research is still in its beginnings, there are already some complementary studies from different working groups who used RRT methods or other indirect questioning. Nevertheless, it will still take many highly sophisticated studies to accumulate an appropriate level of scientific evidence covering individual and collective determinants of doping behavior.

RRT surveys on doping in elite sport

Striegel *et al.* (2010) measured the doping prevalence by using an unrelated question RRT design without cheater detection among members or junior members of national teams from Olympic disciplines from Germany. "The median age was 16 years ... 67.7% practiced individual sports. Altogether, athletes from 43 different sports were questioned, although track and field (19.2%), soccer (9.4%), handball (11.0%), and cycling (8.8%) were the most prevalent sports" (2010: 230). The distribution by gender and by discipline was not compared to the respective distribution in the population. The lifetime doping prevalence was estimated at 6.8 percent with a 95 percent confidence interval ranging from 2.7 up to 10.9. By also using a direct question in a second subsample, they were able to show that the RRT outperforms the classical questioning methods. The difference between 0.2 percent doping users when asked directly and 6.8 percent when asked with an RRT demonstrate the suitability of the RRT also for surveys on doping.

In two independent studies, Pitsch *et al.* (2007) as well as Pitsch and Emrich (2012) measured the prevalence of doping in elite sport. In their first study, they recruited a sample of 448 German squad athletes from 49 different sports in an e-mail pyramid system. They used an asymmetric forced answer method with no-cheater-detection according to Clark and Desharnais (1998). The e-mail pyramid system started from the athletes' speakers in German sports associations as seed persons. Due to the uncontrolled sampling process, the return differed heavily in the distribution by discipline and by gender from the population of German squad athletes. Cyclists and weightlifters were especially overrepresented in the sample, while track and field athletes were underrepresented. The distribution by squad status differed only marginally between the sample and the population.

They estimated that an overall doping prevalence in the 2005 season was at a minimum of 20.4 percent (rate of "honest yes" responders) and at maximum of 38.1 percent (rate of "honest yes" responders plus cheaters). The lifetime prevalence was estimated at a minimum of 25.8 percent and a maximum of 48.1 percent. Detailed results were also presented by the level of athletic success and for discipline groups (see Table 8.1).

This study was replicated with a different instrument (pencil-and-paper survey instead of online questionnaire) and with a better sampling control by individually addressing a 50 percent random sample of German squad athletes in 2008 (Pitsch and Emrich 2012). The return summed up to 863 records from athletes from 61 different disciplines. It didn't differ distinctly from the population of German squad athletes by gender or by discipline.

For the 2008 season, they measured a doping prevalence of at least 9.6 percent and a maximum of 36 percent. The lifetime prevalence was estimated at

Table 8.1 RRT studies on doping in sport: overall results and identified significant determinants

Study	Sample	Method	Doping prevalence	Significant influence of...
Elite sport				
Pitsch et al. (2007)	448 national squad athletes from 49 different sports	RRT with cheater detection (forced answer)	25.8%–48.1% (lifetime) 20.4%–38.1% (current season)	discipline level of competition
Striegel et al. (2010)	480 members or junior members of national teams in 43 different sports	RRT (unrelated question)	6.8% (lifetime)	
Pitsch and Emrich (2012)	863 national squad athletes from 61 different sports	RRT with cheater detection (forced answer)	10.2%–34.9% (lifetime) 9.6%–360% (current season)	1 discipline 2 level of competition 3 of gender
Breuer and Hallmann (2013)	1,154 elite athletes from all Olympic disciplines	RRT with cheater detection (forced answer)	Maximum: 46.6% "regularly consuming"	
Mass sport/recreational sport				
Dietz et al. (2013b)	2,997 recreational triathletes	RRT (unrelated question)	14.1% (lifetime)	1 training plan 2 recovery habits 3 amount training
Pitsch et al. (2013)	7,252 university students from Belgium, Denmark, Germany, and Switzerland	RRT with cheater detection (forced answer)	5.2%–14.0% (broad doping term, lifetime) 4.8%–29.2% (narrow doping term, lifetime)	1 gender (broad term) 2 faculty (narrow term) 3 level of exertion for success (narrow term) 4 University (both terms)

a minimum value of 10.2 percent and a maximum of 34.9 percent. For single discipline groups and dependent on the level of athletic success, they also found values which differed from this overall estimation, but which widely confirmed the results of the first study (see Table 8.1). Without a predefined hypothesis, they also discovered a significant and large difference between male and female athletes. The lifetime prevalence of female athletes (minimum 2.9 percent, maximum 21.3 percent) ranged far below the respective values for male athletes (minimum 17.1 percent, maximum 47.4 percent). The same pattern also holds for the last year's prevalence.

Breuer and Hallmann (2013) published a research report on dysfunctions of elite sport. Among other negative effects like depression and match fixing, they also asked for doping as a regular habit. They used the cheater detection method in a web-based survey on 1,154 elite athletes from all Olympic disciplines. Unfortunately, they used an inappropriate setting for the RRT questions. The randomization was done based on the respondents' birthday, but the same randomization instruction was used for a series of nine questions. With this setting, some respondents were forced to answer "yes" to all questions. On the contrary, any respondent answering "no" at least once could be clearly identified as belonging to the group of honest answering respondents. With this setting, the sense of the RRT as providing perfect security was not given any more. This resulted in large "cheater" proportions (falsely mentioned as "no answer") and low prevalence estimates. Besides these methodological flaws, the results can still partly be interpreted because of the forced response method which was used. Due to this method, a "no" answer is an unambiguous indicator that the embarrassing property was not present. The rate of 53.4 percent "honest no" responders confirms the result of the studies presented above, which indicated that the majority of elite athletes do not resort to doping.

RRT surveys on doping in mass sport

A basic problem when studying "doping" in mass sport is that participants of these studies often are not familiar with the definition of "doping" in the WADA Code. Therefore, in the instruments which are used the term "doping" must be paraphrased. As a result, the concepts under study may differ from the concept of "doping" as it is defined in elite sport. Nevertheless, the following studies focus on concepts which largely overlap with the "doping" issue.

Dietz et al. (2013b) conducted an unrelated question RRT survey in order to analyze associations between substance use for physical and for cognitive enhancement among 2,997 "recreational triathletes" (2013b: 1). The respondents had participated in three different triathlon events in Germany. The study focused on the usage of "substances which can only be prescribed by a doctor, are available in a pharmacy, or can be bought on the black market (e.g., anabolic steroids, erythropoietin, stimulants, growth hormones)" (Dietz et al. 2013b: 2, Table 2). This concept largely overlaps with the concept of "doping" in elite sport at least as far as the readiness of athletes to use pharmaceuticals in order to enhance their physical performance is addressed. The last year's prevalence was estimated at 14.1 percent for this kind of physical enhancement.

Due to the fact that a large number of other variables such as gender, training habits, and educational qualification were asked in this survey, the authors were also able to calculate for the influence of these variables on "physical doping" (see Table 8.1). Unfortunately, in this concern the study was widely elaborative and the authors did not refer to the available literature on doping decision determinants (e.g., Mazanov 2006; Mazanov *et al.* 2008) when conducting the significance tests. Furthermore, the chosen randomization device was selected in a way which left room for cheating. This might have inflated the prevalence estimation, as demonstrated by James *et al.* (2013). Therefore, the results of this study should be used with caution but, due to its unique sample, also hint at important empirical insights into doping behavior.

In another study, conducted among university students at four European universities (Aarhus, (Denmark), Liège (Belgium), Geneva (Switzerland) and Saarbrucken (Germany), a group of researchers measured the prevalence of willingly illicit substance or methods use to increase sporting performance (Pitsch *et al.* 2013). They used a symmetric forced answer model in the special modification, suggested by Richard Morton (mentioned without citation and reference by Horvitz *et al.* 1975). The randomization was done using a random number generator or, if convenient to the respondents, using the serial number on a euro banknote (for Belgium and Germany) or the number on a license plate (Denmark).

For a sample of 7,252 university students, they estimated the overall lifetime prevalence of doping in a broad sense ("Have you ever used performance-enhancing substances, banned or non-banned, with full intent in order to enhance your sporting performance?") between at least 5.2 percent and at maximum 14.0 percent. For a narrow doping term ("Have you ever used banned substances according to the rules in your sport in order to enhance your sporting performance?") the respective values were 4.8 percent and 29.2 percent. The results of the detailed analyses for different determinants of doping (see Table 8.1) revealed structural differences between doping in elite sport and in mass sport.

Converging evidence from other studies

For elite sport studies showed that the prevalence of doping use estimated with RRT approaches is far above the values which were reported based on the results of official statistics (~2 percent, see e.g., van Eenoo and Delbeke 2003) or based on direct questioning methods (mostly between ~2 percent and ~5 percent, e.g., Lentillon-Kaestner and Ohl 2010, but also up to approx. 10 percent, see Lazuras *et al.* 2010). These differences suggest that the RRT outperforms the direct questioning method in terms of the reliability of the results.

Until now, there has only been one study which used a different indirect questioning method, although it is not perfectly clear if the level of athletic performance is comparable to elite sport. James *et al.* (2013) used the newly developed SSC model, which is a simplified version of the unmatched count technique.

They recruited 513 club-level athletes via personal contacts "from various sports clubs across the UK and southern Ireland." The sample "consisted of track and field events (57.8% ...), followed by football (10.5%), rugby (10.4%), rowing (8.2%), boxing (5.7%), cycling (4.1%) and cricket (3.3%)" (James *et al.* 2013). The doping prevalence was reported to be 19.88 percent, which broadly confirms the prevalence rates reported in the RRT studies.

For mass sport, the differences between RRT surveys and other studies is harder to compare. The most important reason for this difficulty is that many studies have been conducted on special drugs (e.g., anabolic androgenic steroids, Yesalis *et al.* 1988; Kartakoullis *et al.* 2008) or for certain disciplines (e.g., Röggla *et al.* 1993; Perry *et al.* 2005) or age groups (Johnson *et al.* 2007). Nevertheless, the prevalence reported for recreational triathletes by Dietz *et al.* (2013b) of 14.1 percent, as well as the interval of 4.8–29.2 percent for the narrow doping term among university students, reported by Pitsch *et al.* (2013), converge with the values that were reported in some studies (e.g., Kartakoullis *et al.* 2008; Pedersen 2005). Regardless of this convergence, there are more RRT studies on doping needed without limitations on discipline and/or age group or substance to estimate if the RRT will contribute to our knowledge in this distinct population segment (elite sport).

Conclusion

The RRT is a highly sophisticated instrument which is not easy to set up for a survey and it comes at the cost of large sample sizes and limited possibilities for statistical analyses. Moreover, many details which have to be decided upon when planning an RRT survey bear the risk of leading to distorted estimations of the parameters under study. On the other hand, the RRT, like other indirect measurement techniques, provide a possibility to reliably estimate the prevalence of doping in elite sport – at least more reliably than by asking athletes directly. A reliable measurement of the doping prevalence is a necessary precondition for empirical social research in this field, addressing not only theoretical questions but also the efficacy and possible unintended side effects of anti-doping. Therefore, further RRT studies dealing with special groups (e.g., disciplines, national athlete populations, different levels of athletic success) will be necessary to develop and to quantitatively test a sound theoretical framework of doping behavior, which then can hopefully also be used to derive rational anti-doping strategies. Without a reliable technique to measure the prevalence of doping, doping research as well as anti-doping strategies are prone to develop explanations and interventions for conditions without reference to reality.

References

Ahart, A. M. and Sackett, P. R. (2004). A new method of examining relationships between individual difference measures and sensitive behavior criteria. Evaluating the Unmatched Count Technique. *Organizational Research Methods, 7*, 101–114.

Antonak, R. F. and Livneh, H. (1995). Randomized response technique: A review and proposed extension to disability attitude research. *Genetic, Social and General Psychology Monographs*, *121* (*1*), 97.

Bourke, P. D. (1984). Estimation of proportions using symmetric randomized response designs. *Psychological Bulletin*, *96* (*1*), 166–172.

Breuer, C. and Hallmann, K. (2013). *Dysfunktionen des Spitzensports. Doping, Match-Fixing und Gesundheitsgefährdungen aus Sicht von Bevölkerung und Athleten*. Bonn: Bundesinst. für Sportwiss.

Clark, S. J. and Desharnais, R. A. (1998). Honest answers to embarrassing questions: Detecting cheating in the Randomized Response Model. *Psychological Methods*, 3, 160–168.

Coutts, E. and Jann, B. (2011). Sensitive questions in online surveys: Experimental results for the Randomized Response Technique (RRT) and the Unmatched Count Technique (UCT). *Sociological Methods and Research*, *40* (*1*), 169–193.

Dawes, R. M. and Moore, M. (1980). Die Guttman-Skalierung orthodoxer und randomisierter Reaktionen. In F. Petermann (ed.), *Einstellungsmessung, Einstellungsforschung* (S. 117–133). Göttingen, Toronto, Zürich: Verlag für Psychologie Hogrefe.

Dietz, P., Striegel, H., Franke, A. G., Lieb, K., Simon, P., and Ulrich, R. (2013a). Randomized Response Estimates for the 12-month prevalence of cognitive-enhancing drug use in university students. *Pharmacotherapy: The Journal of Human Pharmacology and Drug Therapy*, *33* (*1*), 44–50.

Dietz, P., Ulrich, R., Dalaker, R., Striegel, H., Franke, A. G., Lieb, K., and Simon, P. (2013b). Associations between physical and cognitive doping – A cross-sectional Study in 2,997 triathletes. *PLOS One*, *8* (*11*).

Fidler, D. S. and Kleinknecht, R. E. (1977). Randomized response versus direct questioning. Two data-collection methods for sensitive information. *Psychological Bulletin*, *84* (*5*), 1045–1049.

Frenger, M., Pitsch, W., and Emrich, E. (2013). Ehrliche Antworten auf sensitive Fragen?! – Entwicklung einer Befragungsmethode und erste Anwendungsplanung. In H. Kempf, S. Nagel, and H. Dietl (eds.), *Im Schatten der Sportwirtschaft* (Sportökonomie, 15, 241–252). Schorndorf, Germany: Hofmann.

Greenberg, B. G., Abul-Ela, A.-L. A., Simmons, W. R., and Horvitz, D. G. (1969). The Unrelated Question Randomized Response Model: Theoretical framework. *Journal of the American Statistical Association*, *64*, 520–539.

Greenberg, B. G., Kuebler, R. R., Abernathy, J. R., and Horvitz, D. G. (1977). Respondent hazards in the unrelated question randomized response model. *Journal of Statistical Planning and Inference*, *1* (*1*), 53–60.

Holbrook, A. L. and Krosnik, J. A. (2010). Measuring voter turnout by using the Randomized Response Technique. Evidence calling into question the method's validity. *Public Opinion Quarterly*, *74*, 328–343.

Holbrook, A. L. and Krosnik, J. A. (2012). Social desirability bias in voter turnout reports: Tests using the Item Count Technique. *Public Opinion Quarterly 74*, 37–67.

Horvitz, D. G., Greenberg, B. G., and Abernathy, J. R. (1975). Recent developments in Randomized Response Designs. In J. N. Srivastava (ed.), *A survey of statistical design and linear models* (271–285). Amsterdam: North-Holland.

Horvitz, D. G., Shah, B. V., and Simmons, W. R. (1967). The unrelated question randomized response model. In American Statistical Association (eds.), *Proceedings of the American Statistical Association. Section on Survey Research Methods* (S. 65–72). Washington, DC: American Statistical Association.

James, R. A., Nepusz, T., Naughton, D. P., and Petróczi, A. (2013). A potential inflating effect in estimation models: Cautionary evidence from comparing performance enhancing drug and herbal hormonal supplement use estimates. *Psychology of Sport and Exercise, 14 (1)*, 84–96.

Johnson, M. D., Jay, S., Shoup, B., and Rickert, V. I. (2007). Anabolic steroid use by male adolescents. *Pediatrics, 83 (6)*, 921–924.

Kartakoullis, N. L., Phellas, C., Pouloukas, S., Petrou, M., and Loizou, C. (2008). The use of anabolic steroids and other prohibited substances by gym enthusiasts in Cyprus. *International Review for the Sociology of Sport, 43 (3)*, 271–287.

Lazuras, L., Barkoukis, V., Rodafinos, A., and Haralambos, T. (2010). Predictors of doping intentions in elite-level athletes: A social cognition approach. *Journal of Sport and Exercise Psychology, 32*, 694–710.

Lee, R. M. (1993). *Doing Research on sensitive topics*. London: Sage.

Lee, R. M. (2000). *Unobtrusive methods in social research*. Philadelphia: Open University.

Lensvelt-Mulders, G. J. L. M., Hox, J. J., van der Heijden, P. G. M., and Maas, C. J. M. (2005). Meta-analysis of randomized response research. Thirty-five years of validation. *Sociological Methods and Research, 33*, 315–348.

Lentillon-Kaestner, V. and Ohl, F. (2010). Can we measure accurately the prevalence of doping? *Scandinavian Journal of Medicine and Science in Sports*. http://dx.doi.org/10.1111/j.1600-0838.2010.01199.x.

Mazanov, J. (2006). Measuring athletes' attitudes towards drugs in sport. In *ACSPRI Social Science Methodology Conference 2006*. Sydney.

Mazanov, J., Petróczi, A., Bingham, J., and Holloway, A. (2008). Towards an empirical model of performance enhancing supplement use: A pilot study among high performance UK athletes. *Journal of Science and Medicine in Sport, 11 (2)*, 185–190.

Musch, J., Bröder, A., and Klauer, K. C. (2001). Improving survey research on the World-Wide Web using Randomized Response Technique. In U.-D. Reips and M. Bosnjak (eds.), *Dimensions of Internet Science* (179–192). Lengerich, Germany: Pabst.

Pedersen, I. K. (2005). Doping as a culture-constitutive process: Use of performance-enhancing substances in Danish sports and gyms. In A. R. Hofmann and E. Trangbaek (eds.), *International perspectives on sporting women in past and present* (381–397). Copenhagen: Institute of Exercise and Sport Sciences, University of Copenhagen.

Perry, P. J., Lund, B. C., Deninger, M. J., Kutscher, E. C., and Schneider, J. (2005). Anabolic steroid use in weightlifters and bodybuilders: An internet survey of drug utilization. *Clinical Journal of Sport Medicine, 15 (5)*, 326–330.

Pitsch, W. and Emrich, E. (2012). The frequency of doping in elite sport – Results of a replication study. *International Review for the Sociology of Sport, 47*, 559–580.

Pitsch, W., Emrich, E., and Frenger, M. (2013). Doping im Breiten- und Freizeitsport. Zur Überprüfung von Hypothesen mittels RRT-gewonnener Daten. In H. Kempf, S. Nagel, and H. Dietl (eds.), *Im Schatten der Sportwirtschaft* (Sportökonomie, 15, 253–264). Schorndorf, Germany: Hofmann.

Pitsch, W., Emrich, E., and Klein, M. (2007). Doping in elite sports in Germany: Results of a www survey. *European Journal of Sport and Society, 4 (2)*, 89–102.

Plessner, H. and Musch, J. (2002). Wie verbreitet ist Doping im Leistungssport? Eine www-Umfrage mit Hilfe der Randomized-Response-Technik. In B. Strauß, M. Tietjens, N. Hagemann, and A. Stachelhaus (eds.), *Expertise im Sport. Lehren – lernen – leisten; Bericht über die Tagung vom 9. bis 11. Mai 2002 in Münster* (78–79). Cologne: Bps-Verlag.

Röggla, G., Röggla, M., Zeiner, A., Röggla, H., Deutsch, E., Wagner, A., Hibler, A., Haber, P., and Laggner, A. N. (1993). Amphetamindoping beim Freizeitbergsteigen in mittlerer Höhenlage in den Alpen. *Schweizerische Zeitschrift für Sportmedizin und Sporttraumatologie, 41* (3), 103–105.

Scheers, N. J. (1992). Methods, plainly speaking. A review of randomized response techniques. *Measurement and Evaluation in Counselling and Development, 24*, 27–41.

Stem, D. E. and Steinhorst, K. (1984). Telephone interview and mail questionnaire applications of the Randomized Response Model. *Journal of the American Statistical Association, 79*, 555–564.

Stöber, J. (2001). The social desirability scale-17 (SD-17). *European Journal of Psychological Assessment, 17*, 222–232.

Striegel, H., Ulrich, R., and Simon, P. (2010). Randomized response estimates for doping and illicit drug use in elite athletes. *Drug and Alcohol Dependence, 106* (2–3), 230–232.

Tracy, P. E. and Fox, J. A. (1981). The validity of randomized response for sensitive measurements. *American Sociological Review, 46*, 187–200.

Thompson, E. R. and Phua, F. T. T. (2005). Reliability among senior managers of the Marlowe-Crowne short-form social desirability scale. *Journal of Business and Psychology, 19*, 541–554.

Tourangeau, R. and Yan, T. (2007). Sensitive questions in Surveys. *Psychological Bulletin, 133* (5), 859–883.

van der Heijden, P. G. M., van Gils, G., Bouts, J., and Hox, J. J. (2000). A Comparison of randomized response, computer-assisted self-interview, and face-to-face direct questioning – Eliciting sensitive information in the context of welfare and unemployment benefit. *Sociological Methods and Research, 28*, 505–537.

van Eenoo, P. and Delbeke, F. T. (2003). The Prevalence of Doping in Flanders in Comparison to the Prevalence in International Sports. *International Journal of Sports Medicine, 24* (8), 565–570.

Warner, S. L. (1965). Randomized-response. A survey technique for eliminating evasive answer bias. *Journal of the American Statistical Association, 60*, 63–69.

Yesalis, C. E., Herrick, R. T., Buckley, W. E., Friedl, K. E., Brannon, D., and Wright, J. E. (1988). Self-reported use of anabolic-androgenic steroids by elite power lifters. *The Physician and Sportsmedicine, 16* (12), 91–100.

Part III

Ethical aspects and implications in doping use and control

9 Revisiting values in sports

The case of doping

Lea Cleret

The World Anti-Doping Code, the document regulating the fight against doping on a global level, recently underwent extensive review, and the third version will enter into force in 2015 (WADA 2015). One of the most important amendments was to make anti-doping education mandatory for its stakeholders, with an emphasis on values-based education. This was based on recent evidence suggesting that moral reasoning and related values in sport may have a protective effect against doping use (Melzer *et al.* 2010). Indeed, several studies in the psychology of doping use have emphasized the role of sport values (Smith and Stewart 2010; Mazanov and Huybers Chapter 10, this volume; Mazanov *et al.* 2012). This chapter is written from a philosopher's point of view and, as such, examines the very premises of the arguments about the role of values in sport and doping prevention. By taking one step back, the present chapter looks at *concepts*, and considers questions such as *which sport* and *which values*? With these questions in mind, the chapter will discuss the nature and origin of today's sport, as well as the values that surround it, aiming to provide a basis for the moral reasoning that guides relevant research in the psychological study of doping use.

Values and sport: basic definitions and conceptualization

Conceptualization of values

Etymologically, "value" comes from the Latin *valere* and relates to concepts such as "strong," "brave," and "worthy." The concept was then extended to all traits of a person who commands admiration and respect from his entourage. Therefore, to be *valere* is to be worthy and has, therefore, positive connotations. Conversely, there are traits that should be discouraged, because these will not result in anything positive or worthwhile for humanity. The social context and cultural expectations can shape values. In its plural form, the word "values" refers to a set of emotions (e.g., joy), states of being (e.g., health), behaviors (e.g., courage, commitment) that a community embraces as socially desirable. Put simply, actions that support these values will be seen as good and socially desirable, whereas actions against the values will be perceived as bad and undesirable (McFee 2004).

Values of sport

Values of sport seems to be a widely recognized concept with a sort of universal understanding of what they might entail. The World Anti-Doping Code (WADA 2015) defined the following as the important values that constitute the Spirit of Sport: ethics, fair play and honesty, health, excellence in performance, character and education, fun and joy, teamwork, dedication and commitment, respect for rules and laws, respect for self and other participants, courage, community and solidarity. However, several scholars have criticized the Spirit of Sport and argued that the definition of values described therein can hardly serve as the basis for effective anti-doping policies (Kayser *et al.* 2007; Mazanov 2013). Occurrences of cheating, fighting, and drug-use are not uncommon in sports. A fundamental question that needs to be answered is whether these phenomena reflect the reprehensible conduct of a few "outlier" individuals, or if they are normative practices in a sports system that is shaped by different values than the ones embraced by the Spirit of Sports and the current anti-doping paradigm (Kayser and Broers 2013).

Research has shown that values serve as protective factors against violent (Knafo *et al.* 2008) and doping behaviors (Rodek *et al.* 2009), and more focused studies have addressed the role of values and moral reasoning in doping prevention (Elbe and Brand Chapter 12, this volume; Melzer *et al.* 2010). Thus, values seem to represent a core aspect of anti-doping efforts, albeit a controversial one, that need to be better understood in order to more effectively guide anti-doping policies and interventions. Should these values be unclear or imprecise, athletes and their entourage face the risk of misconduct, despite their intentions or actual efforts to avoid it. For instance, if health is an important value of sport involvement, then practices such as doping use should be prohibited and avoided, because doping jeopardizes athletes' health and is against the Spirit of Sport. In this context, the first assumption that should be explored with respect to "values of sport" is that this concept implies that sport is a unique object, and that there is only one set of values attached to it. However, "sport" is in itself hard to define, because it may be multidimensional with many (rather than a unitary) values systems attached to it.

Conceptualization of sport

McBride (1975) asserted that reaching consensus in the definition of sport is impossible, and that any effort to find a satisfactory definition will be, at best, a waste of time. He concedes that, although a common definition of sport can be drawn for scientific research purposes, the definitions are very different from those of conventional dictionaries, which are also not necessarily consistent with each other. For instance, jogging on a Sunday morning may be perceived as sport by some but not by others. Accordingly chess and bridge players are considered sportsmen and they are campaigning for the inclusion of their sports in the Olympic Games, although these athletes do not get stiff muscles, nor do they improve physical stamina from their sport practice.

In a similar vein, Pearson (1988) suggested that the problem in finding a commonly agreed definition of sport is rooted in the desire to use a term that is accurate and capable of representing all the existing forms of sport. As McBride (1975) pointed out there are indeed almost as many definitions of the word "sport" as people to whom the question is addressed. To avoid such confusion, sport can be broadly defined with respect to the most popular characteristics that are easily recognized by most people, institutions, and regulatory authorities: competition, rules, institutionalization, and physical skills. For example, the Council of Europe, on Article 2 of the revised European Sports Charter, defines sport as "any form of physical activity which, through casual or organized participation, aims to improve fitness and mental well-being, forming social relationships and getting results in competitions at all levels" (www.coe.int/t/dg4/epas/resources/texts/Rec%2892%2913rev_en.pdf). But the way sports can be practiced may run counter to the physical and mental well-being of the participants. For instance, running is a type of physical activity that improves the mental well-being and overall fitness of people who practice it. Nevertheless, being addicted to running – or to any form of physical activity or sport – can pose physical and mental health risks to runners (Aidman and Woolard 2003; Egorov and Szabo 2013).

Contemporary theorists suggest that the word "sport" can be disambiguated and better understood if it is associated with another word (McFee 2004). For instance the term "elite sports" refers to sporting activities practiced at a high level of physical and technical ability, and is distinguished from other types of sport, such as recreational sports (that may be practiced as a way to recover from a difficult week), fitness sports (to keep fit and in shape), leisure sports (often played by children, and increasingly by adults), outdoor sports (such as hiking, mountain biking, and climbing), and extreme sports (in which participants' lives are at stake, for example base jumping – parachuting from the top of a cliff or a building). In all these cases, the goal of sport participation defines the very concept and meaning of sport for those who practice it. However, goals may vary both between and within people – an individual may initially engage in sport to stay fit and in shape, and later decide to do sports for a different goal (e.g., winning a trophy). Accordingly, the same activity may represent two different types of sport: running can be both fitness and elite sport. Hence, recalling McBride's (1975) contention, sport is a concept hard to define, unless the precise details about the goals, practices, and context of sport participation are provided.

Educational vs. high performance sport

The focus of this chapter will be on two types of sport that are easily distinguishable in theory, but less so in practice. More specifically, in theory educational sport is distinct from high performance. This distinction reflects two very different human activities with different objectives and means. Still, bringing the concept of values can make these two different types of sport indistinguishable. Educational sport represents human activities where the discipline (i.e., football, tennis, basketball, baseball, etc.) is used and harnessed for educational and humanistic purposes. The purpose of activity involvement is human development. It aims for the participants to learn about themselves and the community in order to become responsible and autonomous citizens in society (Carpentier 2004). In contrast, high performance sport reflects a human activity with an explicit goal to strive for improved performance (Donnelly 1996). The means to practice the sport can, therefore, be adapted to this goal. Seeking to improve well-being and striving to improve athletic performance are two distinct aims, and the means and the consequences of the implementation of these aims are different. For instance, a high performance athlete may be at risk for using doping substances if he/she develops a mentality that the aim of sports is to enhance performance at any cost. On the other hand, an athlete involved in educational sports is less likely to use doping substances as they don't help him/her achieve his/her objectives from sport participation. However, these two types of sport can be easily confused, as there are occurrences where it would seem that these two activities are identical. So far there have been identified three main reasons that may elicit a confusion regarding the distinction between educational and high performance sport.

First, this confusion may exist in the case of multidisciplinary events where individuals and institutions of different intentionality are brought together under one banner. This was clearly apparent at the Paralympic Games in Beijing in 2008, as evidenced by the president of the French Paralympic sports federation, Gérard Masson, in an interview published on September 17, 2008:

> We could decide to do like the British [102 medals, including 42 gold, the second rank in the medals table] i.e., targeting events where we want medals, influence young people into their choice of discipline, but I don't want that. We currently have 25,000 members who can practice 42 disciplines, and I want to continue along this path.... Elite level is important but medals do not deserve everything to be sacrificed.

It is perfectly clear that, for Gérard Masson, the primary goal is the access to and use of sport by people with disabilities, as a way to become meaningfully reintegrated in the society. Other countries that fixated on winning and sought to produce medal winners used selection methods, either in disciplines or individuals, to increase their chances for goal attainment (win medals). In this respect, the sports and individuals that are unlikely to assist in goal attainment are excluded from sport participation, whereas those who are likely to lead their team to medal winning are selected. Clearly, the British and French approaches to Paralympic sports have different objectives. The French federation preferred fewer medals and were oriented toward attracting more people taking part in grassroots sports, whereas the British were oriented more toward medal winning. This is also the case with doping. For example, an athlete from an underdeveloped country who participates in the Olympic Games for the honor and the experience of participation may be less likely to use doping substances compared to another one who seeks a gold medal, money, and fame. Indeed, Johhson and Ali (2004) indicated that underdeveloped countries participate in Olympic Games, although they don't get any medals.

Second, confusion between educational and high performance sport may also be experienced when individuals compete with different goals in mind. Athletes may practice the same activity, perform the same tasks, and yet derive totally different experiences from sport participation. Fencing in France represents a good example. There is a set of competitions at national level, over a season, which is used to calculate the national ranking. All French fencers are invited to participate. Some come to have fun, be with their teammates, try to find benchmarks to improve, get opportunities to try out their skills and get feedback and compete. Of course, winning can be a goal, and some of these fencers are very competitive and have a clear objective to proceed to international competitions. This is an illustrative example of achievement goals, that is whether fencers feel successful if they win and outperform others (performance orientation), or whether they experience joy and pleasure, and improved their skills (mastery orientation). Research has shown that different types of achievement goals can have differential outcomes on moral beliefs and functioning in sports settings (e.g., Kavussanu and Ntoumanis 2003; Kavussanu and Roberts 2001). With respect to doping use, one study showed that athletes involved in sports in order to improve their abilities and master the event at hand reported lower intentions and self-reported doping use as compared to those aiming to outperform others and demonstrate ability (Barkoukis *et al.* 2011).

Lastly, in some cases high performance sport is a perfect context for some individuals to blossom. In Aristotelian theory, at the beginning of their life, all human beings possess the potential for self-actualization, and a goal in their life can be to realize this potential. Some athletes have everything it takes for them to become high performance athletes, including physical and mental abilities, psychological traits, and all the other elements which compose a high performance athlete. Imagine Roger Federer's mother deciding that he should do weightlifting or equestrian. Therefore, in some cases, there is a perfect match between being a high performing athlete and being a responsible and autonomous citizen. In the case of doping, it is very often that athletes use prohibited substances to expand their physical limits and achieve goals higher than their physical talent. Within this context, sport can serve two objectives. One is a human activity to contribute to the upbringing of responsible and ethical citizens, and the other is to produce high performance, perhaps at the expense of other attributes, such as responsibility and ethics. The role of values is important in disentangling these two objectives.

Values within the context of sport

The view of Pierre de Coubertin

To understand how values can relate to sport, it is important to keep in mind that sport is not a unitary construct (McBride 1975; McFee 2004); accordingly, the identification and definition of values of sport is rather complicated and raises several questions. Is there a set of sport-specific values or a set of values that can be applied across types of sport? Olympism, one of the most important sport movements, and the overarching philosophy of its founder, Pierre de Coubertin, may provide some answers to these overarching questions, and allow us to understand how values are formed within the sport context. The values stated in the World Anti-Doping Code are inspired by those of the Olympic Games. It may be hypothesized that these values were generated by Coubertin's conception of his "ideal man" (Coubertin 1889). Coubertin indeed had a template in mind of what Man should aim to be. After observing his contemporaries, he knew something had to be done in order to draw young people closer to what he believed was an accomplished person. Coubertin had a very clear idea of what Man should be. It stems from two premises: the fact that Man has a will, which makes him different from an animal, and the second is that everything should be aiming to reach one's potential (Coubertin 1889). The purpose of life is to become who we are potentially. According to his theories of education, Coubertin argued that each and every individual has the potential to become one of the "ideal men," and that the purpose of education is to steer individuals in the direction of becoming these "ideal men." Coubertin argued that education is more about not interfering with the natural development of the child rather than a means to make all individuals fit in the same mould (Coubertin 1889).

To achieve this goal of becoming an ideal man, one must consider how Man is structured. According to Coubertin, Man is composed of body, mind, and character. The purpose of a man's life is to exercise his will the best he can. Will vests in one's character, therefore character must be hardened. And as character is connected to the body, the body must be hardened to harden the character. A strong body is a moral body, because it is capable of directing the will and responding to its orders. And we must not forget the place of pleasure: a trained body will enjoy challenging the will, and, reversely, the will shall enjoy challenging the body (Coubertin 1889). If one wanted to draw a portrait of the ideal man of Coubertin, it would be quite similar to that of the self-made man: the harder the adversity, the more merit there is because this means that the will shall have been challenged even more to achieve social success when starting from nothing.

Pierre de Coubertin's system had the aim of developing a new generation of young men, able to put their wills to the task, young men who want to strive and succeed. All the values named as important in sport (ethics, fair play and honesty, health, excellence in performance, character and education, fun and joy, teamwork, dedication and commitment, respect for rules and laws, respect for self and other participants, courage, community and solidarity) seek to allow for this ambition to happen. Therefore, actions following these values should be encouraged, and actions which go against them should be discouraged. In the context of sport, these values reflect the values of Olympism, and everything in Olympism is organized to achieve these values.

Values in educational and high performance sport

Educational sport, as mentioned previously, aims to use activities which require physical movement as tools to help individuals become complete human beings. Performance is not an aim, even though it can be collateral, and victory is not a negated concept. The values of Olympism apply quite nicely to this type of sport, and it is not so surprising after all: the aim of educational sport is quite similar to that of Olympism. It does not aim to produce performance, but a certain type of person who can actively contribute to society. High performance sport, as mentioned previously, aims to produce performance. What helps with achieving performance is valued and what undermines this quest is rejected. Most of the values mentioned previously, such as health, excellence in performance, teamwork, dedication and commitment, courage, will help with performance, but these values are not valued for themselves. The point of high performance is to produce performance, not to uphold these values. Having said that, doping use is not consistent with high performance sports as, although it may help achieve its main objective, it may enhance performance by violating the values of sport (e.g., health).

Still, several athletes perceive doping use as an inevitable means to achieve in performance sports (Petróczi and Aidman 2008). So, what if the current high performance sport system was organized in such a way that these values actually became a hindrance to high performance? Health is an example. Coubertin argued that exercise was a way to get young men healthy, and there was a direct correlation between health and performance. One had to be healthy to be able to run a race. The point of organizing races was therefore to make sure that the population was able to run them, therefore be healthy and fit. In this sense, doping use clearly deviates from this focal value of sports.

Today high performance sport can have a devastating effect on the human body. It can be physiological, through over-training or the female triad. It can be mechanical, with shoulder injuries typically for swimmers, knee and back injuries for skiers, joint problems for runners. It can also be traumatic, through concussions and accidents. There can also be negative health consequences from doping, assuming that high performance sport is a risk factor for doping. In addition, an important risk factor for these health issues is the gruelling sport calendar, which never ceases to expand, or the unreasonable demands for some endurance events. Thus, although health is one of the values of sport according to the World Anti-Doping Code and the IOC, high performance sport in effect would not promote this value as the choices made do not take into consideration the health of the athletes. By making unreasonable demands on the human body, the sport system is creating a big risk factor for doping. Evidence suggests that many athletes use medication and nutritional supplements to protect or cure themselves from the negative health consequences of high performance sport (Tscholl et al. 2008). In fact, Tscholl et al. raised questions about whether the medication reported in this study was used solely for therapeutic reasons. Therefore, a possible solution to protect athletes' health could be to alter the calendar or the distances of some events. A change in the requirements of these events might result in lowering the pressure on athletes.

Should doping use be legalized?

The controversy in the meaning of sport and the role of values in a sport system led to a debate about the legalisation of doping. If we are going to make unrealistic demands on the athletes, shouldn't we allow them to use whatever means they can to meet these demands? In support of this view, several scholars have advocated the legalization of doping use (Kayser *et al.* 2007; Savulescu *et al.* 2004). First, athletes are responsible adults and should have the right to use their bodies in any way they wish. Second, athletes should be given the right to go as far as they wish to transform their bodies and do what it takes to become the super-athlete, or even the superhuman. Third, doping is already happening, so instead of trying to ban it and push athletes even further underground to use performance-enhancing drugs, we should bring it to light and provide doping under medical supervision, which would be safer than doping on their own (Kayser *et al.* 2007; Savulescu *et al.* 2004). In line with the above arguments, some medical practitioners argue that high performance sport itself is bad for health and that some doping substances are actually simply rebalancing the human body: doping would be the medication for the health hazards produced by high performance sport (Hoberman 2002).

However, these arguments show that the debate on the legalisation of doping makes sense only in light of the following assumptions: (1) the nature of sport cannot be changed; (2) sport and the competitive system automatically lead to doping; and (3) we can only rely on the willpower of athletes to resist doping. Notably, the motto of the Olympic Games, "Citius, Altius, Fortius," develops a mentality that performance enhancement is the most important objective of the Games, and, possibly, should be achieved at any cost. Petróczi (2007) argued that some athletes may view doping as a necessary evil: although they do not hold positive attitudes toward doping, they may still endorse doping use to achieve their performance goals. Therefore, if the existing sport movement creates a system where doping appears as a viable performance enhancement strategy, then, indeed, there is room to debate about whether doping should be banned or legalized. In essence, the argument about doping legalization attempts to put the horse (sport values) before the cart (athletes).

Tackling doping in sport: sport system revisited

Values and doping use

Prioritizing sport values in the context of doping prevention leads to questions about the ways sport is promoted and commercialized. If the current system of sport is conducive to a certain type of behavior (high performance at any cost), and this increases the risk for doping use, then the very system of sport should be changed in order to effectively prevent doping. Empirical support for this assertion comes from studies that show a strong positive correlation between performance-oriented goals and doping intentions among athletes (e.g., Barkoukis *et al.* 2011, 2013; Sas-Nowosielski and Swiatkowska 2008), as well as research showing that sport values and pressure for higher performance in light of monetary rewards shape athletes' beliefs toward doping use (Bloodworth and McNamee 2010; Smith and Stewart 2010). Modifying the competitive system in order to foster an environment conducive to mastery orientation (vs. performance orientation) could probably act protectively against doping use. For example, sport organizations/federations could foster a system which rewards skills development and progress (vs. outperforming others).

Toward a global change of the sport system

One of the most prominent aspects of the existing sport "system" relates to reward contingencies, and how these contingencies impact on the value system. In fencing, for instance, winning a match is contingent upon a number of hits within a specific time frame. So it isn't rewarded to have attacked or to have taken risks, but simply to have touched, one time more, one's opponent. The assumption is that in order to have touched at least once more than one's opponent, one would have had to display strategy, ruse, panache, technical ability which comes with hard work, and dedication. Therefore, the first place, the gold medal, is rewarding hard work, dedication, not simply to have touched one time more. However, one possible strategy is to simply defend once the score is in one's favor until time runs out. This can lead to excruciatingly boring matches, where one simply "waits" for the win. During a world cup final, a fencer who was very tall and very strong just stood on the piste after having scored a point and defended until the time run out. The opponent displayed beautiful fencing: strategy, technical ability, remarkable footwork, panache, took risks, played. The reaction of the audience, when the time ran out and the passive fencer won, did not cast a shadow of doubt on whom everyone believed should have won, or, more accurately, deserved to have won.

In this case, it is apparent that there is a disconnection between the value system and the reward system. If the reward system was consistent with the value system which verbally promotes excellence, then the active fencer should have won. A usual reaction to this type of situation is "sport, like life, is sometimes unfair." But what if the reward system was simply obsolete? What if fencing borrowed from boxing or judo a point system and updated the scoring mechanism? What if the outcome of a match depended on the number of attacks, of pares? Or what if fencing borrowed from skating or equestrian dressage evaluations, and included bonuses for fighting spirit, technical ability, and even an esthetic component? The scale would then more accurately reflect the values one tries to promote through sport.

Broadening the discussion on the values of sports, it is evident that athletes may face a contradiction, where on the one hand they are told about values which are the core of sport, and on the other hand they are ranked according to a system which doesn't necessarily reward the behaviors consistent with those values. Could it be that the reward system today rests on the outdated assumption that the final result (i.e., winning or coming first) is in direct correlation with the quality of the performance which in turns is a direct result of the quality of the training? And, actually, it may be this system that leads many athletes to doping use, as the most important outcome from sport participation is winning.

Conclusion

Is the sport movement still interested in the journey of the athlete rather than the destination? The existing sport system heavily emphasizes winning at all cost, and neglects the pursuit of the fundamental values of sport. Within this framework, doping use surfaces as a viable performance enhancement option, and athletes can be tempted to engage in this practice to meet their professional or personal goals. Doping use is against the values of sport and its legalization would not necessarily address the ethical issues attached to it. Rather, a global modification of the sport system is needed to more effectively tackle doping use in sports. A modification that will be aligned with the values of sport and adapted to human nature capacities, and that will encompass changes in the reward system, the sport calendar, and the gigantic lengths of sport events.

References

Aidman, E. V. and Woollard, S. (2003). The influence of self-reported exercise addiction on acute emotional and physiological responses to brief exercise deprivation. *Psychology of Sport and Exercise*, *4* (*3*), 225–236.

Barkoukis, V., Lazuras, L., Tsorbatzoudis, H., and Rodafinos, A. (2011). Motivational and sportspersonship profiles of elite athletes in relation to doping behavior. *Psychology of Sport and Exercise*, *12* (*3*), 205–212.

Barkoukis, V., Lazuras, L., Tsorbatzoudis, H., and Rodafinos, A. (2013). Motivational and social cognitive predictors of doping intentions in elite sports: An integrated approach. *Scandinavian Journal of Medicine and Science in Sports*, *23*, e330–e340. doi: 10.1111/sms.12068.

Bloodworth, A. and McNamee, M. (2010). Clean Olympians? Doping and anti-doping: The views of talented young British athletes. *International journal of drug policy*, *21* (*4*), 276–282.

Carpentier, F. (2004). *Le sport est-il éducatif?(Le)*. Rouen: Publications de l'Université de Rouen.

Coubertin, P. (1889). Compte rendu de la 18ème session de l'Association pour l'Avancement des Sciences. In P. de Coubertin, *Le sport mène tout droit à cet idéal humain: la victoire de la volonté* (15–25). Paris: Masson.

Donnelly, P. (1996). Prolympism: sport monoculture as crisis and opportunity. *Quest*, *48* (*1*), 25–42.

Egorov, A. Y. and Szabo, A. (2013). The exercise paradox: An interactional model for a clearer conceptualization of exercise addiction. *Journal of Behavioral Addictions*, *2* (*4*), 199–208.

Johnson, D. K. and Ali, A. (2004). A Tale of two seasons: Participation and medal counts at the Summer and Winter Olympic Games. *Social Science Quarterly*, 85 (4), 974–993.

Hoberman, J. (2002). Sports physicians and the doping crisis in elite sport. *Clinical Journal of Sport Medicine*, 12 (4), 203–208.

Kavussanu, M. and Ntoumanis, N. (2003). Participation in sport and moral functioning: Does ego orientation mediate their relationship? *Journal of Sport and Exercise Psychology*, 25, 501–518.

Kavussanu, M. and Roberts, G. C. (2001). Moral functioning in sport: An achievement goal perspective. *Journal of Sport and Exercise Psychology*, 23, 37–54.

Kayser, B. and Broers, B. (2013). Anti-doping Policies: Choosing between imperfections. In J. Tolleneer, S. Sterckx, and P. Bonte (eds.), *Athletic enhancement, human nature and ethics* (271–289). Dordrecht, Netherlands and New York: Springer

Kayser, B., Mauron, A., and Miah, A. (2007). Current anti-doping policy: a critical appraisal. *BMC Medical Ethics*, 8 (1), 2.

Knafo, A., Daniel, E., and Khoury-Kassabri, M. (2008). Values as protective factors against violent behavior in Jewish and Arab high schools in Israel. *Child development*, 79 (3), 652–667.

Mazanov, J. (2013). Vale WADA, ave "World Sports Drug Agency". *Performance Enhancement and Health*, 2 (2), 80–83.

Mazanov, J., Huybers, T., and Connor, J. (2012). Prioritising health in anti-doping: What Australians think. *Journal of Science and Medicine in Sport*, 15 (5), 381–385.

McBride, F. (1975). Toward a non-definition of sport. *Journal of the Philosophy of Sport*, 2 (1), 4–11.

McFee, G. (2004). *Sport, rules and values. Philosophical investigations into the nature of sport*. London and New York: Routledge.

Melzer, M., Elbe, A. M., and Brand, R. (2010). Moral and ethical decision-making: A chance for doping prevention in sports? *Nordic Journal of Applied Ethics*, 4, 69–85.

Pearson, K. M. (1988). Deception, sportsmanship, and ethics. In W. J. Morgan and K. V. Meier (eds.), *Philosophic inquiry in sport* (183–184). Champaign, IL: Human Kinetics.

Petróczi, A. (2007). Attitudes and doping: A structural equation analysis of the relationship between athletes' attitudes, sport orientation and doping behaviour. *Substance Abuse Treatment, Prevention, and Policy*, 2 (1), 34.

Petróczi, A. and Aidman, E. (2008). Psychological drivers in doping: The life-cycle model of performance enhancement. *Substance Abuse Treatment, Prevention, and Policy*, 3, 7.

Rodek, J., Sekulic, D., and Pasalic, E. (2009). Can we consider religiousness as a protective factor against doping behavior in sport? *Journal of Religion and Health*, 48 (4), 445–453.

Sas-Nowosielski, K. and Swiatkowska, L. (2008). Goal orientations and attitudes toward doping. *International Journal of Sports Medicine*, 29, 607–612.

Savulescu, J., Foddy, B., and Clayton, M. (2004). Why we should allow performance enhancing drugs in sport. *British Journal of Sports Medicine*, 38 (6), 666–670.

Smith, A. C. and Stewart, B. (2010). The special features of sport: A critical revisit. *Sport Management Review*, 13 (1), 1–13.

Tscholl, P., Junge, A., and Dvorak, J. (2008). The use of medication and nutritional supplements during FIFA World Cups 2002 and 2006. *British Journal of Sports Medicine*, 42 (9), 725–730.

WADA (2015). *The World Anti-Doping Code*. Montreal, Canada.

10 Societal and athletes' perspectives on doping use in sport

The Spirit of Sport

Jason Mazanov and Twan Huybers

Morality is seen as having a central role to play in the psychology of doping in sport. This core assumption is central to some psychological models of athlete doping (e.g., Sports Drug Control Model; Donovan *et al.* 2002). Empirically, there is variability in morality being nominated as a factor influencing the decision to dope in qualitative research by athletes and athlete support personnel (such as coaches, medical practitioners, and trainers), with morality being nominated as a key variable in some studies (e.g., Kirby *et al.* 2011) and absent from others (e.g., Mazanov and Huybers 2010). This suggests that a deeper understanding of the role of morality in the psychology of doping in sport is needed. A key challenge facing research on the role of morality in the psychology of doping in sport is effectively operationalizing morality. This chapter explores operationalizing morality to better understand its role in the psychology of doping in sport using the World Anti-Doping Code's (the Code) Spirit of Sport statement (WADA 2015: 14).

Underlying assumptions

The discussion about the role of morality makes two assumptions. The first is that the term "moral" is used as the default term, although it is acknowledged that it could be used interchangeably with "ethical" as intrinsically interrelated while linguistically separable. The second is that while the discussion is framed in terms of substance use (as does most psychological research in the area), it is acknowledged that the Code governs the use of performance-enhancing technologies beyond substances. Therefore, the generalizability of the discussion to other technologies may be limited.

Morality and moral disengagement

Research on the psychology of doping in sport has typically operationalized morality in terms of moral disengagement. For example, the Moral Disengagement in Sport Scale (MDSS; Boardley and Kavussanu 2007, 2008) has proven to be a psychometrically robust operationalization of Bandura's (1991) approach to moral disengagement in sporting contexts. Moral disengagement seeks to explain the psychological processes that selectively inhibit moral standards from preventing socially stigmatized conduct by disengaging self-reproof when engaging in behavior that contravenes personal moral standards (Boardley and Kavussanu 2011). The empirical evidence suggests that moral disengagement explains some aspect of athletes' intentions to dope (e.g., Hodge *et al.* 2013; Lucidi *et al.* 2013). (Noting the standing critiques of the gap between intention and behavior that plague social-cognitive approaches, see Rhodes and Dickau 2012 for an example in relation to physical activity; and the critiques for reliable measurement of doping behavior, see Petróczi *et al.* 2010.)

Importantly, the use of moral disengagement in relation to the psychology of doping in sport seeks to explain how athletes make sense of doping behavior rather than attempting to measure their morality. For example, when moral disengagement predicts intention to dope, it indicates the extent to which an individual tends to morally disengage, across the range of sporting situations measured by instruments such as the MDSS, influence doping intentions. That is, it predicts the likelihood an athlete will try to explain away their doping behavior based on their self-reported propensity to do so in relation to other sports-related behavior. This is different to measuring the moral stance of the athlete, which may be completely consistent with abstinence from doping. Morality and moral disengagement should therefore be considered separate constructs when seeking to understand the psychology of doping in sport.

Operationalizing morality: the Spirit of Sport

The moral basis for the prohibitionist legalistic approach to drug control in sport, known as anti-doping, comes from the Spirit statement (WADA 2015: 14). The Spirit statement is defined by 11 values representing the essence of Olympism (see Table 10.1). These values are presented as that which makes sport intrinsically valuable. Doping behavior is asserted to be definitionally antithetical to these values (an assertion which has been vigorously challenged; e.g., Møller and Dimeo 2014). In principle, these values are what make athletes and sport worth protecting from doping. In practice, these values are the basis for the third test used to ban substances or methods (Article 4.3.1.3) alongside the performance enhancing (Article 4.3.1.2) and health tests (Article 4.3.1.2). In principle and practice, the Spirit statement is the moral basis for the international effort against doping.

The Spirit statement values are assumed to be universal, which is consistent with the practicalities of the Code's policy harmonization aspirations necessary to enable international sporting competition (Houlihan 1999, 2004). In doing so, they form a set of heuristics that guide decision-making around the use of performance-enhancing technologies by athletes and their support personnel (defined as anyone working with, treating, or assisting an athlete preparing for competition; WADA 2015: 132, see Section 4.2.2). Thus, decisions made following these heuristics are by definition moral. This is consistent with values approaches to ethics commonly used in military contexts, where the application of selected values or virtues defines whether an action is moral (Coleman 2012). It would therefore seem appropriate to use the Spirit statement to operationalize the role of morality in the psychology of doping.

Genesis of the Spirit of Sport statement

Ritchie's (2014) history of the Spirit statement puts its genesis in the infamous 1988 Seoul Olympics Men's 100 m final and the subsequent Dubin Inquiry. Dubin's report cast sport as a public good that compelled a morality well beyond the interests of sport. In 1993, the Canadian Center for Drug Free Sport introduced the "Spirit of Sport Campaign," which became the template for the Spirit statement. Following a range of doping scandals (e.g., the Perth Swimming Championship and 1998 Tour de France), in 2000 a five-member "Code Project Team" was put together to develop the statement by consulting widely across international sport organizations. The Spirit statement was formulated to address four challenges to enacting the anti-doping ideology. The first was to capture the intent of doping. The second was to enable prohibition of performance-enhancing substances that had no particular health implications. The third was to provide a clear definition of doping. The fourth was to provide a catch-all term that enabled prohibition of substances deemed to be contrary to the principles of sport and therefore cheating. The Spirit statement was subsequently formalized in the first version of the Code, and has remained unchanged through to the 2015 version of the Code.

To some degree, the Spirit statement could be considered a grounded theory of morality in sport. Ritchie's (2014) analysis suggests the Spirit statement may better reflect the values of its authors rather than a universally held morality of sport. This observation can be leveled at any grounded theory, which is usually tested with large sample quantitative research aimed at establishing validity and reliability. The authors are unaware of any work that has sought to validate the Spirit statement beyond its initial development.

Definitional issues in the Spirit of Sport

The Spirit statement has received some attention in the general debate about drug control in sport (e.g., Loland and Hoppeler 2012). A particular concern has been the absence of clear definition of the values that make up the Spirit statement (e.g., Mazanov and Connor 2010). For example, when the authors queried the World Anti-Doping Agency (WADA) about the Spirit statement, there were no documents available to explain either the genesis of the Spirit statement or what the values meant (L. Cleret, personal communication, November 3–4, 2010); at the time of writing no such documents had emerged.

McNamee (2012, 2013) argues that clear definition of the Spirit statement's values is unnecessary as it represents a set of principles characterizing that which makes sport valuable. The list is, and never can be, definitive as sport means many things to many people. While this approach may be philosophically satisfactory, it presents problems for operationalizing the Spirit statement. For example, using health as an example, the general population usually follows the dominant medicalized health discourse of disease-free longevity (Lupton 1995). This contrasts with athletes defining health instrumentally – where the body's inability to achieve expected performance is considered a sign of ill health (Møller 2010). Health is also understood differently across different cultural contexts. Haque (2010) provides a useful overview of the important differences in the ways Hindus, Buddhists, and Muslims construct health relative to Christian definitions. This suggests operationalizing morality in sport using the Spirit statement needs to control for potential for intra- and intercultural variation in interpretation, such as stratified sampling or repeated measures designs.

The role of morality in the psychology of doping

Two studies have operationalized the Spirit statement using small, nationally representative samples of the Australian general population. These studies offer an insight into the way the Australian general population thinks about morality in sport. While the original purpose of these studies related to a specific test of drug control policy, they demonstrate morality in sport can be operationalized using the Spirit statement and how morality in sport might evolve, at least in Australia.

Mazanov *et al.* (2012) tested the extent to which Australians agreed or disagreed with harm minimization (prioritizing athlete health as the main focus of drug control for sport) as an alternative to the anti-doping policy (the Code). This was tested by asking $n = 168$ Australians to identify what they prioritized in protecting the integrity of sport by establishing the relative importance of each value in the Spirit of Sport statement using a technique called Best Worst Scaling (BWS) (see Mazanov *et al.* 2012 for an overview of BWS), similar to work assessing how different cultures rank Schwartz's 10 universal values (Lee *et al.* 2011). If Australians prioritized health above other aspects of the Spirit statement, it would suggest that advocates of harm minimization approaches to drug control in sport better reflected the prevailing moral norms for Australian sport.

This work was extended with an additional nationally representative sample of $n = 154$ Australians to determine whether the general population saw any difference in the way the Spirit statement values were prioritized across elite ($n = 77$) and non-elite sport ($n = 77$). This replication and extension was done for two reasons. The first was to determine whether any differences emerged in the way Australians constructed the moral basis for sport across the two levels. The second was to determine whether Mazanov *et al.*'s (2012) model better reflected elite sport (as the default mental model for thinking about sport), was a composite of elite and non-elite sport, or was completely different across sporting frames.

The views arising from the two studies of the Australian general public are given in Table 10.1 in the order the values are presented in the Code. The fact

Table 10.1 BWS ratio scores (in order of WADA's Spirit of Sport statement)

	2012	Non-elite	Elite
N	168	77	77
Ethics, fair play and honesty	4.072 (1)	3.627 (2)	3.642 (1)
Health	1.161 (7)	1.044 (6)	0.942 (7)
Excellence in performance	0.439 (8)	0.342 (10)	1.216 (6)
Character and education	0.426 (9)	0.423 (9)	0.320 (11)
Fun and joy	1.177 (6)	2.163 (3)	0.399 (9)
Teamwork	1.551 (4)	1.591 (4)	1.371 (5)
Dedication and commitment	1.178 (5)	0.874 (7)	2.795 (2)
Respect for rules and laws	1.807 (3)	1.342 (5)	2.556 (3)
Respect for self and other participants	4.024 (2)	3.731 (1)	2.303 (4)
Courage	0.336 (11)	0.331 (11)	0.444 (8)
Community and solidarity	0.378 (10)	0.613 (8)	0.371 (10)

that the values are differentiated in terms of priority shows some values are clearly more important than others to Australians. Mazanov *et al.* (2012) report the initial data clusters around three broad constructs: societal preparation (ranks 1–2), societal consequences (ranks 3–7), and individual benefits (ranks 8–11). They note that the values associated with societal preparation were rated as ten times more important than individual benefits.

Comparing the outcomes of the BWS experiment across the 2012 and the elite/non-elite data shows similarities and differences emerging across independent samples. In terms of societal preparation, the data show the role of "ethics, fair play and honesty" was consistently prioritized across samples whereas "respect for self and others" dropped for elite sport. This suggests elite athletes may be expected to place less emphasis on themselves and others in pursuit of performance. There were three notable differences across the societal consequences construct. First, "respect for rules" was seen as less important in non-elite sport. Second, "dedication and commitment" was seen as the second most important value for elite sport, and one of the less important values for non-elite sport. Third, "fun and joy" was seen as very important to non-elite sport and largely irrelevant to elite sport. There was little difference across the individual benefits of sport, with "excellence in performance" being seen as more important in elite sport the only exception.

This pattern of results suggests there are some important differences in the way Australians construct morality across sporting contexts. Non-elite sport might be better explained regrouping the constructs as societal preparation (ranks 1–2), fun and joy (rank 3), societal consequences (ranks 4–7), and individual benefits (ranks 8–11). The main difference appeared to be the promotion of enjoying sport at the expense of rule-driven performance. By comparison, elite sport was constructed with "ethics, fair play and honesty" (rank 1), what might be called respect for sport (ranks 2–4), societal consequences (ranks 5–7), and individual benefits (ranks 8–11). From this point of view, Australians constructed the morality of elite sport emphasizing formal and informal rule following at the expense of the person's societal and personal development, which is consistent with the performance narrative of elite sport reported by elite athletes (Carless and Douglass 2013).

While the results show Australians consistently prioritized rule-following over health in sport, suggesting a different view to that advocated by harm minimization advocates, it also shows that it is possible to operationalize morality in sport using the Spirit statement. The slight variations in how morality in sport is constructed suggest different moral appeals would resonate at different levels of sport. For example, the Australian general population might expect to see drug control for sport place an emphasis on moral appeals to rules-based approach for elite athletes. By comparison, moral appeals around drug control for non-elite sport may have to augment rules with observations around how substance use can change sporting capital (e.g., fun) (cf. Rowe 2015).

Applying the Spirit of Sport to other contexts

The previous section showed it is possible to operationalize morality using the Spirit statement to conduct meaningful research on the psychology of doping in sport. In doing so, it is relevant to consider how operationalizing morality using the Spirit statement might apply to the main focus of research into the psychology of doping in sport – athletes and their support personnel.

Athletes

A pressing question for athletes is how changes in morality over their career influence the psychology of doping. Like any substance use behavior, all athletes start from a position of sustained abstinence. There is some point at which athletes then move through the typical stages of initial use, trying, occasional use, and regular use. The natural history of doping in cycling (e.g., Ohl *et al.* 2013; Lentillon-Kaestner and Carstairs 2010) suggests junior or early career athletes have little need for exogenous enhancement as they grow toward fulfilling their genetic potential. At this stage, junior elite athletes demonstrate values and arguments consistent with the Code and Spirit statement (Bloodworth and McNamee 2010; Bloodworth *et al.* 2012), despite a system that normalizes performance-based substance use (e.g., supplements and non-prohibited drugs) as part of the broader normalization of sports science in junior sport (Mazanov *et al.* 2015).

The transition to mid- and late-career sport sees athletes change their views, with a far more subtle and nuanced view of the moral implications of doping (e.g., Erickson *et al.* 2015; Overbye *et al.* 2013). For example, there is growing evidence that athletes see substance use as a normal part of sporting practice without any particular moral implications (e.g., Pappa and Kennedy 2012). The evolution of morality of doping across sporting careers therefore represents a potentially important set of questions.

This can be easily assessed with cross-sectional and longitudinal studies examining the stability of the Spirit statement values. This then needs to account for type of sport, to determine whether the Spirit statement is prioritized differently across different types of sport. If conducted on a large enough scale, such a study (or set of studies) gives some indication of the consistency or variation of interpretation in the Spirit statement across sporting contexts. At an aggregate level it means establishing the importance athletes attach to the values given as the basis for Olympism and the moral basis for anti-doping.

Athlete support personnel

The definition of athlete support personnel given in the Code (WADA 2015: 132) includes administrators, coaches, psychologists, and parents. The Code also obliges support personnel to promote the anti-doping ideology (Article 21.2.3). This is based on evidence that support personnel have a key role to play in shaping athlete doping behavior (e.g., see Backhouse and McKenna 2012 for a discussion in relation to coaches). While there is some evidence around the knowledge and attitudes of support personnel (Backhouse and McKenna 2011, 2012; Mazanov et al. 2014), there is very little evidence about the role morality plays for support personnel in relation to doping.

Given the empirical evidence that support personnel start shaping values around doping in junior sport (Mazanov et al. 2015), it would seem prudent to focus attention on the psychology of those individuals to better understand their moral position and what they are promoting. Quantitative evidence from Australian support personnel shows considerable variation in the rationales underlying their practice of anti-doping (Mazanov et al. 2014). For example, while support personnel broadly support the notion of drug control in sport, they appear willing to substitute professional or other moral standards when confronted with doping scenarios (Mazanov et al. 2015).

Like research with athletes, operationalizing morality with the Spirit statement offers an efficient insight into how different support personnel construct morality around doping. Generalizing the arguments arising from the natural history of athletes, there may be significant variation by level of sport, experience in sport, and role in sport. Of significant concern is the psychology of those who make the rules: the architects of the Code and those who implement it. To some degree, those charged with designing and implementing the Code are the moral guardians of sport (at least in terms of doping) and it is relevant to understand their psychology of doping as much as that of the athletes.

Psychological practice

If morality is a central variable in explaining the psychology of doping it is also central to intervening in the behavior. Arguably, the moral basis for sport defined by the Spirit statement represents the mental model athletes use to rationalize their positive or negative views of anti-doping. The role of the psychologist in this context is helping athletes explore variation in how the Spirit statement might be interpreted, informed by research such as that articulated in the Section discussing the Spirit of Sport and the Australian general public.

It is plausible that an athlete might ask a psychologist their views on the Code, perhaps with reference to literature that offers counterarguments to the Code (e.g., Savulescu *et al.* 2004; Waddington *et al.* 2013). Arguably, the psychologist needs to respond effectively with multiple points of view around the moral implications of both doping and other forms of drug use and performance enhancement in sport. This suggests the psychologist needs to critically reflect on his/her own moral position in relation to drug control, performance enhancement in sport, and the Code (which are separate, but related issues; see Mazanov *et al.* 2015) with reference to common counterarguments and contrasting views (e.g., harm minimization; see Kayser and Smith 2008; Kirkwood 2009; or Smith and Stewart 2008). The importance of doing so becomes clear when psychologists work with athletes in the context of psycho-educational interventions aimed at altering athletes' psychology around doping to be consistent with the Code (e.g., Jalleh *et al.* 2012). Being able to conduct such a discussion sees the psychologist help the athlete find the rationale that leads to stable functional behavior in the long term, whether abstinence, uptake, maintenance, or cessation.

Future research on the Spirit of Sport

Given the Spirit statement is likely to persist as the Code evolves beyond the 2015 update, psychological research needs to investigate this construct in much greater depth. As the moral basis for anti-doping, it becomes the anchor by which athletes justify their doping behavior one way or the other. At its core, psychological research on the Spirit statement needs to get back to basics. Qualitative work is needed with the full range of athletes and support personnel across sports to develop a much greater understanding of what the values in the Spirit statement mean. Quantitative work along the lines of the BWS approach with the full range of athletes and support personnel across sports is needed to develop insight into variation in how the Spirit statement is understood. The exploration of variation needs to occur both intra- and interculturally, drawing on large numbers of international studies. Such results provide the foundation to effectively operationalize and then understand the role of morality in the psychology of doping in sport.

Another approach is to conduct qualitative research around what respondents understand the Spirit statement to mean. A broader examination of how the general population understands the Spirit statement would be a worthwhile exercise to progress understanding of the psychology of doping in sport, and perhaps more broadly. With enough replications across different samples, an effective description of variation across social contexts could be built to enable an assessment of the universality or contextuality of the Spirit statement.

It is also worth considering that the psychology of doping extends beyond sport. The role of morality in the psychology of doping in elite performing arts (e.g., Sekulic *et al.* 2010), the military (e.g., Estrada *et al.* 2012) or university education (e.g., Lamkin 2012) also needs to be considered. This serves to potentially inform the broader discussion on the moral implications of human enhancement in a non-elite setting such as the workplace (see Savulescu *et al.* 2011; and Academy of Medical Sciences 2012). From this point of view, sport is a vehicle to understanding the psychology of performance-enhancing technology use in other contexts. It would be worthwhile to determine whether the Spirit statement is a generalizable operationalization of morality for doping in other contexts.

References

Academy of Medical Sciences (2012). *Human Enhancement and the Future of Work.* Available at www.britac.ac.uk/policy/Human-enhancement.cfm (accessed October 23, 2014).

Backhouse, S. H. and McKenna, J. (2011). Doping in sport: A review of medical practitioners' knowledge, attitudes and beliefs. *International Journal of Drug Policy, 22 (3),* 198–202.

Backhouse, S. H. and McKenna, J. (2012). Reviewing coaches' knowledge, attitudes and beliefs regarding doping in sport. *International Journal of Sports Science and Coaching, 7 (1),* 167–176.

Bandura, A. (1991) Social cognitive theory of moral thought and action. In W. M. Kurtines and J. L. Gewirtz (eds.), *Handbook of Moral Behavior and Development: Theory, Research and Applications.* Hillsdale, NJ: Lawrence Erlbaum Associates.

Bloodworth, A. and McNamee, M. (2010). Clean Olympians? Doping and anti-doping: The view of talented young British athletes. *International Journal of Drug Policy, 21,* 276–282.

Bloodworth, A. J., Petróczi, A., Bailey, R., Pearce, G., and McNamee, M. J. (2012). Doping and supplementation: The attitudes of talented young athletes. *Scandinavian Journal of Science and Medicine in Sport, 22,* 293–301.

Boardley, I. D. and Kavassanu, M. (2007). Development and validation of the Moral Disengagement in Sport Scale. *Journal of Sport and Exercise Psychology, 29,* 608–628.

Boardley, I. D. and Kavassanu, M. (2008). The Moral Disengagement in Sport Scale – Short. *Journal of Sports Sciences, 26 (14),* 1507–1517.

Boardley, I. D. and Kavussanu, M. (2011). Moral disengagement in sport. *International Review of Sport and Exercise Psychology, 4 (2),* 93–108.

Carless, D. and Douglas, K. (2013). Living, resisting, and playing the part of athlete: Narrative tensions in elite sport. *Psychology of Sport and Exercise, 14 (5),* 701–708.

Coleman, S. (2012). *Military Ethics: An Introduction with Case Studies.* Oxford: Oxford University Press.

Donovan, R. J., Egger, G., Kapernick, V., and Mendoza, J. (2002). A conceptual framework for achieving performance enhancing drug compliance in sport. *Sports Medicine, 32 (4),* 269–284.

Erickson, K., McKenna, J., and Backhouse, S. H. (2015). A qualitative analysis of the factors that protect athletes against doping in sport. *Psychology of Sport and Exercise, 16 (2),* 149–155.

Estrada, A., Kelley, A. M., Webb, C. M., Athy, J. R., and Crowley, J. S. (2012). Modafinil as a replacement for dextroamphetamine for sustaining alertness in military helicopter pilots. *Aviation, Space, and Environmental Medicine, 83 (6),* 556–567.

Haque, A. (2010). Mental health concepts in Southeast Asia: Diagnostic considerations and treatment implications. *Psychology, Health and Medicine, 15 (2),* 127–134.

Hodge, K., Hargreaves, E. A., Gerrard, D., and Lonsdale, C. (2013). Psychological mechanisms underlying doping attitudes in sport: Motivation and moral disengagement. *Journal of Sport and Exercise Psychology, 35* (*4*), 413–432.

Houlihan, B. (1999). Policy harmonisation: The example of global anti-doping policy. *Journal of Sport Management, 13*, 197–215.

Houlihan, B. (2004). Harmonising anti-doping policy: The role of the WADA. In J. Hoberman and V. Møller (eds.), *Doping and Public Policy* (19–30). Odense, Denmark: University Press of Southern Denmark.

Jalleh, G., Donovan, R., and Gucciardi, D. (2012). Development of a psycho-educational anti-doping intervention program for emerging athletes. *Journal of Science and Medicine in Sport, 15* (*6, Suppl.*), 72–73.

Kayser, B. and Smith, A. C. (2008). Globalisation of anti-doping: The reverse side of the medal. *British Medical Journal, 337* (*7661*), 85–87.

Kirby, K., Moran, A., and Guerin, S. (2011). A qualitative analysis of the experiences of elite athletes who have admitted to doping for performance enhancement. *International Journal of Sport Policy and Politics, 3* (*2*), 205–224.

Kirkwood, K. (2009). Considering harm reduction as the future of doping control policy in international sport. *Quest, 61* (*2*), 180–190.

Lamkin, M. (2012). Cognitive enhancements and the values of higher education. *Health Care Analysis, 20* (*4*), 347–355.

Lee, J., Soutar, G., Daly, T., and Louviere, J. (2011). Schwartz values clusters in the United States and China. *Journal of Cross-Cultural Psychology, 42* (*2*), 234–252.

Lentillon-Kaestner, V. and Carstairs, C. (2010). Doping use among young elite cyclists: A qualitative psychosociological approach. *Scandinavian Journal of Medicine and Science in Sports, 20* (*2*), 336–345.

Loland, S. and Hoppeler, H. (2012). Justifying anti-doping: The fair opportunity principle and the biology of performance enhancement. *European Journal of Sports Science, 12* (*4*), 347–353.

Lucidi, F., Zelli, A., and Mallia, L. (2013). The contribution of moral disengagement to adolescents' use of doping substances. *International Journal of Sport Psychology, 44* (*6*), 493–514.

Lupton, D. (1995). *The Imperative of Health: Public Health and the Regulated Body.* London: Sage Publications.

McNamee, M. (2012). The Spirit of Sport and the medicalisation of anti-doping: Empirical and normative ethics. *Asian Bioethics Review, 4*, 374–392.

McNamee, M. (2013). The spirit of sport and anti-doping policy: An ideal worth fighting for. *Play True, Issue 1 2013*, 14–16.

Mazanov, J. and Connor, J. (2010). Rethinking the management of drugs in sport. *International Journal of Sport Policy, 2* (*1*), 49–63.

Mazanov, J. and Huybers, T. (2010). An empirical model of athlete decisions to use performance enhancing drugs: Qualitative evidence. *Qualitative Research in Sport and Exercise, 2* (*3*), 385–402.

Mazanov, J., Huybers, T., and Connor, J. (2012). Prioritising health in anti-doping: What Australians think. *Journal of Science and Medicine in Sport, 15*, 381–385.

Mazanov, J., Backhouse, S., Connor, J., Hemphill, D., and Quirk, F. (2014). Athlete support personnel and anti-doping: Knowledge, attitudes and ethical stance. *Scandinavian Journal of Science and Medicine in Sport, 24* (*5*), 846–856.

Mazanov, J., Hemphill, D., Connor, J., Quirk, F., and Backhouse, S. (2015). Australian athlete support personnel lived experience of anti-doping. *Sports Management Review*, *18 (2)*, 218–230.

Møller V. (2010). *The Ethics of Doping and Anti-Doping: Redeeming the Soul of Sport.* London and New York: Routledge.

Møller V. and Dimeo, P. (2014). Anti-doping – The end of sport. *International Journal of Sport Policy and Politics*, *6 (2)*, 259–272.

Ohl, F., Fincouer, B., Lentillon-Kaestner, V., Defrance, J., and Brissonneau, C. (2013). The socialisation of young cyclists and the culture of doping. *International Review for the Sociology of Sport*. doi: 10.1177/1012690213495534.

Overbye, M., Knudsen, M. L., and Pfister, G. (2013). To dope or not to dope: Elite athletes' perceptions of doping deterrents and incentives. *Performance Enhancement and Health*, *2 (3)*, 119–134.

Pappa, E. and Kennedy, E. (2012). "It was my thought … he made it a reality": Normalisation and responsibility in athletes' accounts of performance enhancing drug use. *International Review for the Sociology of Sport*, *48 (3)*, 277–294.

Petróczi, A., Aidman, E. V., Hussain, I., Deshmukh, N. Nepusz, T., Uvacsek, M., Tóth, M., Barker, J., and Naughton, D. P. (2010). Virtue or pretense? Looking behind self-declared innocence in doping. *PloS one*, *5 (5)*, e10457.

Rhodes, R. E. and Dickau, L. (2012). Experimental evidence for the intention–behavior relationship in the physical activity domain: A meta-analysis. *Health Psychology*, *31 (6)*, 724.

Ritchie, I. (2014). The construction of a policy: The World Anti-Doping Code's "Spirit of Sport" clause. *Performance Enhancement and Health*, *2 (4)*, 194–200.

Rowe, N. F. (2015). Sporting capital: A theoretical and empirical analysis of sport participation determinants and its application to sports development policy and practice. *International Journal of Sport Policy and Politics*, *7 (1)*, 43–61.

Savulescu, J., Foddy, B., and Clayton, M. (2004). Why we should allow performance enhancing drugs in sport. *British Journal of Sports Medicine*, *38 (6)*, 666–670.

Savulescu, J., ter Meulen, R., and Kahane, G. (2011). *Enhancing Human Capacities.* Chichester, UK: Wiley-Blackwell.

Sekulic, D., Peric, M., and Rodek, J. (2010). Substance use and misuse among professional ballet dancers. *Substance Use and Misuse*, *45 (9)*, 1420–1430.

Smith, A. C. and Stewart, B. (2008). Drug policy in sport: Hidden assumptions and inherent contradictions. *Drug and Alcohol Review*, *27 (2)*, 123–129.

Waddington, I., Christiansen, A. V., Gleaves, J., Hoberman, J., and Møller, V. (2013). Recreational drug use and sport: Time for a WADA rethink? *Performance Enhancement and Health*, *2 (2)*, 41–47.

WADA (2015). *World Anti-Doping Code*. Montreal, Canada: World Anti-Doping Agency.

11 Moral disengagement and doping

Maria Kavussanu

The use of prohibited performance-enhancing drugs (PEDs) or doping is a pervasive phenomenon in sport; doping examples are numerous in elite sport with Lance Armstrong, Marion Jones, and Tyler Hamilton constituting just a few of the many high-profile cases of athletes who have admitted to, or have been found guilty of, doping. Doping constitutes one of the dark sides of sport with potentially important negative consequences not only for athletes' health but also for the integrity of sport. It is a behavior which breaks the rules of sport participation; given that athletes do not openly admit to doping when taking part in sport, doping is cheating, thus it is a moral issue. Its study, like the study of morality, has inherent challenges not present in other areas of inquiry. Specifically, researchers ask people who cheat to tell the truth about cheating. Despite its challenges, this is an important area of research, and understanding why some athletes dope and what enables them to act in this way has received considerable attention in recent years (see Ntoumanis *et al.* 2014).

A number of social psychological factors have been associated with doping. A recent meta-analysis of psychosocial predictors of doping identified moral disengagement as one of the strongest predictors of doping intention (Ntoumanis *et al.* 2014). Moral disengagement is a construct described by Bandura (1991) in his social-cognitive theory of moral thought and action. The focus of this chapter is on this construct as applied to doping. The chapter starts by briefly outlining the main tenets of social-cognitive theory as they pertain to moral disengagement and describes the moral disengagement mechanisms. Next, the instruments that measure this construct and have been used in doping research are briefly discussed, followed by a review of quantitative studies examining moral disengagement and doping variables in athletes. Finally, qualitative studies in bodybuilders are reviewed, and the chapter ends with some concluding remarks.

Mechanisms of moral disengagement

Moral disengagement is a central construct in Bandura's (1986, 1991) social-cognitive theory of moral thought and action. Bandura (1986, 1991) proposed that in the course of socialization, individuals develop moral standards from a variety of influences, such as observation of others, approving and disapproving reactions of their behavior by others, and direct tuition. These moral standards regulate behavior through evaluative self reactions: people feel good when behaving in ways that match their moral standards, and experience self-reproof when their actions violate their moral standards. These evaluative self-reactions regulate conduct anticipatorily: people do things that give them satisfaction and a sense of self-worth and refrain from behaving in ways that bring self-condemnation (Bandura 1991, 2002). Thus, anticipated self-sanctions in reaction to one's behavior keep behavior in line with moral standards.

Even though moral standards are assumed to guide behavior, people do not always act in accordance with these standards. They are able to disengage moral self-sanctions from reprehensible behavior, through the use of one or more of eight psychosocial mechanisms, collectively known as moral disengagement. This allows different types of behavior from individuals with the same moral standards (Bandura 2002). The mechanisms operate by cognitively restructuring transgressive behavior and its consequences, minimizing or obscuring one's role in the harm one causes, disregarding or distorting the detrimental consequences of one's behavior, and dehumanizing or blaming one's victim. The mechanisms act on different aspects of the process of moral control (Bandura 1991), and have been grouped into four sets.

The first set operates on detrimental conduct and includes three mechanisms: moral justification, euphemistic labeling, and advantageous comparison. *Moral justification* entails the cognitive restructuring of a harmful behavior into a praiseworthy one, making it appear acceptable by portraying it as facilitating a valued social or moral purpose (Bandura 1991). For example, doping could be justified as a way of helping one's team. *Euphemistic labeling* involves the use of language to disguise transgressive behavior as less harmful (Bandura 1991). In sport, athletes may talk about "bending the rules" rather than breaking them (Boardley and Kavussanu 2007). An example of this mechanism among athletes who dope is when they refer to illegal substances as "juice" (Boardley and Grix 2014). *Advantageous comparison* involves comparing transgressive behavior with more harmful acts, making the behavior in question appear relatively benign (Bandura 1991). For instance, athletes could compare doping to physical violence and conclude that it is not that bad.

The second set operates on the agency of action by obscuring or minimizing one's role in the harm one causes (Bandura 1999), and includes two mechanisms: displacement and diffusion of responsibility. *Displacement of responsibility* occurs when people view their behavior as resulting from social pressures or dictates of an authority figure rather than something for which they are personally responsible (Bandura 1991). For instance, athletes may displace responsibility for taking illegal substances to their coach, who may have asked them to dope. *Diffusion of responsibility* occurs through: group decision-making (when everyone is responsible, no one feels truly responsible); division of labor for tasks that appear harmless on their own but are harmful in their entirety; and group action, which involves attributing the harm done by the group to the behavior of the other group members (Bandura 2002). An example of group decision-making is when athletes attribute their doping behavior to a collective team decision to engage in such behavior.

The third set of moral disengagement mechanisms operates on the consequences of detrimental behavior and consists of only one mechanism: *distortion of consequences*. This entails avoiding or downplaying the harm caused by the individual's transgressive behavior on others (Bandura 1991). Individuals who can avoid finding out or minimize the harm caused by their behavior, are more likely to continue the harmful behavior. An example of distortion of consequences in sport is when athletes deny the seriousness of the injuries they have caused (Boardley and Kavussanu 2007).

The final set acts on the victim of the act and consists of dehumanization and attribution of blame. *Dehumanization* involves cognitively divesting victims of their human qualities or attributing animal-like qualities to them (Bandura 1991), while *attribution of blame* occurs when people view themselves as faultless victims, who are forced to injurious behavior by their own victim or the circumstances (Bandura 1991). Clearly, these two mechanisms are not relevant to doping: individuals who dope do not actively harm another person, thus in the absence of a victim there is no one to dehumanize or blame for doping behavior. Indeed, these two mechanisms have not emerged in qualitative doping research (e.g., Boardley and Grix 2014; Boardley *et al.* 2014; Lucidi *et al.* 2008).

The construct of moral disengagement was originally developed to explain inhuman acts such as terrorist acts, war atrocities, and aggression (Bandura 1990, 1991; Bandura *et al.* 1996). However, selective disengagement of moral control is not confined to aggression (Bandura 1990). People often experience conflicts when behaviors they do not value can help secure benefits that they value. Often, these conflicts are resolved by selective disengagement of moral self-sanctions thereby enabling otherwise considerate people to act in ways that are self-serving and have detrimental consequences for others (Bandura 1990). This makes doping, a behavior that is intended to benefit oneself but at the same time breaks the rules of sport (and is therefore cheating), a prime candidate for the effects of moral disengagement. Indeed, in previous sport research, moral disengagement has been positively associated with cheating (d'Arripe-Longueville *et al.* 2010). Numerous studies have also reported links with antisocial sport behavior (e.g., Boardley and Kavussanu 2007; Hodge and Lonsdale 2011; Kavussanu *et al.* 2013; Stanger *et al.* 2013; Traclet *et al.* 2011). Thus, moral disengagement is highly relevant to understanding doping behavior in sport.

Measures of moral disengagement

One of the first steps toward examining a new construct is the development of a valid and reliable instrument to assess the construct. Several measures of moral disengagement have been developed over the years. In this section, instruments that have been employed in doping research are reviewed, in the chronological order they have been developed.

The first ever measure of moral disengagement was constructed by Bandura and his colleagues (Bandura *et al.* 1996) to measure the eight mechanisms in schoolchildren. Four items were developed for each mechanism (thus the scale consists of 32 items), and an overall score was computed for moral disengagement and used in this study of aggression and delinquent behavior. Participants are presented with a number of statements and are asked to indicate the extent to which they agree with these statements; this format has been used in the remaining instruments described in this section. Example items are "it is all right to fight to protect your friends" measuring moral justification, and "slapping and shoving someone is just a way of joking" assessing euphemistic labeling. This instrument was used in the first study that examined moral disengagement in relation to doping in sport (Lucidi *et al.* 2004).

Addressing the need for a sport-specific measure of moral disengagement, Boardley and Kavussanu (2007) developed the Moral Disengagement in Sport Scale (MDSS), which, in line with Bandura *et al.* (1996), also consists of 32 items. This was followed by the Moral Disengagement in Sport Scale – Short (MDSS-S), which comprises a subset of eight items from the MDSS, with only one item measuring each mechanism (Boardley and Kavussanu 2008). Example items are "it is okay for players to lie to officials if it helps their team" for moral justification, and "bending the rules is a way of evening things up" for euphemistic labeling. Although these two scales measure moral disengagement in sport, none of their items refer to doping. Nevertheless, the MDSS-S has been used in one doping study (Hodge *et al.* 2013).

An instrument that measures doping moral disengagement was developed by Lucidi and colleagues (Lucidi *et al.* 2008) based on interviews conducted with 35 high school students, who competed in sport regularly; its psychometric properties were assessed in a large sample of high school students, many of whom (55 percent) were active sport participants. The "doping moral disengagement scale" consists of six items tapping the six moral disengagement mechanisms that are relevant to doping. Example items are "compared to the damaging effects of alcohol and tobacco, the use of illicit substances is not so bad," for advantageous comparison; "it is not right to condemn those who use illicit substances to improve their body, since many do the same" for diffusion of responsibility; and "there is no reason to punish those who use illicit substances to improve their physical appearance; after all, they do not hurt anyone," for distortion of consequences. No items assess attribution of blame or dehumanization, the two mechanisms that operate on the victim, as these mechanisms did not emerge in the interviews (Lucidi *et al.* 2008).

Perhaps due to the focus of their research, described in the next section, the scale developed by Lucidi *et al.* (2008) included a variety of items. Specifically, two items explicitly referred to one's body and physical appearance, while only one item referred explicitly to sport. The remaining three items did not specify the doping context (i.e., sport, bodybuilding) but referred to the use of illicit substances in general (e.g., "it is OK to use illicit substances if this can help one to overcome one's own limits"). Thus, this scale measures moral disengagement with respect to doping in bodybuilding *and* sport, and includes some items that can be applied to both contexts. Due to its broad focus, this scale would be less than ideal if one wishes to investigate doping in either sport or bodybuilding.

Finally, Kavussanu *et al.* (in review) developed the Moral Disengagement in Doping Scale, which also consists of items that are specific to sport. The items were developed by academics with expertise in scale development and research experience on moral disengagement and doping. The scale was administered to three samples of athletes competing in a variety of team sports, and evidence for its content, convergent, concurrent, and discriminant validity, was provided (Kavussanu *et al.*, in review). Example items are "Doping is alright because it helps your team" for moral justification and "Doping is a way to maximize your potential" for euphemistic labelling. This scale consists of six items, one for each of the six mechanisms of moral disengagement that are relevant to doping. Similar to Lucidi *et al.* (2008), no items measure dehumanization or attribution of blame. More recently, Lucidi and colleagues (2014) developed a six-item measure of team doping moral disengagement. The items were developed based on focus group interviews, where athletes were provided with sets of distinct circumstances in which doping use could be justified. Team sport athletes evaluated the extent to which the moral disengagement items were clear and pertinent to doping, while experts on social-cognitive theory and research guessed the theoretical moral disengagement mechanism, to which each item referred (at this stage seven items were available), thus supporting the validity of the scale. Example items are "in a team, doping use is just another good way to 'keep the group together'" for euphemistic labeling, and "in a team, a player cannot say 'no' to doping use when the coach or the teammates ask him/her to do it" for displacement of responsibility. Lucidi *et al.* (2014) have provided evidence for the psychometric properties of this scale.

In sum, moral disengagement in doping research has been measured with a variety of instruments, three of which are specific to doping. One of them pertains to both sport and physical appearance (Lucidi *et al.* 2008), while the other two refer to doping in team sports (Kavussanu *et al.* 2014; Lucidi *et al.* 2014). Although an instrument that is specific to individual sports does not currently exist, the latter two measures could be easily adapted for use in these sports.

Moral disengagement and doping in sport

A growing body of work has investigated the role of moral disengagement on doping using a variety of theoretical perspectives. Specifically, a few studies (e.g., Lucidi *et al.* 2004, 2008) have examined moral disengagement alongside constructs from Ajzen's (1991) Theory of Planned Behavior; one study (Hodge *et al.* 2013) has investigated this in conjunction with constructs from self-determination theory (Deci and Ryan 2002); and another (Kavussanu *et al.* 2014) has examined moral disengagement along constructs from social-cognitive theory (Bandura 1991). In some cases, researchers have included constructs from other theoretical perspectives in an effort to better understand doping. These studies are reviewed in this section, with a focus on the primary theory guiding each investigation.

Theory of Planned Behavior

The seminal study of moral disengagement and doping intention was conducted by Lucidi *et al.* (2004) using a cross-sectional design and a sample of 952 Italian high school students, approximately one-third of whom competed regularly (i.e., at least once a month) in sport. Doping intention, a key variable in Ajzen's (1991) theory, was measured by asking participants to indicate how strong was their intention to use illegal substances to improve their sport performance or physical appearance in the next three months, and what was the probability they would do this. Moral disengagement was a positive – albeit weak – predictor of doping intention. One weakness of this study was the use of Bandura *et al.*'s (1996) moral disengagement measure, which is not doping specific; this might explain the weak relationship noted between moral disengagement and doping intention.

This weakness was rectified in subsequent work by Lucidi *et al.* (2008), in 762 Italian high school students, of whom approximately half (i.e., 55 percent) were taking part in some type of sport activity. Moral disengagement was measured with the doping moral disengagement scale (Lucidi *et al.* 2008), while doping intention was assessed with the two items used in the previous study (Lucidi *et al.* 2004). Participants also completed questionnaires assessing other key constructs of the Theory of Planned Behavior, such as subjective norms (i.e., the extent to which significant others would have approved their use of illegal substances to improve sport performance or physical appearance), and attitudes toward doping. Finally, doping self-regulatory efficacy (i.e., individuals' beliefs about their capability to resist use of doping substances) was measured. These assessments represented the Time 1 measures. Three months later, participants were asked to indicate from a list of illegal substances which ones they had used in the last three months (doping use) with the aim of enhancing their athletic performance or improving their physical appearance without a doctor's prescription.

Moral disengagement moderately and positively predicted both intention to dope at Time 1 and reported doping at Time 2. Interestingly, participants with higher scores on moral disengagement also reported more positive attitudes toward doping, perceived that important others would approve of their doping, and were less likely to believe they could resist doping, if the opportunity arose. The latter finding is interesting, and suggests that people, who do not feel capable of resisting temptation tend to justify doping, because they are not psychologically strong enough to say no. Moral disengagement might allow these individuals to minimize negative emotion by justifying their behavior. Thus, the low capability to resist temptation may lead one to morally disengage.

In a study designed to replicate the findings of Lucidi *et al.* (2008), Zelli *et al.* (2010) administered the same instruments to 864 high school students at two time points, 4–5 months apart. Moral disengagement was a weak positive predictor of doping intention (but not doping use), was positively linked to subjective norms and positive doping attitudes, and was inversely and strongly associated with doping self-regulatory efficacy. An interesting aspect of this study was the examination of interpersonal appraisals. Specifically, participants were presented with hypothetical scenarios in which they had to imagine themselves in a situation where someone (a peer, coach, instructor), advised or strongly encouraged them to use a doping substance. Then they indicated the likelihood they thought the counterpart in the scenario acted: (1) in the protagonist's interest and welfare (positive appraisal); (2) for his own personal interest (instrumental appraisal); or (3) to harm the protagonist (negative appraisal). They also indicated the likelihood they would do what the counterpart asked them to do if they were in that hypothetical situation (behavioral appraisal).

Across the two time points, moral disengagement was associated positively with the behavioral and positive appraisals and negatively – albeit weakly – with the instrumental and negative appraisals. The behavioral appraisal variable could be considered a proxy for doping as participants who indicated higher likelihood to dope should be at higher risk for doping. This link was strong and provides further evidence to suggest that moral disengagement plays an important role in facilitating doping (see also Boardley and Grix 2014; Boardley and Kavussanu 2011).

Finally, Lucidi *et al.* (2013) analysed data collected from 1,975 Italian high school students with characteristics very similar to those of Lucidi *et al.* (2008) and Zelli *et al.* (2010) and using the same instruments. Again, doping moral disengagement was positively associated with both doping intention and doping use, and its relationships with the other constructs were similar to those reported by Lucidi *et al.* (2008).

The studies by Lucidi and colleagues have several strengths: they employed impressively large samples; they were the first to apply moral disengagement to doping; they developed the first measure of doping moral disengagement; and most of them used a longitudinal design, which provides stronger evidence – than cross-sectional studies – about the direction of causality between variables. One weakness of this line of work is that many of the participants were not competing regularly in sport. Given that some items explicitly referred to sport performance, greater precision would have been achieved if all participants were athletes. Similarly, a very small percentage (1 to 3.1 percent) of the participants reported having used doping substances. Nevertheless, these studies made a significant contribution to the literature by identifying links between moral disengagement and doping intention as well as other variables within the Theory of Planned Behavior. It would be interesting to examine these variables in individuals who are at higher risk of doping, such as elite athletes, to determine whether the identified relationships are replicated.

Self-determination theory

One study has investigated the effects of moral disengagement on doping susceptibility along constructs of self-determination theory (Deci and Ryan 2002). This theory describes different types of motivation. Of particular relevance to moral disengagement and doping is controlled motivation, which occurs when individuals take part in sport for extrinsic reasons, for example to avoid feelings of shame or guilt, due to pressure from others, or for the extrinsic rewards associated with sport participation (Bartholomew *et al.* 2010). Athletes with controlled motivation strive for ego enhancement, fame, and extrinsic rewards (Deci and Ryan 2002, cited in Hodge *et al.* 2013). As their focus is on winning, which would allow them to achieve these goals, these athletes are more likely to morally disengage and use PEDs (Hodge *et al.* 2013). Indeed, controlled motivation has been positively associated with both moral disengagement (Hodge and Lonsdale 2011) and use of PEDs (Barkoukis *et al.* 2011) in past research. One precursor of controlled motivation is the controlling interpersonal style, which is evident when the coach acts in a coercive, pressuring, or authoritarian way (see Bartholomew *et al.* 2010).

Hodge and colleagues (2013) investigated moral disengagement as a mediator between controlling coach climate, controlled motivation, and doping attitudes and susceptibility. In a sample of 224 competitive athletes, including 81 elite athletes, Hodge *et al.* found that controlling coach climate (i.e., interpersonal style) positively predicted controlled motivation. Importantly, controlled motivation positively – albeit weakly – predicted moral disengagement, which, in turn, was a strong positive predictor of attitudes toward PEDs; the latter variable strongly and positively predicted drug-taking susceptibility (i.e., the amount of consideration athletes would give to using a banned PED). The link between controlled motivation and moral disengagement indicates that athletes who play sport for extrinsic reasons are at risk for morally disengaging; however, the effect was weak, suggesting that self-determination theory (Deci and Ryan 2002) may not be as useful as other theories (e.g., Ajzen 1991; Bandura 1991) in enhancing our understanding of doping behavior in sport. One limitation of this study is that the moral disengagement scale used (Boardley and Kavussanu 2008) was not specific to doping.

Social-cognitive theory

Moral disengagement mechanisms are described in the social-cognitive theory of moral thought and action (Bandura 1991) as the practices that enable individuals to transgress without experiencing negative affect. Kavussanu and colleagues (2014) tested this tenet of the theory in young elite football players ($n=345$). Participants completed the Moral Disengagement in Doping Scale (Kavussanu *et al.*, in review), and were presented with a scenario describing a hypothetical situation in which they had the opportunity to use a banned performance-enhancing substance. Then, they were asked to imagine themselves in the hypothetical situation and indicate the likelihood they would use the substance (doping intention), as well as their anticipated feelings of guilt, if they were to use the substance. Moral disengagement negatively predicted anticipated guilt, which in turn negatively predicted doping intention.

These findings support Bandura's (1991) theory that moral disengagement facilitates transgressive behavior by minimizing the negative affect associated with such behavior, and are consistent with previous research, which has also shown links between moral disengagement and anticipated guilt (Bandura *et al.* 1996; Stanger *et al.* 2013). Guilt is an important adaptive emotion that elicits reparative action. Feeling remorse about one's behavior means that the person is unlikely to repeat the behavior. Indeed, Kirby *et al.* (2011) in their interviews of elite athletes, who admitted doping, found that guilt was one of the most important deterrents of doping. Moral disengagement has the power to reduce this adaptive emotion thereby facilitating doping. Interestingly, moral disengagement also predicted doping intention independently of anticipated guilt (i.e., had a direct effect on doping intention), a finding that is consistent with previous research on both delinquent and antisocial behavior (Bandura *et al.* 1996; Stanger *et al.* 2013). Thus, moral disengagement is an important variable to consider in its own right.

Kavussanu *et al.* (2014) also investigated the conditions that could lead to moral disengagement, that is, its antecedents. Given that doping is a moral issue, performance climate (i.e., coaching behavior that highly values normative success), moral atmosphere (i.e., coach and teammates condoning doping), and moral identity (i.e., placing importance on being a moral person) were examined. This study indicated that performance climate and moral atmosphere positively predicted moral disengagement, whereas moral identity was a negative predictor of this construct. These findings highlight the significance of the team environment in which the athlete operates in facilitating moral disengagement and subsequent doping behavior. However, placing importance on being a moral person could suppress moral disengagement, thereby reducing its effects on doping. Although this study revealed some interesting findings, and is the first study to test Bandura's (1991) theory on doping, it is cross-sectional, which precludes firm conclusions about the direction of causality.

Moral disengagement and doping in bodybuilders

The studies reviewed so far used quantitative methods to examine moral disengagement. Recently, Boardley and his colleagues (Boardley and Grix 2014; Boardley *et al.* 2014) embarked on a venture of qualitative research of moral disengagement and doping. In two studies, they interviewed bodybuilders, a population whose main aim is to build muscle mass, and the use of doping substances can facilitate this aim. Research shows that there is greater prevalence of doping in athletes from sports that require high levels of physical strength such as bodybuilding (e.g., Thiblin and Petersson 2005); thus, understanding this population is important.

In the first study that examined moral disengagement in bodybuilders, Boardley and Grix (2014) conducted semi-structured interviews with 1 female and 8 male bodybuilders aged between 20 and 30 years. All participants were either using PEDs at the time of the interview or had used PEDs previously, but it is unknown whether they competed in sport. The interview protocol included open-ended and targeted questions centered on the eight mechanisms of moral disengagement. For example, a question used to explore moral justification was "do you think there are any ways in which you using PEDs can benefit others?" Content analysis was performed by applying operational definitions of the mechanisms on the data.

This analysis revealed that some mechanisms were clearly evident. For example, euphemistic labeling was evident when participants referred to PEDs as "juice" or "gear," thus they used sanitized language rather than calling them by their actual name. Diffusion of responsibility was also evident when participants felt that most bodybuilders dope, therefore it was okay for them to dope. The presence of bodybuilders in the training environment, who dope, was interpreted as creating pressure to use PEDs thereby enabling individuals to displace responsibility. It was stated that PEDs users did not encourage PEDs explicitly, but did so "by appearance, so maybe by someone looking at them and going 'yeah'" (Boardley and Grix 2014: 428). However, Bandura (2002) clearly refers to *social pressure* and the presence of an authority figure to whom responsibility for one's actions is displaced, and who is viewed as dictating harmful behavior: under displaced responsibility, people "view their actions as stemming from the dictates of authorities" (Bandura 2002: 106). In this study, more experienced bodybuilders (who could be seen as authority figures) did not explicitly encourage doping and were not perceived as putting explicit pressure on young bodybuilders to dope.

Boardley and Grix (2014) stated that advantageous comparison was evident when participants compared doping to other unhealthy practices, such as drinking alcohol or smoking. They also refer to evidence of moral justification when one participant indicated that if he tried the PEDs himself, he could give people feedback on it.

Boardley and Grix (2014) also interpreted some quotes as reflecting the distortion of consequences mechanism because participants downplayed the consequences of PEDs on their health and did not consider the psychological harm their potentially ill health in the future could cause to others who care about them. Although PEDs could have health consequences for the user, participants felt that, based on the research they did, if PEDs was done properly, it looked like it was okay and safe. Perhaps these bodybuilders did downplay the health consequences of doping, but it is also possible that they used substances in a manner that was not harmful to them (e.g., small quantities, not too frequently, etc). Psychological harm can be caused to others if a loved one's health deteriorates (Boardley and Grix 2014), but this assumes that their health will indeed deteriorate in the future, and participants have friends and family who truly care about them; this may not always be the case.

Boardley *et al.* (2014) extended this work to an impressive sample of 64 male bodybuilders, who had admitted using doping substances. They used the same approach as Boardley and Grix (2014) and reported similar findings. For example, professional bodybuilders mentioned that PEDs allowed them to financially support their family, thus they justified their behavior in pursuit of a valued social or moral purpose (moral justification); they pointed out that compared to alcohol and smoking, PEDs use is not that bad (advantageous comparison); they used the terms "juice" and "gear" to refer to PEDs (euphemistic labeling); and they felt that everybody uses PEDs, so it is okay to use them (diffusion of responsibility).

There was also more clear evidence of displacement of responsibility in this second study. For instance, the culture of bodybuilding whereby more experienced bodybuilders typically encourage new young bodybuilders to "maximize their potential" was interpreted as displacement of responsibility (Boardley *et al.* 2014). This mechanism was less clear in the quote "You see people doing what you want to do, and if you know that they are doing certain things [using PEDs], that's the route to get there … definitely," which was also interpreted as indicating displacement of responsibility (Boardley *et al.* 2014). Specifically, it is not clear from this quote to which authority figure bodybuilders displaced responsibility.

These two studies by Boardley and colleagues have provided interesting information regarding the way male (and one female) bodybuilders think about PEDs. An important strength of this work is the recruitment of participants, who were either current or past users of doping substances. However, some simply used PEDs in order to build muscle mass, and did not formally compete, thus they did not try to deceive others. It can be argued that these bodybuilders' behavior is similar to street drug users: it has the potential to cause harm *to them*, but not necessarily to others, a view that was shared by some participants (Boardley *et al.* 2014). Moral disengagement in individuals who use banned substances to build muscle mass (e.g., Boardley *et al.* 2014) or improve physical appearance (e.g., Lucidi *et al.* 2004, 2008) is somewhat different from the practices originally described by Bandura (1990, 1991, 1999, 2002), who has explicitly and repeatedly referred to the consequences of one's behavior *for others*. Even though PEDs are often illegal, their use by bodybuilders who do not compete, does not involve direct consequences for other people. Nevertheless, the two studies by Boardley and colleagues have provided interesting insights into the way bodybuilders think, and the moral disengagement mechanisms they use, and have undoubtedly enhanced our understanding of doping practices and justifications in this population.

Conclusion

In conclusion, moral disengagement has been positively associated with doping variables (i.e., doping intention, use, susceptibility, and attitudes), in several studies, using a variety of measures, samples, and designs. The evidence is clear that athletes who contemplate using doping substances are also prone to morally disengage. Importantly, moral disengagement may be a key mediator of the influence of both social environmental and personal variables, stemming from different theoretical perspectives, on doping behavior. That is, other factors may influence doping through their effects on moral disengagement. This underlines the need to include moral disengagement in interventions that are aimed at reducing doping in sport.

It is also important to note that although a variety of research designs have been used to date, experimental research is lacking. This means that the evidence for a *causal* relationship between moral disengagement and doping is not unequivocal. Longitudinal (e.g., Lucidi *et al.* 2008), cross-sectional (e.g., Hodge *et al.* 2013; Kavussanu *et al.* 2014), and qualitative (Boardley and Grix 2014; Boardley *et al.* 2014) studies have provided a good foundation for experiments and interventions to begin. For example, interventions that challenge moral disengagement practices in athletes who are tempted to dope could be promising in the fight against doping. The evidence outlined in this chapter is clear that intervening on moral disengagement has potential to reduce doping in sport.

References

Ajzen, I. (1991). The theory of planned behavior. *Organizational Behavior and Human Decision Processes, 50*, 179–211.
Bandura, A. (1986). *Social foundations of thought and action: A social cognitive theory.* Englewood Cliffs, NJ: Prentice-Hall.
Bandura, A. (1990). Selective activation and disengagement of moral control. *Journal of Social Issues, 46*, 27–46.
Bandura, A. (1991). Social cognitive theory of moral thought and action. In W. M. Kurtines and J. L. Gewirtz (eds.), *Handbook of moral behavior and development: Theory, research, and applications* (71–129). Hillsdale, NJ: Lawrence Erlbaum Associates, Inc.
Bandura, A. (1999). Moral disengagement in the perpetration of inhumanities. *Personality and Social Psychology Review, 3*, 193–209.
Bandura, A. (2002). Selective moral disengagement in the exercise of moral agency. *Journal of Moral Education, 31*, 101–119.
Bandura, A., Barbaranelli, C., Caprara, G. V., and Pastorelli, C. (1996). Mechanisms of moral disengagement in the exercise of moral agency. *Journal of Personality and Social Psychology, 71*, 364–374.
Barkoukis, V., Lazuras, L., Tsorbatzoudis, H., and Rodafinos, A. (2011). Motivational and sportspersonship profiles of elite athletes in relation to doping behavior. *Psychology of Sport and Exercise, 12*, 205–212.
Bartholomew, K. J., Ntoumanis, N., and Thogersen-Ntoumani, C. (2010). The controlling interpersonal style in a coaching context: Development and initial validation of a psychometric scale. *Journal of Sport and Exercise Psychology, 32*, 193–216.
Boardley, I. D. and Grix, J. (2014). Doping in bodybuilders: A qualitative investigation of facilitative psychosocial processes. *Qualitative Research in Sport, Exercise, and Health, 6* (3), 422–439.

Boardley, I. D. and Kavussanu, M. (2007). Development and validation of the moral disengagement in sport scale. *Journal of Sport and Exercise Psychology*, *29*, 608–628.

Boardley, I. D. and Kavussanu, M. (2008). The moral disengagement in sport scale short. *Journal of Sports Sciences*, *26*, 1507–1517.

Boardley, I. D. and Kavussanu, M. (2011). Moral disengagement in sport. *International Review of Sport and Exercise Psychology*, *4* (*2*), 93–108.

Boardley, I. D., Grix, J., and Dewar, A. J. (2014). Moral disengagement and associated processes in performance enhancing drug use: A national qualitative investigation. *Journal of Sports Sciences*, *32*, 836–844.

d'Arripe-Longueville, F., Corrion, K., Scoffier, S., Roussel, P., and Chalabaev, A. (2010). Sociocognitive self-regulatory mechanisms governing judgments of the acceptability and likelihood of sport cheating. *Journal of Sport and Exercise Psychology*, *32*, 595–618.

Deci, E. L. and Ryan, R. M. (2002). *Handbook of self-determination research*. Rochester, NY: University of Rochester Press.

Hodge, K. and Lonsdale, C. (2011). Prosocial and antisocial behavior in sport: The role of coaching style, autonomous vs. controlled motivation, and moral disengagement. *Journal of Sport and Exercise Psychology*, *33*, 527–547.

Hodge, K., Hargreaves, E. A., Gerrard, D., and Lonsdale, C. (2013). Psychological mechanisms underlying doping attitudes in sport: Motivation and moral disengagement. *Journal of Sport and Exercise Psychology*, *35*, 419–432.

Kavussanu, M., Stanger, N., and Boardley, I. D. (2013). The Prosocial and Antisocial Behavior in Sport Scale: Further evidence for construct validity and reliability. *Journal of Sports Sciences*, *31*, 1208–1221.

Kavussanu, M., Ring, C., Saunders, E., Hatzigeorgiadis, A., and Elbe, A. M. (2014). *Socio-moral predictors of doping intentions in football: The mediating role of moral disengagement and anticipated guilt*. Paper presented at the Fifth International Sport Psychology Conference, University of Sophia-Antipolis, Nice.

Kirby, K., Moran, A., and Guerin, S. (2011). A qualitative analysis of the experiences of elite athletes who have admitted to doping for performance enhancement. *International Journal of Sport Policy and Politics 3*, 205–224.

Lucidi, F., Zelli, A., and Mallia, L. (2013). The contribution of moral disengagement to adolescents' use of doping substances. *International Journal of Sport Psychology*, *44*, 331–350.

Lucidi, F., Grano, C., Leone, L., Lombardo, C., and Pesce, C. (2004). Determinants of the intention to use doping substances: An empirical contribution in a sample of Italian adolescents. *International Journal of Sport Psychology*, *35*, 133148.

Lucidi, F., Zelli, A., Mallia, L., Brand, R., Tsorbatzoudis, H., and Barkoukis, V. (2014). *A European analysis of young team athletes' beliefs about doping and appraisals of others encouraging substance use*. Report submitted to World Anti-Doping Agency.

Lucidi, F., Zelli, A., Mallia, L., Grano, C., Russo, P. M., and Violani, C. (2008). The social cognitive mechanisms regulating adolescents' use of doping substances. *Journal of Sports Sciences*, *26*, 447–456.

Ntoumanis, N., Ng, J. Y., Barkoukis, V., and Backhouse, S. (2014). Personal and psychosocial predictors of doping use in physical activity settings: A meta-analysis. *Sports Medicine*, *44* (*11*), 1603–1624.

Stanger, N., Kavussanu, M., Boardley, I. D., and Ring, C. (2013). The influence of moral disengagement and negative emotion on antisocial sport behavior. *Sport, Exercise and Performance Psychology*, *2*, 117–129.

Thiblin, I. and Petersson, A. (2005). Pharmacoepidemiology of anabolic androgenic steroids: A review. *Fundamental and Clinical Pharmacology, 19,* 27–44.

Traclet, A., Romand, P., Moret, O., and Kavussanu, M. (2011). Antisocial behavior in soccer: A qualitative study of moral disengagement. *International Journal of Sport and Exercise Psychology, 9 (2),* 143–155.

Zelli, A., Mallia, L., and Lucidi, F. (2010). The contribution of interpersonal appraisals to a social-cognitive analysis of adolescents' doping use. *Psychology of Sport and Exercise, 11,* 304–311.

12 Ethical dilemma training – a new approach to doping prevention?

Anne-Marie Elbe and Ralf Brand

Many moral and ethical values are ascribed to sport due to the fact that it is rule-based (e.g., Alderson and Crutchley 1990). Consequently, sport is often seen as the embodiment of ethical behavior (McFee 1998). This idealistic ascribing of moral meaning to sport is called *sport ethos* (Kuchler 1969). In many cases the terms "morality" and "ethics" are used interchangeably as they both refer to behavior that is judged as being either "right" or "wrong." Morality refers to personal principles created and upheld by the individuals themselves. An individual's moral code is usually stable and consistent across contexts but can change if the individual has a radical change in personal beliefs and/or values. Ethics are external standards, provided by institutions, groups, or a culture to which an individual belongs. Ethics are very consistent within a certain context but can vary greatly between contexts. Today ethics often refers to the systematic study of morality. In this chapter we will discuss moral development in sport, the relevance of moral reasoning for anti-doping prevention, and we will present novel findings from a training program aiming to increase young athletes' moral reasoning in order to prevent doping.

Ethical issues in sports

The realm of sport is closely tied to ethical questions, due to the fact that human behavior in sport is characterized by the interaction with other individuals (McFee 1998). However, a meaningful discussion of morality and ethics in sports can take place only by carefully analyzing the term "sport" (Steenbergen and Tamboer 1998). The idea of limitless achievement present in sport poses many ethical and moral questions. As McFee (1998: 5) points out, "ethical issues arise ... from the nature of sport." Franke (1978) describes sport as "a world in itself" due to two opposing principles: on the one hand, athletes have to defeat their opponents, while, on the other hand, they should show utmost fairness. Franke (1988) states this as a "system of immanent tension" (cited in Steenbergen and Tamboer 1998: 36). The question arises as to what degree a balance between these opposing principles can exist in modern sport.

Concepts such as *fair play*, *playing by the rules* and *sportspersonship*, have been associated with morality in sport and can be seen as characterizations of behaviors that might orient athletes in their efforts to cope with these sport-immanent tensions. The psychological construct of *sportspersonship* broadly refers to a sportsperson's understanding of, and respect for, the rules, rituals, and traditions of sports, as well as to the ability to distinguish between good and bad practices in sports (Siedentop *et al.* 2004). According to Ommundsen *et al.* (2003), examples of sportspersonship exist when athletes avoid taking an unfair advantage over an opponent, when they play fairly according to the rules, and when they try to play well.

Considering the aspirations connected with this idea of sportspersonship, it is not surprising that the occurrence of unethical behavior weighs even more heavily because it attacks sport's innermost values. Ethical problems addressed in relation to sports are, for example, those of equity, access to sports, deviant subcultures and behaviors, or exploitation (Morgan 2007). In sports, the ethics discourse is associated with the discipline of sports philosophy and refers to the study of ethically problematic behavior, persons, or policies. Doping in sports, which can be categorized as a deviant behavior, is a topic that has thus received increased interest from sport philosophy. Doping can be seen as a phenomenon conflicting with the values of sport since consumption of banned performance-enhancing substances or the use of a forbidden method in order to win or defeat an opponent goes against the rule of fairness and creates an unlevel playing field. Sports ethics sees its most urgent task in presenting problem-focused solutions for the doping discussion (Pawlenka 2004). Ethical considerations about the use of performance-enhancing substances in sport are widely discussed (see Bockrath and Franke 1995; Hemphill 2009; Volkwein 1995). Schneider and Butcher (2000) categorize the arguments on doping under four headings: cheating and unfairness, harm, perversion of sport, and unnaturalness and dehumanization.

Development of moral behavior in sports

Given that ethical issues are related to the consumption of illegal performance-enhancing substances, the question arises how an athlete's sense of what is right and wrong in sports develops. The *sport ethos* alone does not guarantee that athletes will show moral behavior. A close connection between sport participation and moral development has only weak empirical support (Kavussanu and Ntoumanis 2003). In general, sport does not automatically turn individuals into moral people. In contrast, unethical behavior seems to be even more accepted in sports than in daily life (Bredemeier and Shields 1984). For example, Long *et al.* (2006) showed that athletes view rule transgression as a legitimate tactical method. As a possible explanation for this behavior, athletes state the desire to win and consider forms of "modest" rule violation as part of the game (see Pilz 1995). Consequently, sport will contribute to the moral development of children and young adults only to a certain degree. In general, ethical and moral behavior can be learned only in a more general societal context. Sport represents only one subcontext in which ethical values and principles can be taught and sport can facilitate their acceptance. It is therefore important to understand how moral reasoning principally develops in individuals in order to understand how morality can be developed in the sport context.

Moral development

Following Piaget (1932) moral development occurs in line with a child's general cognitive development that evolves with age. Children develop from an *amoral stage* to a stage of *simple moral realism*. In this stage children believe that everything that is not punished is allowed, and everything that is punished is not allowed. In the following *heteronomous stage* of morality (around the ages of four to eight years) children's moral beliefs are based on relations of constraints. Morality is seen as something predetermined by others, and everything that others accept is allowed, and what others do not accept is not permitted. The final stage, the *autonomous morality stage* (after about nine years of age) occurs when morality is perceived as something based on relations to others and something that can be negotiated through mutual agreement with others.

Lawrence Kohlberg built on Piaget's theory, but in contrast to it, Kohlberg (1964) identified six developmental stages, which are divided into three levels. Each of the stages allows for a more sophisticated moral behavior than the preceding one. The tempo of ascending these stages, or whether (especially higher) stages are reached at all, differs from individual to individual. In contrast to Piaget, Kohlberg describes moral development as something very individual and not as something that automatically develops in line with general cognitive development. Kohlberg's three levels are *pre-conventional*, *conventional* and *post-conventional morality*. The two stages of the pre-conventional level focus on obedience and punishment as well as on individualism and exchange. In these stages, which mainly pertain to children, rules are seen as fixed absolutes and obeying them is a way to avoid punishment. In the second stage of the pre-conventional level, actions are judged on how they serve individual needs. In the second level (the conventional morality level) others and society play a more important role. The individual focuses more on living up to society's expectations, doing one's duty and respecting authority. The focus is on following the rules in order to maintain law and order. In the final level of post-conventional morality, one allows for differing values, beliefs, and opinions. In the final stage, moral reasoning is based on abstraction, applying universal ethical principles.

Ethical dilemmas

Kohlberg used these different stages as a basis for assessing an individual's level of moral reasoning. His assessment method is to let individuals discuss ethical dilemmas, the most famous being the "Heinz dilemma." This dilemma describes a situation in which a husband contemplates stealing expensive cancer medicine in order to save his wife's life. He feels compelled to steal the medicine because he does not have the financial resources to buy the medicine, while time for his wife is running out. Kohlberg uses the individual's level of sophistication in discussing this situation to determine into which of the six distinct stages a person belongs. Following this rationale of discussing ethical dilemmas, Blatt (1969) and Lind (2009) used this method not only for categorizing an individual's level of moral development, but also as a tool to promote the development of moral skills. Blatt (1969) focused on the dialog of "for and against" (cf. Blatt and Kohlberg 1975). Decades later Lind (2009) developed a comprehensive method in order to train moral abilities. The effectiveness of dilemma discussions for enhancing moral skills, for example, has been shown in the business context (e.g., Lerkiatbundit *et al.* 2006).

In the past, the dilemma technique has also been used in several studies to determine athletes' moral views. The most widely used dilemma in relation to doping in sports is the Goldman dilemma. It raises the question whether or not athletes would take a drug that would guarantee them an Olympic medal but would result in their death in five years' time (Connor *et al.* 2013; Goldman *et al.* 1984). The Goldman dilemma was applied to investigate athletes' moral views, but dilemmas like this were not used in a way to enhance moral skills as proposed by Lind, for example, or as previously applied in the business context.

Promoting ethical behavior with regard to doping

In the past, the most common procedure to ensure that athletes adhere to anti-doping regulation has been that of regular doping controls and punishments for positive tests (*detection and deterrence approach*, Houlihan 2002). For more than ten years organizational structures and standard operating procedures have been in place to ensure compliance with the anti-doping regulations as stated in the Code of the World Anti-Doping Agency (WADA 2009). The underlying assumption is that the detection and deterrence approach might indirectly promote athletes' ethical behavior.

There are, however, several indicators that speak against the practice of the detection and deterrence policy. This practice is very costly due to the large number of controls that have to be conducted and also due to the constant development of new technologies to account for newly developed drugs and methods (Trout and Kazlauskas 2004). Furthermore, there are banned substances for which no tests are available. Haugen (2004) argues that in order to make testing effective as a deterrence method, either the volume of tests conducted or the sanctions imposed has to be increased significantly, potentially to the level that doing so becomes practically unfeasible. Furthermore, Overbye *et al.*'s (2014) study suggests that social and self-imposed (moral) sanctions have a stronger deterring effect than the legal banning from sports for Danish elite athletes.

Therefore more recent approaches to combatting doping in sports have focused on the *educational approach*. Within this approach educational tools are utilized to educate young athletes so that they do not use performance-enhancing drugs. The most common education approach in the past has been of a knowledge-based approach (Hanson 2009; Backhouse *et al.* 2009). The basic idea behind such an approach is that if there is enough information on the risks and dangers of the deviant behavior, then contradictory intentions will be formed and the respective behavior will recede. With respect to the field of anti-doping this means that information about what doping is, that it is forbidden, and that it is unhealthy is presented to the athletes. The focus of many prevention programs seems to be mainly on conveying necessary knowledge which is then expected to lead to changes in doping attitudes and/or decrease the intention to dope (e.g., Goldberg *et al.* 2000; Laure and Lecerf 2002). The underlying assumption is that promotion of knowledge, similar to the detection and deterrence approach, could indirectly lead to enhancing athletes' ethical behavior. However, these and some other doping prevention programs, which have been shown to be only partly effective (for a review see Backhouse *et al.* 2009), are criticized for a number of reasons. These programs have been shown to enhance knowledge about doping, but empirical studies have overwhelmingly illustrated that simple knowledge transfer is not enough (Laure & Lecerf 1999, 2002). Hanson (2009) points out that it is insufficient to focus merely on teaching if one wants to change behavior. Traditional ways of educating about the negative effects of doping produce knowledge is difficult to apply when the actual situation arises. Furthermore, decisions to dope are sometimes characterized by spontaneous and weakly evaluated cognitive processes (Petróczi *et al.* 2008). The majority of prevention programs might thus be following a suboptimal approach when assuming that doping is always a forecasted and rational or even "planned" action (Ajzen 1991). Abstract knowledge, for example of its health dangers or ethical caveats, might form a basis for an athlete's decision, but it is not sufficient by itself to prevent doping.

Following Backhouse *et al.* (2009), the optimal prevention program, according to modern standards, should be a mixture of conveying knowledge, skills, and adequate affection (values, self-awareness, and self-worth). Singler and Treutlein (2010) define these skills as observing, reflecting, deciding, and acting. They further state that a good prevention program should not take a moral high ground with the participant(s) nor try to convince them by inducing fear. It should, instead, "empower" the existing resources and competencies of the young adult (Singler 2011). Louveau *et al.* (1995) propose including the discussion of opposing arguments in a prevention program in order to foster the development of one's own opinion. Hanson (2009) suggests that interventions should be designed to question the validity of athletes' existing beliefs. Prevention programs should therefore aim at changing cognitive structures to incorporate interpersonal control processes that are deeply rooted in one's own subjective disposition.

Training ethical decision-making in sports

This is where our approach of discussing ethical dilemmas comes into play. Respective interventions have to step away from mere knowledge building, but focus the trainees' skills in making *ethical decisions* with regard to concrete situations related to doping behavior. Our method uses the dilemma discussion technique as its theoretical background. Based on the proposed concepts of Blatt,

Kohlberg, and Lind, we developed a training program geared toward doping prevention in sports, as part of a WADA-funded social science research project (Elbe and Brand 2013).

The basis of this *ethical decision-making training program* is the dilemma technique in which participants have to tackle different sport-specific dilemma situations related to doping. The athletes are confronted with specific ethical dilemma situations which they have to contemplate and need to find a "solution" to. The idea is not to focus on the learning of rules but to actively involve participants by letting them re-enact difficult situations that require them to make their own, however subjectively well-founded, decision. It is expected that this method furthers the development of a personal, value-based conviction toward doping. Following Barry's (1979) analytical framework for ethical decision-making, our participants are confronted with pro-doping and contra-doping arguments (and/or have to produce their own) that focus on specific ethical principles, connected with sports-related (sub)culturally determined rules or norms (for a review see Gandz and Hayes 1988).

Empirical investigation of an anti-doping ethical decision-making program

Elbe and Brand's study (2014) aimed at establishing and evaluating the effectiveness of a training program to enhance athletes' ethical anti-doping decision-making skills. The underlying assumption was that the process of cognitive appraisal and the evaluation of supporting and opposing arguments require strong mental skills and capacities that may not be intuitively available. Moral abilities require a process of intensive learning and training (cf. Wright 1995; Lind 2009), which is enforced by the constant confrontation with everyday ethical problems. The innovative aspect of this training program, for which more detailed information can be retrieved from the report published on the WADA website (Elbe and Brand 2013), is that the program is geared toward suggesting to the athlete that knowledge, ethics, or rules will not release an athlete from making his/her own "right" decisions. So, during the course of this training, athletes are confronted with very challenging scenarios in which they might even make a decision that involves taking illegal substances. These decisions, which might involve deviant behavior, are not corrected but are instead intended to show the athlete how difficult some situations can be. The underlying assumption of the program is that athletes, through being confronted with these scenarios, are reminded of the *sport ethos* and, possibly, after a phase of deliberation, will remember to adhere to it. The program deliberately does not take a moral high ground or try to influence the athletes to decide in a certain way. The program design further suggests that one believes in the athletes and does not patronize them. It is assumed that by designing the program in this way rather than prescribing what "wrong" and what "right" behavior is, one can instill confidence, promote self-determination, empower existing resources, and motivate athletes to refrain from doping.

Participants, intervention, study design

Sixty-nine young elite athletes (34 male, 35 female; 15.5±2.4 years old) were recruited for participation in our first attempt to empirically evaluate this training's outcomes. The study was performed in a controlled pre- and post-measurement design (two-week interval). Participants were randomly assigned into either an ethical decision-making training group or to a comparison group, in which a standard anti-doping education program was completed (knowledge-based approach). Participants in the no-treatment control group were recruited separately and not allocated randomly. Training as well as measurement of the dependent variables was conducted in a fully automated online setup. Participants began the study by (1) logging into the pre-test; (2) completing the informed consent form; and (3) completing the tests for measuring the dependent variables. In step 4 participants were randomly assigned to one of the two experimental conditions: ethical training (ET) or knowledge training (KT). The ethical training entailed six sessions with three dilemmas each. All dilemmas dealt with fictitious young athletes in the early stage of their careers. Each of the six training sessions included one dilemma focusing on a female athlete, one on a male athlete, and one on a social group (e.g. team, athlete and coach, athlete and parent, athlete and physiotherapist, etc.). The 18 dilemmas were equal in length (5–10 sentences). An example of a dilemma and a screenshot is presented in Figure 12.1. Each session entailed tasks of varying difficulty in order to motivate sustained attention. Tasks included in each individual session were (1) reading the dilemma; (2) making a decision; (3) creating individual arguments; and (4) ordering them according to one's own liking. There was a progression in the six training sessions concerning (1) increasing difficulty of task; (2) increasing complexity of arguments; and (3) increasing density of difficult tasks.

The knowledge-based approach, which was also comprised of six training sessions, contained six different parts that were each split into two subsections: (1) introduction (famous doping cases & FAQs about doping); (2) precursors and consequences of doping; (3) forbidden substances and methods; (4) the doping control system (introduction to the control system and doping control procedure); (5) law, duty, and punishment (law and punishment and personal rights and duties); and (6) anti-doping on the Internet (NADO online and other anti-doping pages). The structure and content of this training were based on the German NADO's High-Five Program (NADA 2010). In order to encourage reading and processing of the information, brief knowledge rehearsals were conducted at the end of every subsection.

Separate from this study, the effects of an additional combined training (CT) group were explored. This group received a combination of the ET and KT. This combined training (pre-test, six training sessions, post-test) was made up of Training Session 1 from the knowledge training (KT-1; Introduction to doping), followed by Session 1 as presented to the ethical training group (ET-1; three dilemmas), followed by the KT-session on forbidden substances and methods, ET Session 2 (three dilemmas), the KT session on the idea and procedures of the

Murat is one of the top talents in the minor league. From time to time he is nominated for the national U-16 squad. By now, almost every weekend in the year he has got a game or a training camp. Murat does not want to abandon his home club so he plays in all the games of the season. He feels close to his friends in the club, but he also wants to take his chances in the national team and so he wants to go through with both. However, the tight schedule is getting to him. There is little time to recover between events and going on vacation is almost impossible due to the long journeys, the training camp or the games for his home club.
Similarly, some of the other players of the national team suffer from the practice load. One team member suggests taking a substance that increases the rate of recovery. Murat begins to think.

(1) Would you take the substance?

◯ Yes. ⦿ No.

(2) Now please write down as many arguments as possible (to a maximum of 6) that support your decision. If the space is insufficient, just continue in the next row.

Murat should not take the substance, because ...

1) ... | If he can't adjust, he is not strong enough. Doping won't change that.
2) ... | Why trust a teammate so easily?
3) ... | His teammate might not know what he is talking about.
4) ... | This will only postpone a decision between career and friends.
5) ... | He could try something else first. Altered nutrition for example.
6) ... | He's in the national team, not some circus show.

(3) Once more, here are your arguments, which you are now supposed to rank; those that you like the most go on the top, those that you like the least go on the bottom. Drag the arguments (keep the left mouse button pushed) from left to right. If needed, you can rearrange the arguments within the blue box.

BEST ARGUMENT

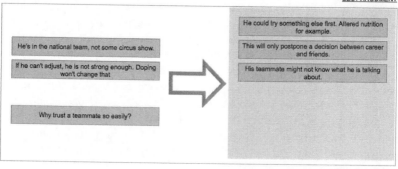

WORST ARGUMENT

Figure 12.1 Example of a dilemma used in the training.

doping control system, and a final session of ethical decision-making training (ET-3; three dilemmas). All other aspects of the training were identical to the trainings described in the previous sections.

The main variable used in these investigations to assess the effect of the training programs was a shortened version of the Performance Enhancement Attitude Scale (PEAS; Petróczi and Aidman 2009). Positive doping attitudes, which have been shown to be the strongest predictors of the intention to dope (Tsorbatzoudis 2009), seem to reflect the prevalence of doping better than results taken from doping controls (Striegel *et al.* 2010). In this study's sample, before the intervention, the mean score of this 6-item PEAS version was 8.77 (*SD*=3.68), with a theoretical scale range from 6 to 36. The higher the score, the more positive an athlete's doping attitude was. The internal consistency of this short scale was $\alpha=0.70$.

Results

Prior to, as well as after, the intervention, the mean doping attitudes of the young athletes were low to very low, indicating that doping was evaluated negatively in all groups (ET, KT, CG, and CT). Multivariate Analyses of Variance showed a significant omnibus effect (Elbe and Brand 2014). *Post hoc* contrast analyses revealed a significant yet marginal increase (+2.6 scoring points on average) in the doping attitude in the ethical training group (ET), compared with the control group (CG). All other contrasts did not show statistical significance. This gives evidence that an intervention effect was not reached in either the knowledge-based treatment (KT) or in the control (CG) or combined training group (CT).

Discussion

The project results were not in line with the assumption that the ethical decision-making training would decrease positive attitudes toward doping. Instead the study showed a significant effect in the opposite direction than what was expected, i.e., an unexpected increase in PEAS doping attitude scores. No significant findings were revealed for the other groups, i.e., PEAS scores remained unchanged in athletes that participated either in the standard educational program, the combined training, or in the control group, showing no respective changes. Despite the increased PEAS values in the ethical decision-making training group all measured scores remained very low and indicated that participants strongly renounced doping, i.e., showed a clear anti-doping attitude.

These results allow the interpretation that the athletes' stereotypical answering behavior has changed (only) in the ethical decision-making group. One explanation is that through the decision-making training with doping related dilemma situations, the athletes have become aware that doping is not a clear "yes" or "no" issue but that many factors influence one's pro or contra decisions when reality becomes more complex. In the light of this interpretation these results also suggest that the athletes have further developed their own opinions by questioning the validity of their prior beliefs. This is primarily supported by standardized interviews we conducted with some of the participants after the completion of the training. One participant stated:

> I had to think about things and find my own answer to doping.... I liked that I had to make up my own mind about what was good and bad and that I had to express this in my own words ... plus, I did not have to accept someone else's opinion but had to decide for myself. Now I have my own opinion about doping.

This statement can be interpreted as that the athletes, after having completed the ethical decision-making training, are better prepared if/when they encounter a realistic dilemma situation.

The combined training, which included three ethical training sessions, showed no effect. It can be assumed that the number of sessions was too low to achieve an effect. In conclusion it can be stated that this study was a first empirical investigation on the effects of a doping-related ethical decision-making training to a sample of young elite athletes, which in some ways still had pilot-study character.

Practical implications and directions for future research

The results from our first application of this ethical decision-making training program offer the opportunity to deduct practical recommendations as well as to suggest ideas for future research. A surprising aspect of the results is that these were achieved in a training program that was conducted entirely online. Online training is not an optimal learning environment. This setting does not offer the trainees opportunities to interact with an instructor (or, for example, peers), and all information, tasks, and instructions are presented in written form. This requires a lot of self-control and disciplined self-study by the participants; all skills need to be acquired alone by the athletes themselves. On the other hand, an online learning tool is very convenient for athletes as they can access it from anywhere and at any time that suits their busy schedules. Future research, therefore, should investigate whether or not training effects would change if online training was supplemented by real-life interactions with a teacher or coach. Regarding that, we developed a training handbook for teachers and coaches[1] which includes exercises and training examples for the classroom and athletic training settings in elite sport (Brand *et al.* 2012). This manual is currently available only in German but could easily be translated into further additional languages, making it available to a larger population of teachers and coaches.

Further, the ethical decision-making training could be integrated into already existing prevention measures and campaigns of national anti-doping organizations. The ethical dilemmas and related exercises are currently available in German and English; a Greek version is in preparation. An advantage of translation into additional languages is that further empirical testing of the effectiveness of the training program could be conducted. Furthermore, the developed handbook (Brand *et al.* 2012) gives many examples of activities and exercises that can be easily integrated into the athletes' daily training. It can also form a solid basis from which teachers and coaches could be further educated.

The described program represents an alternative concept of doping prevention interventions. Results from the empirical study have to be interpreted with caution. There are several limitations, for example, with regard to the chosen sample size and cell distributions. Nevertheless, we believe that the training program itself is a step in the right direction; it has the potential to at least inspire future educational anti-doping programs. We therefore encourage replications of this preliminary effect study, using larger and more diverse samples. Further studies could also investigate whether or not effects can be achieved with shorter or fewer training sessions since the intervention poses demands on the athletes' limited free time (six sessions of about 30 minutes). A general limitation, not only of the study described above, is the fact that a direct measure of doping attitude was included. Self-report questionnaires, however, might be affected by strategical responding. We recommend that future studies co-include measures of implicit attitude (Brand *et al.* 2014a; Brand *et al.* 2014b; Petróczi *et al.* 2008; Petróczi *et al.* 2011) and, for example, employ objective criteria for sampling participants with more significant prevention requirements (Musshoff *et al.* 2006). Finally, we recommend including follow-up katamnestic investigations of mid- and long-term training effects, for example, after six months or a year.

Conclusion

Ethical decision-making training is a new form of an educational approach to doping prevention. In comparison to the predominant knowledge-based educational anti-doping programs, it does not patronize athletes by prescribing what right and wrong doping-related behavior is. Instead, this training program places athletes in a situation in which they need to make and substantiate their own decisions according to their own level of moral reasoning. The decisions they make are left unjudged. By designing the program in this way, the athletes' individual moral resources can be strengthened. This chapter explained the relevance of moral reasoning for anti-doping prevention and demonstrated how the idea of training ethical skills can be implemented in an educational anti-doping approach and how it can be applied to practice. As presented, our training program is still at the beginning. It is our hope that future studies will be able to further investigate the effects of this training concept and elaborate on our initial empirical findings.

In conclusion, our suggestion is not to discontinue already established programs that focus on promoting knowledge about doping, but to complement them with actual training of *skills*. This chapter gives an example of how morality and a specific related skill (ethical reasoning) can be trained. Future research needs to show how this training can be used to enhance existing programs and how it can contribute to a sustainable success of prevention programs.

Note

1 This part of the project was funded by the Federal Institute of Sport Science, Germany (IIA1–080306/10–11).

References

Ajzen, I. (1991). The theory of planned behaviour. *Organizational Behaviour and Human Decision Processes*, *50*, 179–211.

Alderson, J. and Crutchley, D. (1990). Physical education and the national curriculum. In N. Armstrong (ed.), *New directions in physical education* (37–62). Champaign, IL: Human Kinetics.

Backhouse, S., McKenna, J., and Patterson, L. (2009). *Prevention through education: A review of current international social science literature*. Montreal, Canada: World Anti-Doping Agency.

Barry, V. (1979). *Moral issues in business*. Belmont, CA: Wadsworth.

Blatt, M. M. (1969). *The effects of classroom discussion upon children's level of moral reasoning* (unpublished doctoral dissertation). University of Chicago.

Blatt, M. M. and Kohlberg, L. (1975). The effect of classroom moral discussion upon children's level of moral judgment. *Journal of Moral Education*, *4*, 129–161.

Bockrath, F. and Franke, E. (1995). Is there any value in sports? About the ethical signifi-cance of sport activities. *International Review for the Sociology of Sport*, *30* (*3–4*), 283–310.

Brand, R., Heck, P., and Ziegler, M. (2014a). Illegal performance enhancing drugs and doping in sport: A picture-based brief implicit association test for measuring athletes' attitudes. *Substance Abuse Treatment, Prevention, and Policy*, *9* (*7*). doi: 10.1186/1747–597X-9–7.

Brand, R., Wolff, W., and Thieme, D. (2014b). Using response-time latencies to measure athletes' doping attitudes: The brief implicit attitude test identifies substance abuse in bodybuilders. *Substance Abuse Treatment, Prevention, and Policy*, *9* (*36*). doi:10.1186/1747–597X-9–36.

Brand, R., Berding, A., Schlegel, M., and Elbe, A.-M. (2012). Doping – soll ich oder soll ich nicht? Ethiktraining für Sportler, Trainer und Lehrer [Doping – should I or shouldn't I? Ethical training for athletes, coaches, and teachers]. Stuttgart: NeuerSportverlag.

Bredemeier, B. J. and Shields, D. L. (1984). Divergence in moral reasoning about sport and life. *Sociology of Sport Journal*, *1*, 348–357.

Connor, J., Mazanov, J., and Woolf, J. (2013). Would they dope? Revisiting the Goldman dilemma. *British Journal of Sports Medicine*, *47* (*11*), 697–700.

Elbe, A.-M. and Brand, R. (2013). Being a fair sportsman: Ethical decision making as a chance for doping prevention? Final Report for the World Anti-Doping Agency Social Science Research Grant (2008–2011). Available at www.wada-ama.org/Documents/Education_Awareness/SocialScienceResearch/Funded_Research_Projects/2008/ELBE%20-%20%282008%29%20Final_report.pdf.

Elbe, A.-M. and Brand, R. (2014). The effect of an ethical decision-making training on young athletes' attitudes towards doping. *Ethics and Behavior*. doi: 10.1080/10508422.2014.976864.

Franke, E. (1978). *Theorie und Bedeutung sportlicher Handlungen. Voraussetzungen und Möglichkeiten einer Sporttheorie aus handlungstheoretischer Sicht* [Theory and meaning of sport actions – Conditions and possibilities of a sport theory from an action-theoretical perspective]. Schorndorf, Germany: Hofmann.

Franke, E. (1988). *Ethische Aspekte des Leistungssports* [Ethical aspects of high-performance sport]. Clausthal-Zellerfeld, Germany: Deutsche Vereinigung für Sportwissenschaft.

Gandz, J. and Hayes, N. (1988). Teaching business ethics. *Journal of Business Ethics*, 7, 657–669.

Goldberg, L., MacKinnon, D. P., Elliot, D., Moe, E., Clarke, G., and Cheong, J. (2000). The adolescents training and learning to avoid steroids program: Preventing drug use and promoting health behaviors. *Archives of Pediatric and Adolescent Medicine*, 154, 332–338.

Goldman, B., Bush, P. J., and Klatz, R. (1984). *Death in the locker room: Steroids and sports*. South Bend, IN: Icarus Press.

Hanson, J. M. (2009). Equipping athletes to make informed decisions about performance-enhancing drug use: A constructivist perspective from educational psychology. *Sport in Society*, 12, 394–410.

Haugen, K. K. (2004). The performance-enhancing drug game. *Journal of Sports Economics*, 5 (5), 67–86.

Hemphill, D. (2009). Performance enhancement and drug control in sport: Ethical considerations. *Sport in Society*, 12 (3), 313–326.

Houlihan, B. (2002). Managing compliance in international anti-doping policy: The world anti-doping code. *European Sport Management Quarterly*, 2, 188–208.

Kavussanu, M. and Ntoumanis, N. (2003). Participation in sport and moral functioning: Does ego orientation mediate their relationship? *Journal of Sport and Exercise Psychology*, 25 (4), 1–18.

Kohlberg, L. (1964). Development of moral character and moral ideology. In M. L. Hoffman and L. W. Hoffman (eds.), *Review of child development research*, (381–431). New York: Russel Sage Foundation.

Kuchler, W. (1969). *Sportethos. Eine moraltheologische Untersuchung des im Lebensbereich Sport lebendigen Ethos als Beitrag zu einer Phänomenologie der Ethosformen* [Sportethos. A moral-theological investigation of the Ethos alive in sport as a contribution to a phenomenology of Ethos forms]. München: Barth.

Laure, P. and Lecerf, T. (1999). Prevention of doping in sport in adolescents: Evaluation of a health education based intervention. *Archive Pediatrics*, 6, 848–854.

Laure, P. and Lecerf, T. (2002). Doping prevention among young athletes: Comparison of a health education-based intervention versus information-based intervention. *Science and Sports*, 17, 198–201.

Lerkiatbundit, S., Utaipan, P., Laohawiriyanon, C., and Teo, A. (2006). Randomized controlled study of the impact of the Konstanz method of dilemma discussion on moral judgment. *Journal of Allied Health*, 35, 101–108.

Lind, G. (2009). *Moral ist lehrbar. Handbuch zur Theorie und Praxis moralischer und demokratischer Bildung* [Morality can be taught. Handbook on theory and practice of moral and democratic education]. München: Oldenbourg.

Long, T., Pantaléon, N., Bruant, G., and d'Arripe-Longueville, F. (2006). A qualitative study of moral reasoning of young elite athletes. *The Sport Psychologist*, 20, 330–347.

Louveau, C., Augustini, M., Duret, P., Irlinger, P., and Marcellini, A. (1995). *Dopage et performance sportive. Analyse d'une pratique prohibée* [Doping and Sports. Analysis of a prohibited practice]. Paris: INSEP-Publications.

McFee, G. (1998). Are there philosophical issues in respect of sport (other than ethical ones)? In M. J. McNamee and S. J. Parry (eds.), *Ethics and sport* (3–18). London: Routledge.

Morgan, W. J. (2007). *Ethics in Sport*. Champaign, IL: Human Kinetics.

Musshoff, F., Driever, F., Lachenmeier, K., Lachenmeier, D. W., and Banger, M. (2006). Results of hair analyses for drugs of abuse and comparison with self-reports and urine tests. *Forensic Science International, 156 (2–3)*,118–123.

NADA (2010). *High Five. Gemeinsam gegen Doping – Ein Ratgeber für junge Sportlerinnen und Sportler* [High Five. Together against doping. A guide for young athletes]. Bonn: NADA.

Ommundsen, Y., Roberts, G. C., Lemyre, P. N., and Treasure, D. (2003). Perceived motivational climate in male youth soccer: Relations to social-moral functioning, sportspersonship and team norm perceptions. *Psychology of Sport and Exercise, 25*, 397–413.

Overbye, M., Elbe, A.-M., Knudsen, M., and Pfister, G. (2014). Athletes' perceptions of anti-doping sanctions: The ban from sport vs. social, financial and self-imposed sanctions. Manuscript submitted for publication.

Pawlenka, C. (2004). *Sportethik. Regeln – Fairneß – Doping* [Sport ethic. Rules – fairness – doping]. Paderborn, Germany: Mentis.

Petróczi, A. and Aidman, E. V. (2009). Measuring explicit attitude toward doping: Review of the psychometric properties of the Performance Enhancement Attitude Scale. *Psychology of Sport and Exercise, 10*, 390–396.

Petróczi, A., Aidman, E. V., and Nepusz, T. (2008). Capturing doping attitudes by self-report declarations and implicit assessment: A methodology study. *Substance Abuse Treatment, Prevention, and Policy, 3 (9)*, 1–12.

Petróczi, A., Uvacsek, M., Nepusz, T., Deshmukh, N., Shah, I., Aidman, E. V., Barker, J., Tóth, M., and Naughton, D. P. (2011). Incongruence in doping related attitudes, belief and opinions in the context of disconcordant behavioural data: In which measures do we trust? *PloS One, 6 (4)*, 1–10.

Piaget, J. (1932). *The moral judgment of the child*. London: Kegan Paul, Trench, Trubner and Co.

Pilz, G. A. (1995). Performance sport: Education in fair play? *International Review for the Sociology of Sport, 30 (3–4)*, 391–418.

Schneider, A. J. and Butcher, R. B. (2000). A philosophical overview of the arguments on banning doping in sport. In T. Tännsjö and C. M. Tamburrini (eds.), *Values in sport: Elitism, nationalism, gender equality and the scientific manufacture of winners* (185–99). London: E & FN Spon.

Siedentop, D., Hastie, P., and van der Mars, H. (2004). *Complete guide to sport education*. Champaign, IL: Human Kinetics.

Singler, A. (2011). *Dopingprävention – Anspruch und Wirklichkeit* [Doping prevention – Claims and reality]. Aachen, Germany: Shaker Verlag.

Singler, A. and Treutlein, G. (2010). *Doping – von der Analyse zur Prävention* [Doping – From analysis to prevention]. Aachen, Germany: Meyer & Meyer.

Steenbergen, J. and Tamboer, J. W. I. (1998). Ethics and the double character of sport: An attempt to systematize the discussion on the ethics of sport. In M. J. McNamee and S. J. Parry (eds.), *Ethics and sport* (35–53). London: Routledge.

Striegel, H., Ulrich, R., and Simon, P. (2010). Randomized response estimates for doping and illicit drug use in elite athletes. *Drug and Alcohol Dependence, 106 (2–3)*, 230–232.

Trout, G. J. and Kazlauskas, R. (2004). Sports drug testing – An analyst's perspective. *Chemical Society Reviews, 33*, 1–13.

Tsorbatzoudis, H. (2009). *Determinants of doping intentions in sport*. Montreal, Canada: World Anti-Doping Agency.

Volkwein, K. A. (1995). Ethics and top-level sport – A paradox? *International Review for the Sociology of Sport, 30 (3–4),* s. 311–321.

WADA (2009). *The World Anti-doping Code.* Montreal, Canada: WADA.

Wright, M. (1995). Can moral judgment and ethical behavior be learned? A review of the literature. *Management Decision, 33 (10),* 17–28.

Part IV

Doping research and prevention

Where we stand, and where we need to go

13 Nutritional supplements in sport

Prevalence, reasons for use, and relation to doping

Susan Backhouse and Lisa Whitaker

The use of nutritional supplements (NS) is ubiquitous in sport with athletes looking for performance gains or ways to cope with heightened training demands. Such use involves a balance between potential benefits (e.g., through a carefully monitored NS program) and potential risks (e.g., inadvertent doping). Misinformed practice has raised serious concerns at a global level and there have been a growing number of claims of inadvertent doping through the use of NS (e.g., NS containing 1,3-dimethylamylamine or DMAA; "Rule Violations" n.d). Yet, risk does not stop at the possibility of a doping sanction. In the UK alone NS use has been cited as a factor in a number of deaths involving young and apparently healthy men and women. For example, an inquest concluded that DMAA found in Jack-3D was a contributory factor in the death of a 30-year-old runner during the 2012 London Marathon ("Claire Squires inquest" 2013). However, in the absence of clinical trials evidencing the side effects of these substances on human health, we must be cautious and avoid causal claims. Instead, supplement use risk, athletes' reasons for using NS, and the proposition that NS use can act as a gateway to doping are the focus of the chapter. Additionally, we support calls for increased regulation of the industry and research on functional alternatives to NS.

Definitions and prevalence estimates

The use of NS is more prevalent among sportsmen and women than in the general population (Rock 2007), where the smallest of margins can differentiate between winning and losing. In elite sport, estimated prevalence of NS use ranges from 57 percent to 94 percent (Huang *et al.* 2006; Petróczi and Naughton 2007; Suzic Lazic *et al.* 2009) with large proportions of university athletes (Burns *et al.* 2004) and junior athletes (Engelberg *et al.* 2014; Nieper 2005) also declaring use. Despite their popularity, no universally accepted definition of NS exists (Van Thuyne *et al.* 2006), which makes it difficult to accurately assess the prevalence of NS use amongst athletes (Maughan *et al.* 2011). In the 1994 Dietary Supplement Health and Educations Act, the US Food and Drug Administration (FDA) defined NS as "a product taken by mouth which contains substances like vitamins, minerals, herbs, or other botanical products, amino acids, enzymes, glandulars, metabolites and tissue extracts" (FDA 2009, "What is a dietary supplement?" para. 1). NS are intended to supplement the diet and are found in pill, tablet, capsule, powder, gel, or liquid form (FDA 2009). More succinctly, Schröder (2002) defined NS as foods that provide nutrients in a concentrated form which are present in a balanced diet such as vitamins, minerals, and trace elements. Although sports drinks, gels, and energy bars are often used by athletes, these products are usually excluded from definitions of NS (Maughan *et al.* 2011). In terms of a practical application, the nutrition expert group at the Australian Institute of Sport (AIS) ("Classification" n.d., para. 5) define sports foods and supplements into the following categories:

1   Sports foods – specialized products used to provide a practical source of nutrients when it is impractical to consume everyday foods (e.g., sports drink, sports gels).
2   Medical supplements – used to treat clinical issues, including diagnosed nutrient deficiencies and should be used under the supervision of a medical professional (e.g., iron supplement).
3   Performance supplements – used to directly contribute to optimal performance, but should be used under the direction of an appropriate sports medicine/science practitioner (e.g., caffeine, creatine).

Assessing the evidence base

Whilst it is beyond the scope of this chapter to review the evidence base regarding NS effects,[1] it is important to acknowledge that the ergogenic effects of many NS are contested and good evidence for efficacy is rare (Castell *et al.* 2009). Put simply, researchers have been unable to demonstrate that the use of some NS matches their bold marketing claims (Heikkinen *et al.* 2011b). Despite the lack of evidence, and the assertions that NS use is unnecessary when combined with a balanced diet (Sundgot-Borgen *et al.* 2003), many athletes use NS (Bishop 2010; Dascombe *et al.* 2010). Typically use occurs without clinical guidance from trained sports nutrition professionals (Waddington *et al.* 2005) or without considering adequate product information (Petróczi *et al.* 2007b). Moreover, reports of NS use amongst athletes often indicate overconsumption (Carlsohn *et al.* 2011), which could lead to adverse side effects and possibly long-term health concerns.

NS are considered to be foodstuffs rather than medicines (Maughan 2005) and this leads to an industry with a lack of regulation and accountability. Unlike medicines which have to be proven safe before being released onto the market, NS have to be proven unsafe before they are removed from the market (Cohen 2009). Subsequently, products may contain unlisted ingredients or doses of ingredients that exceed the amounts listed on the label (Geyer *et al.* 2008). Recognizing the challenges faced by athletes in identifying a safe, legal, and effective NS, the AIS were proactive in launching an athlete-centered Sports Supplement Framework in February 2014, which followed on from the Sports

Supplement Program initiated in 2000 ("Background" n.d., para. 1). A key goal of the Framework is to minimize the risk of an anti-doping rule violation which might arise through the use of NS ("Classification" n.d., para. 2). The Framework includes, amongst other things, a simple classification system (ABCD) which ranks NS ingredients according to the scientific evidence base ("Supplements" n.d.). Importantly, underpinning the Framework is a coordinated research program which aims to ensure that best practice protocols for the use of NS supplements evolve over time. This proactive approach has merit because the very nature of sport means that athletes are constantly in search of performance gains (Hawley *et al.* 2007). Therefore, NS will continue to occupy athletes' kit bags for the foreseeable future and we need to be pragmatic in designing education programs around this issue as "just say no" campaigns are likely to be counterproductive.

Possible risks of misinformed NS use

Potential side effects that may occur as a result of overconsumption of NS or the ingestion of potentially harmful substances include renal failure (Stickel *et al.* 2011), seizures following high consumption of energy drinks (Duchan *et al.* 2010), caffeine intoxication (Reissig *et al.* 2009), iron toxicity (Papanikolaou and Pantopoulos 2005), and hepatotoxicity (Navarro 2009). As already highlighted, the use of NS has also been identified as a contributory factor in a number of deaths involving young men and women. For example, the use of NS containing the now banned DMAA ("Claire Squires inquest" 2013) and 2, 4-dinitrophenol which is used in pesticides but banned for human consumption (Dixon 2013). Further investigation with large randomized controlled studies is required to provide more definitive evidence of health risk; especially studies involving young and apparently healthy males and females.

In addition to the possible health concerns associated with NS use, athletes also face the possibility of certain NS being contaminated with prohibited substances. This can occur due to the manufacturing process (e.g., using machinery which is also used to prepare prohibited substances) or unscrupulous practice by manufacturers (e.g., adding an active ingredient not listed on the label). Evidence suggests that NS cannot be guaranteed to be 100 percent free from prohibited substances (Geyer *et al.* 2008). For example, out of 634 samples, Geyer *et al.* (2004) found 14.8 percent of non-hormonal NS contained one or more androgenic anabolic steroids not identified on the label. If a product contains a prohibited substance, an athlete could inadvertently dope and produce a positive drug test.

The World Anti-Doping Agency (WADA), and signatories to the World Anti-Doping Code, adopts a strict liability stance. This means that an athlete is solely responsible for any banned substance they use, attempt to use, or is found in their system, regardless of how it got there and whether there was an intention to cheat or not ("2015 World Anti-Doping Code" 2014). Consequently, inadvertent doping through the use of contaminated NS could have implications for an athlete and his/her career. Indeed, Brand *et al.* (2011) noted that participants in their implicit attitude study made numerous mistakes when it came to distinguishing doping substances from NS. They posit that in recent years, and with the growing awareness of NS contamination risk, international sports federations have adopted a strong stance to deter NS use in sports. In turn, this could have elicited insecurity in the athlete population regarding the use of NS, which was subtly evidenced by descriptively longer response times in the "doping vs. supplement" IAT (Brand *et al.* 2011).

From January 2015, such insecurities may be exacerbated because an athlete with a presence finding will have to demonstrate that they have taken every reasonable step to ensure the purity of their supplement prior to use. Failure to do so will result in an automatic four-year ban from sport. In light of the concept of strict liability there is a growing recognition of the need for comprehensive third-party NS quality assurance programs. Established in the UK in 2008, the Informed-Sport certification program tests products for banned substances and ensures that they are made in accordance with good manufacturing practices. NS that go through this certification process then bear the Informed-Sport logo, which gives athletes greater confidence that the batch of NS that they have purchased has been tested for banned substances by a leading anti-doping laboratory. Whilst athletes would be taking steps to minimize the risk of a positive drugs test by using this service, it still does not offer a 100 percent guarantee. Supplement certification processes also invariably lead to a higher price tag, which, in turn, may influence consumer decision-making as price can be a factor when choosing and comparing NS. Furthermore, a risk management system of this kind arguably favors athletes and countries with sufficient funds to access these risk minimization processes. Thus, more needs to be done to regulate the manufacturing of NS at a global level. Black market supplies that can be easily obtained via the Internet, and shipped worldwide, represent a significant and growing concern (Anti Doping Danmark, Dopingautoriteit, STAD, Instytut Sportu, and CyADA 2012).

NS as a gateway to doping in sport

Not only are there contamination and health risks involved in the misuse of NS, an association between ingesting NS and the use of prohibited substances also exists. This relationship suggests NS use may act as a gateway to doping (Backhouse *et al.* 2013; Petróczi and Aidman 2008; Petróczi *et al.* 2011a). The gateway theory (Kandel 2002) proposes a positive relationship between legal and illegal substances, which lends itself to substance use being sequential. Similarly, the incremental-functional model of doping suggests gradual involvement with assisted performance enhancement moving from conscious diet to habitual NS use to potential doping (Petróczi 2014). However, this is not to say that all NS have the same likelihood of leading to doping. Some NS may be more likely (e.g., prohormone NS) to lead to illegal performance-enhancing substance (PES) use than others, dependent on an athlete's reasons for using them.

Supporting the theory, empirical research has demonstrated that doping coincides with NS use (Backhouse *et al.* 2013; Barkoukis *et al.* forthcoming; Lucidi *et al.* 2008; Papadopoulos *et al.* 2006) and studies indicate that athletes who use NS are two to four times more likely to dope than nonusers (Backhouse *et al.* 2013; Papadopoulos *et al.* 2006).

Backhouse and colleagues (2013) also noted significant differences in doping attitudes and beliefs between NS users and nonusers. Equally, Barkourkis *et al.* (forthcoming) found that NS users displayed biased normative beliefs related to doping use (i.e., they perceived doping as more prevalent in fellow athletes and socially approved). Furthermore, the assertion that NS users are at a much higher risk of using illegal substances was supported by the findings of a recent meta-analysis which examined 63 independent data sets (Ntoumanis *et al.* 2014). Although the findings should be interpreted with caution due to the small number of studies examined, the use of legal NS was found to have a large positive effect on doping intentions and behavior (Ntoumanis *et al.* 2014). Although causality has yet to be established due to the cross-sectional nature of previous research, these findings – combined with the widespread use of NS across all levels of sport (Hoffman *et al.* 2008; Tscholl *et al.* 2010) – highlight the importance of examining athletes' current NS practices and supplementation outcome expectancies. Athletes who engage in NS use may become accustomed to the use of chemical substances to enhance performance and see prohibited substances as a natural progression from habitual NS use (Petróczi 2014). This could be explained by operant conditioning as the consequence (perceived or real) of supplementation influences the repeatability of this behavior. In this context, our current program of research speaks of the importance of social rewards (e.g., praise on progression/changes in physique) serving as a source of positive reinforcement for NS use.

With a lack of primary prevention of NS use in place (Petróczi *et al.* 2011a), it is important to understand the reasons why athletes are willing to overlook the potential risks highlighted earlier in the chapter. With the gateway theory in mind, examining athletes' self-reported reasons for consuming NS may provide insight into why athletes take banned substances. A review of the literature demonstrates that they can be broadly categorized under the headings of (1) therapeutic control; and (2) performance enhancement. These categories are based upon the idea that therapy can involve curing disease and/or improving human functioning within its normal variations (Tannsjo 2008), whereas enhancement is seen as increasing functioning above its natural limits (Garcia and Sandler 2008). Some reasons vary with gender, nationality, type of sport, and level of competition, whereas other reasons are prevalent across a range of athletes.[2] These reasons evidence social-cognitive processes, which can emerge from biased and ill-informed pro-supplementation beliefs, which in turn might lead to pro-doping beliefs.

Reasons for using NS

Therapeutic control reasons can be broken down into the use of NS to (1) aid recovery; (2) optimize health; (3) prevent illness; and (4) compensate for an inadequate diet. Whilst performance enhancement related reasons are less cited in the literature and typically refer to (1) general performance enhancement; (2) weight control; (3) strength/muscle size; and (4) increasing energy. These reasons for NS use will be considered in turn.

Aid recovery

Athletes have reported the use of NS to aid recovery from both training and injury, though the former appears more common. Sixteen percent of British athletes (Petróczi *et al.* 2007a) and 26 percent of athletes competing in the 2004 World Masters Athletics Championships used NS as a way to overcome an injury (Striegel *et al.* 2006). In comparison, between 30 and 80 percent of elite athletes reported using NS to enhance recovery from training (Erdman *et al.* 2006; Heikkinen *et al.* 2011a; Kim *et al.* 2011a; Petróczi *et al.* 2008; Sousa *et al.* 2013). Yet only 16 percent of elite athletes working with a dietician used NS for recovery (Lun *et al.* 2012). To date, the focus has been on elite athletes and therefore it is unclear if athletes across all levels of competition use NS to aid recovery. Equally, Sousa and colleagues (2013) found 31 percent of under-18s reporting NS use to accelerate recovery compared to 72 percent of athletes over the age of 18 indicating that age may also influence athletes' reasons for use.

Optimize health

Health is regarded as one of the main reasons for NS use and has been associated with both recreationally active and competitive athletes (McDowall 2007). Typically, females associate NS use with health more frequently than males, who tend to cite athletic performance as their main reason for use (Froiland *et al.* 2004; McDowall 2007). Research suggests that 44 to 70 percent of young athletes (including adolescents and college athletes) use NS for health-related reasons (Braun *et al.* 2009; Kiertscher and DiMarco 2013; Nieper 2005) while 19 to 75 percent of elite athletes use NS to optimize their health (Dascombe *et al.* 2010; de Silva *et al.* 2010; Erdman *et al.* 2006; Heikkinen *et al.* 2011a; Lun *et al.* 2012; Sousa *et al.* 2013). In particular, vitamins and minerals were used by 30 percent of Finnish athletes (Heikkinen *et al.* 2011a) and 75 percent of Portuguese athletes (Sousa *et al.* 2013) to stay healthy. In contrast, only 7 to 15 percent of Korean elite athletes reported using NS for health maintenance (Kim *et al.* 2011a, 2011b, 2013). Given the interest in health enhancement and maintenance, education programs may wish to tailor education programs to ensure healthy living practices are disseminated (e.g., eating a balanced diet, getting enough sleep, optimizing mental preparation), attractive alternatives to NS use are offered and evidence-based risks are highlighted.

Prevent illness

As well as wanting to maintain health, athletes have been interested in using NS to prevent illness. However, many NS do not claim to treat illness because manufacturers cannot make this claim without valid proof (Maughan *et al.* 2011). Despite this, a number of studies – focusing mainly on young high performance athletes – have reported the use of NS to prevent illness. Findings indicate that over 30 percent of athletes have used NS either to boost their immune system or avoid sickness (Kiertscher and DiMarco 2013; Nieper 2005; Petróczi *et al.* 2007a; Tian *et al.* 2009). In particular, vitamins and minerals have once again been identified as being used to prevent illness (Heikkinen *et al.* 2011a; Petróczi *et al.* 2007a, 2008; Tian *et al.* 2009). Yet incongruence between the types of NS used and the reasons for use is evident (Petróczi *et al.* 2007a, 2008) suggesting that rather than using vitamins and minerals, some athletes may be using other types of NS which could be inappropriate for preventing illness. In light of this lack of knowledge, the potential side effects of the substances athletes choose to ingest and the unregulated nature of the NS industry (Baume *et al.* 2006), athletes are always encouraged to consult with a qualified sports nutritionist in order to prevent NS misuse.

Inadequate diet

NS have also been used as a way to compensate for an inadequate diet, with females reporting the use of NS to balance out a poor diet more frequently than males (McDowall 2007). Corroborating this assertion, Tian and colleagues (2009) found that one of the most common reasons for using NS by Singaporean university athletes was to supplement a poor diet. Yet in comparison to using NS for other therapeutic purposes, the proportion of athletes reporting the use of NS because of an inadequate diet was much lower. Typically, the use of NS to combat an imbalanced diet is reported by 15 to 18 percent of athletes (Froiland *et al.* 2004; Nieper 2005; Ziegler *et al.* 2003) with Ziegler *et al.* (2003) noting a slightly higher prevalence rate of 28 percent of female elite figure skaters. A lack of time to prepare meals was also reported as a reason for NS use by 19 percent of British athletes (Petróczi *et al.* 2007a). However, this evidence base contains conflicting accounts as one study found that only 3 percent of young elite UK athletes used NS to combat an imbalanced diet (Petróczi *et al.* 2008). Therefore, further research is warranted before clear conclusions can be drawn.

General performance enhancement

Performance enhancement as a general reason for NS use tends to only be cited by athletes competing at a high level. In addition, the prevalence of using NS for performance-related reasons appears to differ with sporting culture. In general, 21 to 43 percent of athletes have reported that they use NS to enhance their performance (Braun *et al.* 2009; Kiertscher and DiMarco 2013; Nieper 2005;

Zaggelidis *et al.* 2005; Ziegler *et al.* 2003). However, higher percentages were observed amongst Portuguese national level athletes (62 percent; Sousa *et al.* 2013) and Sri Lankan national-level athletes (79 percent; de Silva *et al.* 2010). In contrast, only 9 percent of Australian elite athletes (Dascombe *et al.* 2010) and 6 percent of female figure skaters (Ziegler *et al.* 2003) self-reported NS use to improve performance. Acknowledging the limitations of self-report surveys, the differences between nationalities suggest the context within which an athlete is situated could be influential in the use of NS and further research into these dynamic factors is warranted.

Weight control

Some athletes have declared the use of NS to lose weight, whilst others have used NS to gain weight. However, these reasons for using NS are infrequent compared to reasons associated with therapeutic control. Only three studies utilizing multiple-choice question responses included reasons associated with weight control. Ziegler *et al.* (2003) found 3 percent of elite female figure skaters used NS to lose weight whilst 7 percent of elite gymnasts used NS to reduce body fat (Zaggelidis *et al.* 2005). In contrast, Froiland *et al.* (2004) found college athletes use NS to gain weight. Indeed, weight gain was more popular amongst male college athletes compared with females (37 percent versus 5 percent). In addition, athletes from track and field, American football, wrestling, and soccer were significantly more likely to identify weight/muscle gain as their reason for NS use, compared to sports such as golf, tennis, bowling, gymnastics, and basketball (Froiland *et al.* 2004). As a result, weight control as a reason for NS use may not be generalizable across all sports but rather unique to specific sports. Similarly, it is unknown whether weight control is prevalent as a reason for older adults to use NS, as both studies including weight control as a possible response focused on young athletes.

Strength/muscle size

The desire to increase strength/muscle size permeates the literature as a reason for NS use. Studies reporting strength/muscle size have involved either high performance athletes or university athletes. Of those studies involving the use of NS to increase muscle size, 3 to 23 percent of high performance athletes declared use (Heikkinen *et al.* 2011a; Kiertscher and DiMarco 2013; Lun *et al.* 2012; Sousa *et al.* 2013; Zaggelidis *et al.* 2005; Ziegler *et al.* 2003), with the reason for use being higher amongst males than females (Sousa *et al.* 2013; Zaggelidis *et al.* 2005; Ziegler *et al.* 2003). This gender difference was also seen when athletes reported using NS to increase strength (Froiland *et al.* 2004; Kim *et al.* 2011a) with the proportion of athletes reporting this reason for use tending to be higher. Specifically, two studies involving American collegiate athletes demonstrated that 36 to 43 percent of athletes used NS to increase strength (Froiland *et al.* 2004; Kiertscher and DiMarco 2013) while the proportion of high performance athletes using NS to increase strength typically ranged from 10 to 38 percent (Kim, *et al.* 2011a, 2011b, 2013; Nieper 2005; Petróczi *et al.* 2007b; Sousa *et al.* 2013). Two studies exceeded the high performance range with 45 percent of Korean judoists (Kim *et al.* 2013) and 72 percent of UK elite athletes involved in power sports (Petróczi *et al.* 2008) declaring the use of NS to increase strength. In stark contrast, only two out of 58 elite Australian athletes identified strength as a reason for NS use (Dascombe *et al.* 2010). This discrepancy might be explained by the fact that sports where strength may be perceived as less important (e.g., hockey, netball) were the focus of the study. As a result, education which targets males and highlights alternative methods and practices to increase strength and muscle size (e.g., guided strength and conditioning programs) seems an important avenue of development to help stem the misuse of NS to bulk up.

Increase energy

As with increasing strength/muscle size, athletes' desire to increase their energy levels is a pertinent reason for NS use. Four studies involving university athletes from either the United States or Asia noted that between 18 and 43 percent of athletes surveyed had used NS to increase energy (Froiland *et al.* 2004; Kiertscher and DiMarco 2013; Kim *et al.* 2011b; Tian *et al.* 2009). In comparison, 15 to 60 percent of elite athletes, representing a variety of nationalities, reported using NS to increase their energy levels (Erdman *et al.* 2006; Heikkinen *et al.* 2011a; Kim *et al.* 2013; Lun *et al.* 2012; Sousa *et al.* 2013; Ziegler *et al.* 2003). However, only 5 percent of UK junior athletes (Nieper 2005) and two out of 58 elite Australian athletes (Dascombe *et al.* 2010) reported using NS to increase energy. Whilst the evidence base is somewhat equivocal, findings consistently indicate that males are more likely to report NS use to increase energy than females (Heikkinen *et al.* 2011a; Kim *et al.* 2011b; Ziegler *et al.* 2003) with the exception to this trend being noted by Froiland *et al.* (2004) in a study on American collegiate athletes.

In sum, these studies highlight the need to educate athletes, and their support network, on the importance of a balanced diet and the use of functional foods. Put simply, NS cannot be used as substitutes for a poor diet in the long run (International Olympic Committee 2010). Whilst there may be times when NS are necessary to provide essential nutrients to athletes (e.g., when food intake is restricted due to the need to control weight, a vegan diet, travel; International Olympic Committee 2010) it is imperative that the decision to use NS is informed (i.e., assess the need, assess the risk, assess the consequence) and made with the support of a qualified professional. Similarly, athletes need to adopt the same approach if they already consume a balanced diet but are seeking out strategies to enhance their performance or aid recovery.

Source of information regarding NS use

Athletes often look to significant others such as coaches, team mates, trainers, and medical staff for information and guidance related to their performance and potential ways to improve it (Bonci 2009). Studies show that while some athletes do seek information from reputable sources such as allied health professionals or medical doctors (e.g., Dascombe *et al.* 2010) the vast majority identify peers, coaches, and family members as their dominant source of NS information (Bonci 2009; Erdman *et al.* 2006; Kim *et al.* 2011a; Nieper 2005). Research also suggests that sources of information may be influenced by an individual's age, gender, and level of performance. Kim and colleagues (2011a) found that amongst Korean Olympic athletes, males and older athletes were more likely to seek information from their coach, while females and younger athletes approached their parents. In contrast, Erdman *et al.* (2006) found college athletes were least likely to be influenced by a coach or dietician, whilst international/professional performance athletes were more likely to receive NS information from strength trainers than athletes representing other performance levels. Thus, in general educated professionals in the field are not systematically guiding athletes' choices (Nieper 2005). Therefore, research is needed to determine what prevents athletes from discussing their nutritional practice with allied health professionals so that changes can be made to increase accessibility and reach of sound dietary advice. It may be that athletes are not aware of a nutritionist to approach for information or that access to nutritional support is limited because of the associated costs. Sport and exercise nutritionists may need to promote their profession and services more widely to athletes and their entourage so that access to this important source of support is increased. Educational efforts should also target current information sources (e.g., coaches) so that they are better equipped to prevent the misuse of NS by their athletes.

Conclusions and future directions

There are a number of reasons why athletes choose to use NS despite the potential risk of compromised health or inadvertent doping. These reasons vary with sport, gender, and level of competition. Consequently, a "one size fits all" approach to education appears to be unfeasible. NS use can provide benefits to some individuals but athletes need to be better informed of the risks of using certain NS as well as alternative ways to enhance performance without using NS (e.g., importance of a balanced diet and optimized strength and conditioning training). This paradigm shift in educational efforts may help prevent overuse of legitimate and illegitimate NS and curb the forming of a belief system in which performance enhancement is associated with some form of chemical assistance.

It is therefore important to promote practices that can enhance performance without the ingestion of a chemical substance (e.g., sport psychology, performance analysis, sleep). Furthermore, it is vital that further investment is committed to studies that examine the ergogenic and recovery-enhancing effects of naturally rich foodstuffs (e.g., beetroot juice, cherries, milk) as evidence-based alternatives to NS use may assist in creating abstinence-oriented norms. However, we must also acknowledge that providing fact-based information on the comparable physiological effects of naturally rich foods with their synthetic alternatives could raise awareness of the potentially performance-enhancing effects of the synthetic drug (James *et al.* 2010).

Critically, attention needs to turn toward the NS industry as a whole. The industry markets products with unsubstantiated claims and coercive images to lure athletes and the general population into using their products. The lack of scientific evidence to support such claims is serious (Lieberman 2007) and athletes' NS outcome expectancies are grounded upon such dubious claims (James *et al.* 2010). Therefore, stricter regulation is required to ensure that NS are marketed in a safe and ethical manner, similar to medicines. The possibility of inadvertent doping and negative health consequences will also continue to exist unless legislative and regulatory change occurs. Further, a greater debate on the blurred boundaries between legal NS and banned substances should be encouraged.

Evidence continues to suggest that NS use may act as a gateway to doping, but we are unaware of why some athletes move from NS to ingesting prohibited substances. The types of NS athletes are using and their rationale for use may provide insight into this. Not only does prospective research need to identify the factors that prevent athletes from progressing on to prohibited substances from NS, it also needs to ascertain whether opportunities for prevention targeting NS use exist. Shifting the focus from anti-doping to Clean Sport education could provide greater opportunities for more positive behavior reinforcement. In turn, this might facilitate engagement by the wider sporting community and increase the reach and accessibility of sound advice from qualified professionals, rather than the current reliance on misinformed peers, coaches, and the Internet.

Notes

1 The reader is referred to the British Journal of Sports Medicine A–Z of Nutritional Supplements as this presents an edited series on this topic.
2 Different self-report questionnaires have been used in published studies. Therefore, athletes' responses may have differed depending on the type of question used (e.g., multiple-choice versus open-ended questions).

References

2015 World Anti-Doping Code (2014). In UK Anti-Doping website. Available at www. ukad.org.uk/assets/uploads/Files/2014/2015_code_athletes.pdf (accessed November 20, 2014).

Anti Doping Danmark, Dopingautoriteit, STAD, Instytut Sportu, & CyADA (2012). *Strategy for Stopping Steroids*. Copenhagen: Anti-Doping Danmark.

Background (n.d.). In Australian Institute of Sport website. Available at www.ausport. gov.au/ais/nutrition/supplements/background (accessed June 27, 2014).

Backhouse, S. H., Whitaker, L., and Petróczi, A. (2013). Gateway to doping? Supplement use in the context of preferred competitive situations, doping attitude, beliefs, and norms. *Scandinavian Journal of Medicine and Science in Sports*, 23 (2), 244–252. doi: 10.1111/j.1600–0838.2011.01374.x.

Barkoukis, V., Lazuras, L., Lucidi, F., and Tsorbatzoudis, H. (forthcoming). Nutritional supplement and doping use in sport: Possible underlying social cognitive processes. *Scandinavian Journal of Medicine and Science in Sports*.

Baume, N., Mahler, N., Kamber, M., Mangin, P., and Saugy, M. (2006). Research of stimulants and anabolic steroids in dietary supplements. *Scandinavian Journal of Medicine and Science in Sports*, 16 (1), 41–48.

Brand, R., Melzer, M., and Hagemann, N. (2011). Towards an implicit association test (IAT) for measuring doping attitudes in sports. Data-based recommendations developed from two recently published tests. *Psychology of Sport and Exercise*, 12 (3), 250–256.

Bishop, D. (2010). Dietary supplements and team-sport performance. *Sports Medicine*, 40, 995–1017.

Bonci, L. (2009). Supplements: help, harm or hype? How to approach athletes. *Current Sports Medicine Reports*, 8 (4), 200–205.

Braun, H., Koehler, K., Geyer, H., Kleinert, J., Mester, J., and Schänzer, W. (2009). Dietary supplement use among elite young German athletes. *International Journal of Sport Nutrition and Exercise Metabolism*, 19 (1), 97–109.

Burns, R. D., Schiller, M. R., Merrick, M. A., and Wolf, K. N. (2004). Intercollegiate student athlete use of nutritional supplements and the role of athletic trainers and dietitians in nutrition counseling. *Journal of the American Dietetic Association*, 104 (2), 246–249.

Carlsohn, A., Cassel, M., Linne, K., and Mayer, F. (2011). How much is too much? A case report of nutritional supplement use of a high-performance athlete. *British Journal of Nutrition*, 105 (12), 1724–1728.

Castell, L. M., Burke, L. M., and Stear, S. J. (2009). BJSM reviews: A–Z of supplements: Dietary supplements, sports nutrition foods and ergogenic aids for health and performance Part 2. *British Journal of Sports Medicine*, 43 (11), 807–810.

Claire Squires inquest: DMAA was factor in marathon runner's death. (January 30, 2013). Available at www.bbc.co.uk/news/uk-england-london-21262717 (accessed June 27, 2014).

Classification. (n.d.). In Australian Institute of Sport website. Available at www.ausport. gov.au/ais/nutrition/supplements/classification (accessed June 27, 2014).

Cohen, P. A. (2009). American roulette – Contaminated dietary supplements. *New England Journal of Medicine*, 361 (16), 1523–1525. doi: 10.1056/NEJMp0904768.

Dascombe, B. J., Karunaratna, M., Cartoon, J., Fergie, B., and Goodman, C. (2010). Nutritional supplementation habits and perceptions of elite athletes within a state-based sporting institute. *Journal of Science and Medicine in Sport*, 13 (2), 274–280.

de Silva, A., Samarasinghe, Y., Senanayake, D., and Lanerolle, P. (2010). Dietary supplement intake in national-level Sri Lankan athletes. *International Journal of Sport Nutrition and Exercise Metabolism*, 20 (1), 15–20.

Dixon, H. (2013). Teenage rugby star killed by online diet pills. *The Telegraph*. Available at www.telegraph.co.uk/news/uknews/law-and-order/10310834/Teenage-rugby-star-killed-by-online-diet-pills.html (accessed June 27, 2014).

Duchan, E., Patel, N. D., and Feucht, C. (2010). Energy drinks: A review of use and safety for athletes. *The Physician and Sportsmedicine*, 38 (2), 171–179.

Engelberg, E. T., Moston, S., and Skinner, J. (2014). Tracking the development of attitudes to doping: A longitudinal study of young elite athletes. *A report submitted to the Australian Government's Anti-Doping Research Program, Department of Health.*

Erdman, K. A., Fung, T. S., and Reimer, R. A. (2006). Influence of performance level on dietary supplementation in elite Canadian athletes. *Medicine and Science in Sports and Exercise, 38* (*2*), 349–356.

FDA (2009). Consumer information: Overview of dietary supplements. Available at www.fda.gov/Food/DietarySupplements/ConsumerInformation/ucm110417.htm#what.

Froiland, K., Koszewski, W., Hingst, J., and Kopecky, L. (2004). Nutritional supplement use among college athletes and their sources of information. *International Journal of Sport Nutrition and Exercise Metabolism, 14* (*1*), 104–120.

Garcia, T. and Sandler, R. (2008). Enhancing justice? *Nanoethics, 2* (*3*), 277–287.

Geyer, H., Parr, M. K., Koehler, K., Mareck, U., Schänzer, W., and Thevis, M. (2008). Nutritional supplements cross-contaminated and faked with doping substances. *Journal of Mass Spectrometry, 43* (*7*), 892–902.

Geyer, H., Parr, M. K., Mareck, U., Reinhart, U., Schrader, Y., and Schänzer, W. (2004). Analysis of non-hormonal nutritional supplements for anabolic-androgenic steroids: Results of an International study. *International Journal of Sports Medicine, 25* (*2*), 124–129.

Hawley, J., Gibala, M. J., and Bermon, S. (2007). Innovations in athletic preparation: Role of substrate availability to modify training adaptation and performance. *Journal of Sports Science, 25* (*Suppl. 1*), S115–124.

Heikkinen, A., Alaranta, A., Helenius, I., and Vasankari, T. (2011a). Dietary supplementation habits and perceptions of supplement use among elite Finnish athletes. *International Journal of Sport Nutrition and Exercise Metabolism, 21* (*4*), 271–279.

Heikkinen, A., Alaranta, A., Helenius, I., and Vasankari, T. (2011b). Use of dietary supplements in Olympic athletes is decreasing: A follow-up study between 2002 and 2009. *Journal of the International Society of Sports Nutrition, 8* (*1*), 1–8.

Hoffman, J. R., Faigenbaum, A. D., Ratamess, N. A., Ross, R., Jie, K., and Tenenbaum, G. (2008). Nutritional supplementation and anabolic steroid use in adolescents. *Medicine and Science in Sports and Exercise, 40* (*1*), 15–24.

Huang, S.-H., Johnson, K., and Pipe, A. (2006). The use of dietary supplements and medications by Canadian athletes at the Atlanta and Sydney Olympic Games. *Clinical Journal of Sport Medicine, 16* (*1*), 27–33.

International Olympic Committee (2010). Consensus Statement on Sports Nutrition. Available at www.olympic.org/Documents/Reports/EN/CONSENSUS-FINAL-v8-en. pdf.

James, R., Naughton, D. P., and Petróczi, A. (2010). Promoting functional foods as acceptable alternatives to doping: Potential for information-based social marketing approach. *Journal of the International Society of Sports Nutrition, 7*, 37. doi: 10.1186/1550–2783–7–37.

Kandel, D. B. (2002). Examining the gateway hypothesis stages and pathways of drug involvement. In D. B. Kandel (ed.), *Stages and pathways of drug involvement: Examining the gateway hypothesis* (3–15). New York: Cambridge University Press.

Kiertscher, E. and DiMarco, N. M. (2013). Use and rationale for taking nutritional supplements among collegiate athletes at risk for nutrient deficiencies. *Performance Enhancement and Health, 2* (*1*), 24–29. doi: http://dx.doi.org/10.1016/j.peh.2013.04.002.

Kim, J., Kang, S.-K., Jung, H.-S., Chun, Y.-S., Trilk, J., and Jung, S. H. (2011a). Dietary supplementation patterns of Korean Olympic athletes participating in the Beijing 2008 summer Olympic Games. *International Journal of Sport Nutrition and Exercise Metabolism, 21* (*2*), 166–174.

Kim, J., Lee, N., Kim, E.-J., Ki, S.-K., Yoon, J., and Lee, M.-S. (2011b). Anti-doping education and dietary supplementation practice in Korean elite university athletes. *Nutrition Research And Practice, 5* (*4*), 349–356. doi: 10.4162/nrp. 2011.5.4.349.

Kim, J., Lee, N., Lee, J., Jung, S.-S., Kang, S.-K., and Yoon, J.-D. (2013). Dietary supplementation of high-performance Korean and Japanese Judoists. *International Journal of Sport Nutrition and Exercise Metabolism, 23* (*2*), 119–127.

Lieberman, H. R. (2007). Achieving scientific consensus in nutrition and behaviour research. *Nutrition Bulletin, 32* (*8*), 100–106.

Lucidi, F., Zelli, A., Mallia, L., Grano, C., Russo, P. M., and Violani, C. (2008). The social-cognitive mechanisms regulating adolescents' use of doping substances. *Journal of Sports Sciences, 26* (*5*), 447–456. doi: 10.1080/02640410701579370.

Lun, V., Erdman, K. A., Fung, T. S., and Reimer, R. A. (2012). Dietary supplementation practices in Canadian high-performance athletes. *International Journal of Sport Nutrition and Exercise Metabolism, 22* (*1*), 31–37.

Maughan, R. J. (2005). Contamination of dietary supplements and positive drug tests in sport. *Journal of Sports Sciences, 23* (*9*), 883–889.

Maughan, R. J., Greenhaff, P. L., and Hespel, P. (2011). Dietary supplements for athletes: Emerging trends and recurring themes. *Journal of Sports Sciences, 29* (*Suppl. 1*), 57–66. doi: 10.1080/02640414.2011.587446NS.

McDowall, J. A. (2007). Supplement use by young athletes. *Journal of Sports Science and Medicine, 6*, 337–342.

Navarro, V. (2009). Herbal and dietary supplement hepatotoxicity. *Seminars in Liver Disease, 29* (*4*), 373–382.

Nieper, A. (2005). Nutritional supplement practices in UK junior national track and field athletes. *British Journal of Sports Medicine, 39* (*9*), 645–649.

Ntoumanis, N., Ng, J. Y., Barkoukis, V., and Backhouse, S. (2014). Personal and Psychosocial predictors of doping use in physical activity settings: A meta-analysis. *Sports Medicine, 44* (*11*), 1603–1624. doi: 10.1007/s40279–014–0240–4.

Papadopoulos, F. C., Skalkidis, I., Parkkari, J., and Petridou, E. (2006). Doping use among tertiary education students in six developed countries. *European Journal of Epidemiology, 21* (*4*), 307–313. doi: 10.1007/s10654–006–0018–6.

Papanikolaou, G. and Pantopoulos, K. (2005). Iron metabolism and toxicity. *Toxicology And Applied Pharmacology, 202* (*2*), 199–211.

Petróczi, A. (2014). The doping mindset – Part 1: Implications of the functional use theory on mental representations of doping. *Performance Enhancement and Health, 2* (*4*), 153–163.

Petróczi, A. and Aidman, E. (2008). Psychological drivers in doping: The life-cycle model of performance enhancement. *Substance Abuse Treatment, Prevention, and Policy, 3* (*7*). doi: 10.1186/1747–597X-3–7.

Petróczi, A. and Naughton, D. P. (2007). Supplement use in sport: Is there a potentially dangerous incongruence between rationale and practice? *Journal of Occupational Medicine and Toxicology, 2* (*4*).

Petróczi, A., Mazanov, J., and Naughton, D. (2011a). Inside athletes' minds: Preliminary results from a pilot study on mental representation of doping and potential implications for anti-doping. *Substance Abuse Treatment, Prevention, and Policy, 6* (*10*).

Petróczi, A., Naughton, D. P., Mazanov, J., Holloway, A., and Bingham, J. (2007a). Limited agreement exists between rationale and practice in athletes' supplement use for maintenance of health: a retrospective study. *Nutrition Journal, 6* (*34*).

Petróczi, A., Naughton, D. P., Mazanov, J., Holloway, A., and Bingham, J. (2007b). Performance enhancement with supplements: Incongruence between rationale and practice. *Journal of International Society of Sports Nutrition, 4 (19)*.

Petróczi, A., Naughton, D. P., Pearce, G., Bailey, R., Bloodworth, A., and McNamee, M. (2008). Nutritional supplement use by elite young UK athletes: Fallacies of advice regarding efficacy. *Journal of International Society of Sports Nutrition, 5 (22)*.

Reissig, C. J., Strain, E. C., and Griffiths, R. R. (2009). Caffeinated energy drinks – A growing problem. *Drug and Alcohol Dependence, 99 (1–3)*, 1–10. doi: 10.1016/j.drugalcdep. 2008.08.001.

Rock, C. L. (2007). Multivitamin-multimineral supplements: Who uses them? *The American Journal of Clinical Nutrition, 85* (1), 277S–279S.

Rule Violations: Historical sanctions (n.d). In UK Anti-Doping website. Available at www.ukad.org.uk/anti-doping-rule-violations/historical-sanctions/ (accessed November 20, 2014).

Schröder, U. (2002). Health effects of nutritional supplements. In W. Schänzer, F. T. Delbeke, A. Deligiannis, G. Gmeiner, R. J. Maughan, and J. Mester (eds.), *Health and doping risks of nutritional supplements and social drugs* (11–15). Cologne: Sport and Buch Strauß.

Sousa, M., Fernandes, M. J., Moreira, P., and Teixeira, V. H. (2013). Nutritional supplements usage by Portuguese athletes. *International Journal for Vitamin and Nutrition Research, 83 (1)*, 48–58.

Stickel, F., Kessebohm, K., Weimann, R., and Seitz, H. K. (2011). Review of liver injury associated with dietary supplements. *Liver International, 31 (5)*, 595–605. doi: 10.111 1/j.1478–3231.2010.02439.x.

Striegel, H., Simon, P., Wurster, C., Niess, A. M., and Ulrich, R. (2006). The use of nutritional supplements among master athletes. *International Journal of Sports Medicine, 27 (3)*, 236–241.

Sundgot-Borgen, J., Berglund, B., and Torstveit, M. K. (2003). Nutritional supplements in Norwegian elite athletes – Impact of international ranking and advisors. *Scandinavian Journal of Medicine and Science in Sports, 13*, 138.

Supplements (n.d.). In Australian Institute of Sport website. Available at www.ausport. gov.au/ais/nutrition/supplements (accessed June 27, 2014).

Suzic Lazic, J., Dikic, N., Radivojevic, N., Mazic, S., Radovanovic, D., Mitrovic, N., Lazic, M., Zivanic, S., and Suzic, S. (2009). Dietary supplements and medications in elite sport – Polypharmacy or real need? *Scandinavian Journal of Medicine and Science in Sports.* doi: 10.1111/j.1600–0838.2009.01026.x.

Tannsjo, T. (2008). Medical enhancement and the ethos of elite sport. In J. Savulescu and N. Bostrom (eds.), *Human enhancement* (315–326). Oxford: Oxford University Press.

Tian, H. H., Ong, W. S., and Tan, C. L. (2009). Nutritional supplement use among university athletes in Singapore. *Singapore Medical Journal, 50 (2)*, 165–172.

Tscholl, P., Alonso, J. M., Dolle, G., Junge, A., and Dvorak, J. (2010). The use of drugs and nutritional supplements in top-level track and field athletes. *The American Journal of Sports Medicine, 38 (1)*, 133–140. doi: 10.1177/0363546509344071.

Van Thuyne, W., Van Eenoo, P., and Delbeke, F. T. (2006). Nutritional supplements: Prevalence of use and contamination with doping agents. *Nutrition Research Reviews, 19 (1)*, 147–158.

Waddington, I., Malcolm, D., Roderick, M., and Naik, R. (2005). Drug use in English professional football. *British Journal of Sports Medicine, 39 (e18)*.

Zaggelidis, S., Martinidis, K., Zaggelidis, G., and Mitropoulou, T. (2005). Nutritional supplements use in elite gymnasts. *Physical Training*. Available at http://ejmas.com/pt/2005pt/ptart_zaggelidis_0305.html.

Ziegler, P. J., Nelson, J. A., and Jonnalagadda, S. S. (2003). Use of dietary supplements by elite figure skaters. *International Journal of Sport Nutrition and Exercise Metabolism, 13*, 266–276.

14 Parent-based interventions

Implications for doping prevention

Tonya Dodge, Paige Clarke, and Steffi Renninger

Performance-enhancing substances (PES) are used to help improve athletic performance or physical appearance. Two types of PES used by adolescents are anabolic steroids (AS) and performance-enhancing nutritional supplements. AS are synthetic derivatives of testosterone with the potential to improve muscle mass (Strauss and Yesalis 1991). Although there are a number of legitimate medical uses for AS, these substances may be misused by adolescents (i.e., used without oversight from a physician to treat a medical condition) as a way to increase athletic or physical performance. Between 1 and 5 percent of adolescents in the United States (US) report having tried AS during their lifetime (Dodge and Jaccard 2006; Hoffman *et al.* 2008), and these estimates are comparable to those documented in other countries (Mattila *et al.* 2010; Pallesen *et al.* 2004). This chapter highlights the potential utility of developing parent-based interventions to reduce use of PES among adolescents.

Misuse of AS is associated with numerous health and social consequences including cardiovascular problems, endocrine dysfunction, increases in aggression, and use of alcohol and other drugs (Casavant *et al.* 2007; Dodge and Hoagland 2011; Dunn and White 2011; Lumia and McGinnis 2009). The potential of health problems posed by the misuse of AS has led to a general consensus among the medical community and other organizations that efforts be made to prevent adolescents' misuse of these substances (Committee on Sports Medicine and Fitness 2005; National Federation of State High School Associations 2013).

Performance-enhancing nutritional supplements are marketed in the United States (US) as dietary supplements. These supplements include products such as creatine and whey protein and may be purchased over the counter. There is considerable variability in the US with respect to the safety of nutritional supplements because of the way in which these supplements are regulated. This means that while some performance-enhancing nutritional supplements are relatively safe (e.g., creatine, whey protein) others can be dangerous. Take ephedrine, for example. Ephedrine was an ingredient in a number of performance-enhancing nutritional supplements sold in the US, but in 2004 the US Food and Drug Administration pulled ephedrine and products containing the substance from the market. This is because ephedrine was linked to a number of very serious negative health outcomes including nausea, vomiting, increased autonomic activity, and heart palpitations (Shekelle *et al.* 2003). The variability in safety of dietary supplements is concerning because adolescents may come to view performance-enhancing nutritional supplements as a safer alternative to AS use, yet there are some nutritional supplements that pose significant health risks.

Given that performance-enhancing nutritional supplements are readily available, it is unsurprising that rates of nutritional supplement use are considerably higher than AS use with estimates of adolescent lifetime use ranging between 4 and 71 percent (Frison *et al.* 2013; Hoffman *et al.* 2008; Šterlinko *et al.* 2011; Dodge and Jaccard 2008). The variability in prevalence estimates reflects heterogeneity in the way nutritional supplement use has been measured with the lower end focusing on a single supplement (e.g., amino acids; Frison *et al.* 2013) and the higher end encompassing multiple supplements (e.g., vitamins, minerals, or high-energy drinks; Hoffman *et al.* 2008).

Risk factors for performance-enhancing substances

AS and performance-enhancing nutritional supplements are taken to help improve muscularity, physical appearance, athletic performance, or some combination thereof. Research has found that males are more concerned with enhancing their muscularity than females (Brunet *et al.* 2010; McCreary and Sasse 2000; Zelli *et al.* 2010) and this concern with muscularity is associated with more positive expectancies about PES (Dodge *et al.* 2008). Therefore it is not surprising that males are more likely to use AS and nutritional supplements than are females (Dodge and Jaccard 2006; Hoffman *et al.* 2008). When females do use performance-enhancing nutritional supplements it may be as a way to control or lose weight especially in sports where weight is critical (Stirling *et al.* 2012). In addition, use of both AS and performance-enhancing nutritional supplements is often more common among athletes than non-athletes (Dodge and Jaccard 2006), among those involved in weightlifting (Dodge and Jaccard 2006), and among those who are highly concerned with improving their muscular appearance (Hildebrandt *et al.* 2012; Kanayama *et al.* 2006; Litt and Dodge 2008).

The most effective prevention programs targeting PES use will be those that can reach a wide range of adolescents who are at increased risk and that can be tailored to target the underlying motivations (e.g., improved athletic performance or better appearance). A parent-based intervention is one approach that would allow content to be tailored to meet the needs of each individual adolescent. An additional advantage of parent-based approaches is that parents may be viewed by their adolescents as both expert (i.e., knowledgeable) and trustworthy (i.e., having the best interests of their adolescent at heart). Frameworks focusing on persuasive communication (e.g., Elaboration Likelihood Model; Petty and Cacioppo 1979, 1986) specifically identify these source characteristics (expertise and trustworthiness) as important for success. Indeed there is evidence showing that adolescents view their parents, and especially mothers, as an important source of information with respect to health behaviors (Baheiraei *et al.* 2014;

Whitfield *et al.* 2013). This is likely because adolescents view their parents as holding knowledge about the topic at hand and having their best interests at heart (Jaccard *et al.* 2002).

Extending this to building a prevention program to target use of PES, we can expect that parents have the potential to serve as an effective source of information. In the following sections we provide a brief review of existing programs that target PES use, identify the limitations of such approaches, and then describe how a parent-based approach can complement these existing approaches.

Existing interventions

Nearly all of the interventions targeting PES focus on the misuse of AS specifically. Few, if any, target the use of performance-enhancing nutritional supplements. Furthermore, a majority of AS intervention programs are team-centered. Team-centered programs are those that are developed for groups of athletes and delivered in the context of the team, rather than targeting individual athletes. Two notable examples of team-centered prevention programs that target AS misuse are the Adolescent Training and Learning to Avoid Steroids (ATLAS; Goldberg *et al.* 1996a, 1996b) and the Athletes Targeting Healthy Exercise and Nutrition Alternatives (ATHENA; Elliot *et al.* 2004).

Team-centered approaches

ATLAS is a seven- to eight-week program that was initially designed to target AS misuse among high school football players in the US (Goldberg *et al.* 1996a). The ATLAS program features weekly class sessions delivered by team coaches and adolescent team leaders as well as weekly weight-room sessions delivered by ATLAS staff. The multi-component program addresses a number of topics including AS effects, drug refusal role-play exercises, sports nutrition and strength-training alternatives to AS use, and anti-AS media campaigns. An evaluation of the ATLAS program found that when compared with controls, athletes that received the intervention had statistically significantly lower intentions to use AS, greater knowledge about AS and alternatives to AS use, more negative attitudes toward AS use, and improved body image. Long-term follow-ups demonstrated that many of ATLAS's positive outcomes were sustained over the period of one year (Goldberg *et al.* 1996a).

Based loosely on ATLAS, the ATHENA program is a team-based prevention program developed in the US to target the eating, dieting, and weight management strategies used by female athletes (Elliot *et al.* 2004). ATHENA's eight-week program consists of peer-led discussions on effective exercise training, healthy sport nutrition, negative effects of drug use and other unhealthy behaviors on sport performance, depression prevention, and female media images. An evaluation of the ATHENA program found that when compared with controls, athletes that received the ATHENA intervention reported significantly less new use of PES (including AS) and diet pills (Elliot *et al.* 2004).

While the evaluations of these programs imply that the programs are relatively effective at reducing the use of AS among males and females, it is important to acknowledge that the evaluations of the ATLAS and ATHENA programs were conducted by the researchers who developed the programs, and to date there have been no published evaluations of the programs that were conducted by independent investigators. Furthermore, a recent meta-analysis conducted found that the programs were effective at reducing intentions, but not use (Ntoumanis *et al.* 2014).

School-centered approaches

Whereas team-based approaches focus on developing content specifically for adolescent athletes and delivering the program to teams, school-centered approaches deliver content to a much larger number of adolescents, which could result in establishing a general norm or culture against PES use. A program developed by Nilsson and colleagues (2004) exemplifies this type of intervention. Nilsson and colleagues' (2004) AS prevention intervention utilized peer-led discussions. The intervention targeted 16- and 17-year-old male students (*n*=451) and involved having male and female adolescents engage in discussions about their attitudes toward appearance and behavior. The goal of these discussions was to raise the self-confidence and awareness of appearance ideals among adolescent males. The results demonstrated that among 16-year-old males in the sample, the misuse of injections of AS, but not the misuse of AS pills, significantly decreased after the intervention. Among males in the sample who were 17 years old, there were no significant changes after the intervention. Thus, Nilsson and colleagues' (2004) school-centered intervention may be more effective for certain age groups than others and for targeting certain forms of AS.

Limitations of team-centered and school-centered approaches

Despite evidence pointing to the effectiveness of team- and school-centered programs, there are several limitations with these approaches. One limitation of team-centered programs is that adolescent sports teams are often transient. In other words, many adolescent athletes play different sports during different seasons and increase sport level with time; thus, new teammates and coaches are often encountered. As a result, although a team-centered intervention may be successful in creating a team norm opposed to the use of PES, adolescent athletes often encounter new teams with different norms throughout their athletic experiences. A second limitation of team-centered programs is that they may fail to reach other adolescents at risk for using PES, including males involved in weightlifting (Bahrke *et al.* 2000), sexual minority youth, and those who have a strong desire to improve their physical appearance (Lorang *et al.* 2011; Kindlundh *et al.* 1999; Tanner *et al.* 1995).

Although school-centered interventions have the ability to reach a wide range of adolescents at risk for using PES, such programs are typically unable to adapt content to reach the specific needs of the adolescents. For example, non-athletes may benefit most from content focusing on appearance, whereas athletes may benefit more from content focusing on sport performance. Thus, although school-based interventions, as opposed to team-based interventions, may be able to reach more students at risk for PES use, the inability to match the program content to the motivations of adolescents may limit their success.

Effectiveness of team- and school-centered interventions may also be dampened by the fact that the content must be delivered during the school year. Because adolescents only attend school for a certain part of the calendar year, the interventions fail to provide information during extended periods of time, leaving large gaps of time when an adolescent will be left without exposure to a prevention message.

A final limitation of both team- and school-centered interventions is that such interventions, if designed to include performance-enhancing nutritional supplements, would likely send a single message: that all performance-enhancing nutritional supplements should be avoided. Although we can speculate that few parents would condone their child using AS, parents likely differ in their beliefs regarding performance-enhancing nutritional supplements. Because some performance-enhancing nutritional supplements may be relatively safe, parents may be indifferent or even support their adolescent using one. Thus, team- and school-centered interventions may run the risk of delivering a message that is inconsistent with parental beliefs, which could limit the success of the intervention.

Conclusions

Although team- and school-centered programs targeting misuse of AS and performance-enhancing nutritional supplements may be effective, there are several gaps in relying exclusively on such programs. These gaps include the potential to miss some adolescents who are at risk, the inability to adapt content to the needs of the adolescent, constraints on the timing of when the program is delivered, and the possibility that the content of the program conflicts with parental beliefs. One approach to address these limitations is to develop a parent-based intervention that can be used either as a stand-alone program or could be used in conjunction with team- and school-centered approaches (Dodge and Clarke 2014).

Parent-based interventions

Developing a parent-based program to target the use of PES might be one way to meet the limitations of team- or school-based programs. This is because parents are in a position to tailor the content to match the needs of the child and to match the values of the family. For example, a parent-based intervention (PBI) would allow parents to decide on which type of message is likely to resonate best with their child. While messages about speed and athleticism may resonate with an adolescent athlete, a message about body image and muscularity might be more effective for an adolescent involved in weightlifting. Another aspect of tailoring the message that is important to recognize is that parents can deliver the content in a way that is consistent with family values, and this may be particularly relevant when discussing performance-enhancing nutritional supplements. In this case some parents may, for example, be uniformly opposed to their adolescent using any of these substances, whereas other parents may feel certain performance-enhancing nutritional supplements are acceptable. A PBI provides the opportunity for parents to match the content with the specific needs and motivations of their child; something that team- or school-based programs cannot do. Furthermore, these messages can be delivered consistently over time and have the chance to transcend changes in teams or other social contexts. Although parents with particular parenting styles (e.g., authoritative) may be more effective at delivering messages than parents with other parenting styles (e.g., authoritarian) (Becoña *et al.* 2011; Calafat *et al.* 2014), parents, in general, are in a unique position to deliver messages consistently over time and have the chance to transcend changes in teams or other social contexts.

PBIs and adolescent health

Parent-based interventions have a rich and successful tradition in the literature on adolescent health. These types of programs have been used with considerable success to prevent a wide range of adolescent risk-taking and associated outcomes (Doumas *et al.* 2013; Guilamo-Ramos *et al.* 2011; Turrisi *et al.* 2004).

In one example of a parent-based intervention, Guilamo-Ramos and colleagues (2011) developed and implemented a PBI for African American and Latino adolescents (aged 11–14 years) in the US with the goal of reducing sexual risk-taking behaviors. Mother-adolescent dyads were randomly assigned to receive the PBI or to a standard care control condition. The PBI targeted the mothers and included four components: a face-to-face session with mothers, written materials (that explained how to begin conversations about sex), booster phone calls (at one month and five months), and support of the program from the child's physician. Social workers met individually with mothers of adolescents to outline strategies for effective parent–child communication in general, and specifically about preventing risky sexual behaviors. Mothers in the control group completed baseline questionnaires and follow-up assessments only. Results indicated that adolescents whose mothers received the PBI reported no increase in vaginal intercourse at the nine-month follow-up, whereas the percentage of adolescents in the control group that reported engaging in sexual intercourse increased from 6.4 percent to 22 percent. Additionally, adolescents in the control group reported more frequent sexual intercourse in the past 30 days than adolescents in the PBI group.

There is also evidence that PBI can be effective at increasing sun protection behaviors in young adolescents (aged 9–12 years). Turrisi and colleagues (2004) developed, implemented, and tested the efficacy of a PBI delivered in the US to adolescents aged 9–12 years. The intervention, delivered via a handbook, was designed to promote parent–child communication regarding the risks of sun exposure and to encourage safe sun practices. Parents in the control group received the same handbook intervention; however, it was administered after the post-test. Results suggest that adolescents in the intervention reported fewer sunburns and burns that were less severe relative to the control group approximately one month later. Additionally, those in the intervention reported significantly fewer sunbathing behaviors compared to their non-intervention counterparts. Finally, those children receiving the intervention regarded sunscreen as more effective in sunburn and skin cancer prevention than children in the control group (Turrisi *et al.* 2004).

While the above PBIs documented that such programs are better than standard care or no interventions (Guliamo-Ramos *et al.* 2011; Turrisi *et al.* 2004), there is also evidence indicating that when a PBI is used in tandem with an existing student-based intervention, better outcomes are achieved. Koning and colleagues (2009) tested whether parent-based interventions are most effective in reducing heavy alcohol use among Dutch adolescents (aged 12 years at baseline) when used alone or when used simultaneously with a student intervention. Participants were randomly assigned to one of four intervention conditions: parent intervention (PI), student intervention (SI), combined parent-student intervention (CI), and control (CC). The PI occurred during the first week of school, as part of a larger school meeting. Parents listened to a presentation on the negative health consequences of alcohol use and then participated in small group meetings, aimed at establishing a set of rules they could implement regarding alcohol use. Informational packets were sent home to encourage and remind parents to communicate with their adolescents. Participants in the SI group completed an established alcohol prevention program that incorporated lessons on education, school regulations, and parental involvement related to alcohol use. Participants in the control condition did not receive an intervention; however, basic alcohol education is part of the standard school curriculum in the Netherlands, which continued during the study.

At a ten-month follow-up fewer adolescents in the CI had started to drink heavily compared to the control group, but these effects were no longer statistically significant at a 22-month follow-up (Koning *et al.* 2009). However, at both the ten-month and 22-month follow-up significantly fewer students in the CI reported drinking on a weekly basis compared to the controls (Koning *et al.* 2009). At a four-year follow-up results indicated that students receiving the CI were less likely to report heavy weekend drinking, and reported lower amounts of alcohol use compared to those students in the control condition (Koning *et al.* 2013). Furthermore, adolescents in the CI reported greater perceived parental strictness and greater self-control than adolescents in the control condition. Thus, using a PBI in conjunction with an existing student-centered intervention aimed at reducing alcohol use may lead to better long-term outcomes than when using the student intervention alone.

Finally, there is evidence to suggest that an existing intervention that targets tobacco use among adolescents can lead to better outcomes when supplemented with a PBI (Guilamo-Ramos *et al.* 2010). African American and Latino mother-adolescent dyads participated in an intervention for tobacco use prevention. All adolescents (grades 6–8; age $M = 12.1$ years) received the Toward No Tobacco use (TNT) intervention, which was delivered via two in-person sessions. Additionally, some parent-adolescent dyads were randomly assigned to receive an additional PBI, Linking Lives. The TNT component taught adolescents refusal skills, effective communication (with parents and peers), and health consequences associated with tobacco use. Simultaneously, mothers randomly assigned to the Linking Lives intervention received a handbook outlining effective parent–child communication strategies and monitoring tips (i.e., setting restrictions) for preventing tobacco use, as well as information about the consequences of smoking. The contents of this handbook were reviewed and discussed during two in-person meetings. Upon completion of the second session, mothers were given booklets to give to their adolescent about not smoking and received booster calls (one and six months later). At a 15-month follow-up, mothers in the intervention were more likely than mothers in the control condition to set limits on their adolescents' behaviors that had the potential to promote smoking. Additionally, adolescents whose mothers received Linking Lives were more likely to view their mothers as trustworthy, easier to talk to, and reported significantly more frequent communication regarding smoking.

In sum, there is evidence indicating that PBIs are successful at reducing adolescent risk-taking behaviors across a wide range of behaviors. Furthermore, these studies suggest that PBIs are effective either as stand-alone programs (Doumas *et al.* 2013; Guilamo-Ramos *et al.* 2011; Turrisi *et al.* 2004) or when used in conjunction with other existing programs (Guilamo-Ramos *et al.* 2010; Koning *et al.* 2009). Finally, the effectiveness of such approaches has been demonstrated in the US with diverse samples (Guiliamo-Ramos *et al.* 2010) and in the Netherlands (Koning *et al.* 2009, 2013).

PBI as an approach to prevent use of PES in adolescents

There are several key features of the successful PBI reviewed above. One is that these interventions aimed to promote better parent–child communication about the risk behavior (Guilamo-Ramos *et al.* 2010, 2011; Koning *et al.* 2009; Turrisi *et al.* 2004). A second key feature is that the programs trained parents to be more vigilant about factors that promote risk-taking (Guilamo-Ramos *et al.* 2010; Koning *et al.* 2009). Finally, booster calls to remind and encourage parents to communicate with their adolescent were incorporated (Doumas *et al.* 2013; Guilamo-Ramos *et al.* 2010, 2011). Therefore, a PBI targeting use of PES among adolescents is likely to benefit from incorporating these features.

In particular, the program should educate parents about the topic of PES and train parents to be vigilant about factors that may place their adolescent at risk for use of PES (e.g., using a commercial gym). Finally, the intervention should incorporate booster calls to encourage parents to engage in discussions with their adolescent and to remind them to be mindful of contexts that might promote use of PES.

Next steps for building a PBI about PES

There are several next steps that should be considered prior to building a PBI. These include (1) identifying how comfortable and capable parents feel about discussing the topic of PES with their adolescent; (2) understanding whether adolescents believe their parents are an appropriate source for delivering information about PES; and (3) identifying the content that should be conveyed to parents. Each of these next steps is discussed in the paragraphs below.

Parents as an information source: parent and adolescent perspectives

Before embarking on developing a PBI targeting PES use, it would be helpful to know whether parents feel capable of engaging in these discussions and whether adolescents perceive their parents to be an appropriate source of information about PES. In our lab, several studies have been designed to examine this issue (Dodge 2008, 2010; Dodge and Clarke 2014).

In one such study (Dodge 2008) data were collected from parent-son dyads. Sixty-seven adolescents (age $M=15.02$ years, $SD=1.50$) and at least one parent (mothers $n=48$, fathers $n=42$) were recruited from adolescent sporting events (e.g., soccer teams, baseball teams,) or parent groups in the US. In some cases both parents completed a questionnaire, but in other cases only one parent chose to participate. Parents responded on a scale from 1 (*strongly disagree*) to 5 (*strongly agree*), the extent to which they felt (1) they would give helpful advice to their adolescent about illegal and legal PES; (2) were knowledgeable about the side effects of illegal PES; and (3) whether it would be easy to talk with their son about illegal PES. Adolescents completed comparable items using the same five-point scale where they reported the extent to which they felt their parents would give helpful advice about illegal and legal PES and were knowledgeable about illegal PES.

Mean responses for items about illegal PES are shown in Figure 14.1. Figure 14.2 shows the mean responses for items about legal PES. In general, these data indicate that mothers and fathers felt like they could provide some helpful advice to their sons about both illegal and legal PES. However, these data also suggest that both mothers and fathers felt they lacked, to some degree, knowledge about the side effects associated with illegal and legal PES. Furthermore, paired samples t-tests revealed that mothers felt more helpful and more knowledgeable about illegal PES than they did about legal PES. Fathers felt more knowledgeable about the side effects of illegal PES than about side effects of legal PES. In general, adolescents' reports tended to reflect those of their parents.

In a separate study (Dodge 2010), data were collected from 118 male adolescent athletes. Adolescents were recruited from a variety of sports teams in the northeastern US (e.g., football, soccer, baseball) to complete a self-report questionnaire. Adolescents reported the extent to which they: (1) would go to their mothers [fathers] for advice about AS; and (2) believed their mothers [fathers] would provide good advice about AS. Identical items were asked for

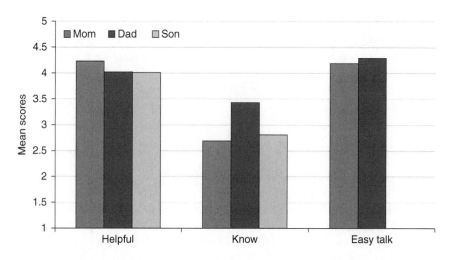

Figure 14.1 Reports of helpful, knowledgeable, and easy to talk about illegal PES.[1]

Note

1 Y-Axis reflects responses which ranged from 1 (strongly disagree) to 5 (strongly agree); Helpful=I [my parent] would give helpful advice; Know=I [my parent is] am knowledgeable about side effects; Easy talk=It would be easy to talk with my son.

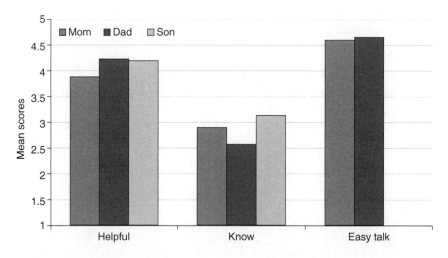

Figure 14.2 Reports of helpful, knowledgeable, and easy to talk about legal PES.[1]

Note

1 Y-Axis reflects responses which ranged from 1 (strongly disagree) to 5 (strongly agree); Helpful=I [my parent] would give helpful advice; Know=I [my parent is] am knowledgeable about side effects; Easy talk = It would be easy to talk with my son.

legal performance-enhancing nutritional supplements. The response scale ranged from 1 (*strongly disagree*) to 7 (*strongly disagree*). Mean responses are shown in Figure 14.3. Overall, adolescents reported some degree of willingness to go to their mothers and fathers for advice about AS and performance-enhancing nutritional supplements. Adolescents also believed to some degree that their mothers and fathers would provide good advice about these topics.

Together these studies suggest that adolescents may perceive their parents to be relatively good sources of information about illegal PES and legal PES. These data also highlight some deficits in parents' self-reported knowledge about the side effects of illegal and legal PES. To the extent that parents wish to convey the potential dangers of these substances, a PBI should be designed to improve parents' knowledge in these areas. A point of promise from these data is that both mothers and fathers reported it would be relatively easy to start conversations with their sons about illegal and legal PES. The next step for building a PBI is to help parents with the content of those communications.

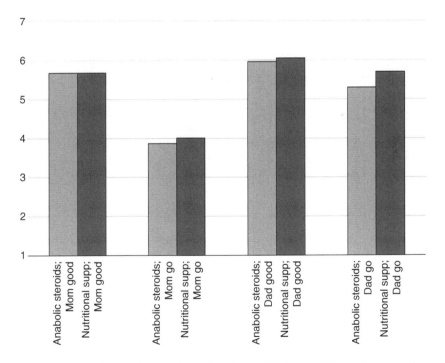

Figure 14.3 Adolescents' perceptions of mothers and fathers as information source.[1]

Note
1 Y-Axis reflects responses which ranged from 1 (strongly disagree) to 5 (strongly agree); Mom [Dad] Good=My mom [dad] is a good source of advice; Mom [Dad] Go=I would go to my mother [father] for advice.

The content of PBI targeting PES

Another step for building a PBI is to identify the specific content that parents should convey to their adolescent. To accomplish this, a focus group study with a sample of adolescents and parents could be conducted. The adolescent focus group should emphasize what type of information is most relevant to their decisions to try PES. The parental focus group should concentrate on identifying where parents feel inadequate or unprepared with respect to PES. The adolescent and parent focus groups should be tailored to elicit information about both illegal and legal PES. Information from these focus groups would be used to help inform the content of the intervention.

In some of our own work, we found adolescent athletes' reports of communication with their parents about the performance outcomes and protective factors of AS to be statistically significant predictors of their willingness to use a newly developed, potentially illegal PES (Dodge and Clarke 2014). Specifically, the more adolescents reported discussing with their parents the performance benefits of AS, the more willing the adolescents were to try a newly developed, potentially illegal PES. In contrast, the more adolescents reported discussing with their parents protective factors associated with AS (e.g., refusal skills), the less willing the adolescents were to try the PES. Thus, the results suggest that communication about performance benefits may increase willingness to use a newly developed PES. This finding highlights an important role for focus groups in developing content: focus groups might help us better appreciate how adolescents might perceive messages that deliver information about why individuals might consider using PES.

Another approach to identifying content to be included in the intervention would be to conduct a systematic literature review to identify those factors that emerge as consistent and reliable predictors of PES use. This has the potential to provide additional insights with respect to specific content about PES that can be delivered by parents to their adolescent.

Policy implications of PBI

The development of PBI may play a role in wider policymaking regarding doping in sports. For example, the World Anti-Doping Agency (WADA) has established the World Anti-Doping Code (WADC) which outlines the rules, policies, and procedures governing anti-doping in sports. Under the WADC athlete support personnel (ASP) are individuals who provide assistance to athletes including coaches, trainers, managers, and parents (WADA 2009: 113). ASP are obligated to encourage athletes to adopt anti-doping attitudes (WADC 21.2.2). Developing PBIs offer one mechanism through which ASP in general, and parents in particular, can be used to help increase adolescent athletes' knowledge about the WADC and in developing stronger anti-doping attitudes in general.

Conclusion

There is ample evidence pointing to the success of using PBI to help reduce adolescent risk-taking and its associated outcomes across a wide range of health behaviors (Doumas *et al.* 2013; Guilamo-Ramos *et al.* 2011; Turrisi *et al.* 2004). Because of the success in utilizing PBI in other areas of adolescent health, it seems reasonable to believe a similar approach may be useful in the prevention of PES. Incorporating PBI into efforts to prevent use of PES has a number of advantages. Parents can emphasize the content to match the needs of the child and to match the values of the family. A PBI also provides the opportunity for parents to adapt content to meet the specific needs of their child (e.g., for some adolescents a message about speed will resonate whereas for others it might be fairness that is most influential). Finally, with PBI parents can send messages consistently over time that have the chance to transcend changes in teams or other social contexts. In sum, we feel that PBI are a largely understudied approach to targeting PES. Incorporating parents into prevention efforts via PBI holds considerable promise. These PBI can be developed as stand-alone programs or add-ons to existing programs. We are hopeful that the field recognizes the potential of PBI and can move toward incorporating parents in efforts to reduce the use of PES among adolescents.

Acknowledgments

Some of the research presented in this chapter was supported by a Social Science Research Grant from the World Anti-Doping Agency.

References

Baheiraei, A., Khoori, E., Foroushani, A. R., Ahmadi, F., and Ybarra, M. L. (2014). What sources do adolescents turn to for information about their health concerns? *International Journal of Adolescent Medicine and Health*, *26*, 61–68.

Bahrke, M. S., Yesalis, C. E., Kopstein, A. N., and Stephens, J. A. (2000). Risk factors associated with anabolic-androgenic steroid use among adolescents. *Sports Medicine*, *29*, 397–405.

Becoña, E., Martínez, U., Calafat, A., Juan, M., Fernández-Hermida, J. R., and Secades-Villa, R. (2012). Parental styles and drug use: A review. *Drugs: Education, Prevention and Policy*, *19*, 1–10.

Brunet, J., Sabiston, C. M., Dorsch, K. D., and McCreary, D. R. (2010). Exploring a model linking social physique anxiety, drive for muscularity, drive for thinness and self-esteem among adolescent boys and girls. *Body Image*, *7*, 137–142.

Calafat, A., Garcia, F., Juan, M., Becoña, E., and Fernandez-Hermida, J. R. (2014). Which parenting style is more protective against adolescent substance use? Evidence within the European context. *Drug and Alcohol Dependence*, *138*, 185–192.

Casavant, M. J., Blake, K., Griffith, J., Yates, A., and Copley, L. M. (2007). Consequences of anabolic androgenic steroids. *Pediatric Clinics of North America*, *54*, 677–690.

Committee on Sports Medicine and Fitness (2005). Use of performance-enhancing substances. *Pediatrics*, *115*, 1103–1106.

Dodge, T. (2008). Parent-teen communication about performance enhancing substances. Unpublished raw data.

Dodge, T. (2010). Incorporating parents in the anti-doping fight: A test of the viability of a parent-based prevention program. Unpublished raw data.

Dodge, T. L. and Clarke, P. (2014). Influence of parent-adolescent communication about anabolic steroids on adolescent athletes' willingness to try performance enhancing substances (under review).

Dodge, T. L. and Jaccard, J. J. (2006). The effect of high school sports participation on the use of performance enhancing substances in adulthood. *Journal of Adolescent Health, 39*, 367–373.

Dodge, T. and Jaccard, J. J. (2008). Is abstinence an alternative? Predicting adolescent athletes' intentions to use performance enhancing substances. *Journal of Health Psychology, 13*, 703–711.

Dodge, T. and Hoagland, M. (2011). The use of anabolic androgenic steroids and polypharmacy: A review of the literature. *Drug and Alcohol Dependence, 114*, 100–109.

Dodge, T., Litt, D., Seitchik, A., and Bennett, S. (2008). Drive for muscularity and beliefs about legal performance enhancing substances as predictors of current use and willingness to use. *Journal of health psychology, 13* (8), 1173–1179.

Doumas, D. M., Turrisi, R., Ray, A. E., Esp, S. M., and Curtis-Schaeffer, A. K. (2013). A randomized trial evaluating a parent based intervention to reduce college drinking. *Journal of Substance Abuse Treatment, 45*, 31–7.

Dunn, M. and White, V. (2011). The epidemiology of anabolic-androgenic steroid use among Australian secondary school students. *Journal of Science and Medicine in Sport, 14*, 10–14.

Elliot, D. L., Goldberg, L., Moe, E. L., Defrancesco, C. A., Durham, M. B., and Hix-Small, H. (2004). Preventing substance use and disordered eating: Initial outcomes of the ATHENA (athletes targeting healthy exercise and nutrition alternatives) program. *Archives of Pediatrics and Adolescent Medicine, 158*, 1043–1049.

Frison, E., Vandenbosch, L., and Eggermont, S. (2013). Exposure to media predicts use of dietary supplements and anabolic-steroids among Flemish adolescent boys. *European Journal of Pediatrics, 172*, 1387–1392.

Goldberg, M. D., Elliot, D., Clarke, G. N., MacKinnon, D. P., Moe, E., Zoref, L., Green, C., Wolf, S. L., Greffrath, E., Miller, D. J., and Lapin, A. (1996a). Effects of a multidimensional anabolic steroids program intervention: The adolescent training and learning to avoid steroids (ATLAS) program. *The Journal of the American Medical Association, 276*, 1555–1562.

Goldberg, M. D., Elliot, D., Clarke, G. N., MacKinnon, D. P., Zoref, L., Moe, E., Green, C., and Wolf, S. L. (1996b). The adolescent training and learning to avoid steroids (ATLAS) prevention program: Background and results of a model intervention. *Archives of Pediatrics and Adolescent Medicine, 150*, 713–721.

Guilamo-Ramos, V., Bouris, A., Jaccard, J., Gonzalez, B., McCoy, W., and Aranda, D. (2011). A parent-based intervention to reduce sexual risk behavior in early adolescence: Building alliances between physicians, social workers, and parents. *Journal of Adolescent health, 48*, 159–163.

Guilamo-Ramos, V., Jaccard, J., Dittus, P., Gonzalez, B., Bouris, A., and Banspach, S. (2010). The Linking Lives Health Education Program: A randomized clinical trial of a parent-based tobacco use prevention program for African American and Latino youths. *American Journal of Public Health, 100*, 1641–1647.

Hildebrandt, T., Harty, S., and Langenbucher, J. W. (2012). Fitness supplements as a gateway substance for anabolic-androgenic steroid use. *Psychology of Addictive Behaviors*, *26*, 955–962.

Hoffman, J. R., Faigenbaum, A. D., Ratamess, N. A., Ross, R., Kang, J., and Tenenbaum, G. (2008). Nutritional supplementation and anabolic steroids use in adolescents. *Medicine and Science in Sport and Exercise*, *40*, 15–24.

Jaccard, J., Dodge, T., and Dittus, P. (2002). Parent adolescent communication about sex and birth control: A conceptual framework. In S. Feldman and D. A. Rosenthal (eds.), *Out in the open: Parent-teen communication about sexuality. New Directions in Child and Adolescent Development*. Series Editor W. Damon. San Francisco: Jossey-Bass.

Kanayama, G., Barry, S., Hudson, J. I., and Pope, H. G. (2006). Body image and attitudes toward male roles in anabolic-androgenic steroid users. *The American Journal of Psychiatry*, *163*, 697–703.

Kindlundh, A. M., Isacsson, D. G., Berglund, L., and Nyberg, F. (1999). Factors associated with adolescent use of doping agents. *Anabolic Androgenic Steroids Addiction*, *94*, 543–545.

Koning, I. M., van den Eijnden, R. J. J. M., Verdurmen, J. E. E., Engels, R. C. M. E., and Vollebergh, W. A. M. (2013). A cluster randomized trial on the effects of a parent and student intervention on alcohol use in adolescents four years after baseline; No evidence of catching-up behavior. *Addictive Behaviors*, *38*, 2032–2039.

Koning, I. M., Vollebergh, W. A. M., Smit, F., Verdurmen, J. E. E., Eijnden, R. J. J. M., van den Bogt, T. F. M., Stattin, H., and Engels, R. C. M. E. (2009). Preventing heavy alcohol use in adolescents (PAS): Cluster randomized trial of a parent and student intervention offered separately and simultaneously. *Addiction*, *104*, 1669–1678.

Litt, D. and Dodge, T. (2008). A longitudinal investigation of the drive for muscularity scale: Predicting use of performance enhancing substances and weight lifting among males. *Body Image*, *5*, 346–351.

Lorang, M., Callahan, B., Cummins, K. M., Achar, S., and Brown, S. A. (2011). Anabolic androgenic steroid use in teens: Prevalence, demographics, and perception of effects. *Journal of Child and Adolescent Substance Abuse*, *20*, 358–369.

Lumia, A. R. and McGinnis, M. Y. (2009). Impact of anabolic androgenic steroids on adolescent males. *Physiology and Behavior*, *100*, 199–204.

Mattila, V. M., Rimpelä, A., Jormanainen, V., Sahi, T., and Pihlajamäki, H. (2010). Anabolic-androgenic steroid use among young Finnish males. *Scandinavian Journal of Medicine and Science in Sports*, *20*, 330–335.

McCreary, D. R. and Sasse, D. K. (2000). An exploration of the drive for muscularity in adolescent boys and girls. *Journal of American College Health*, *48*, 297–304.

National Federation of State High School Associations (2013). Position statement on anabolic, androgenic steroids. Available at https://nsaahome.org/textfile/spmeds/steroids.pdf (accessed September 26, 2013).

Nilsson, S., Allebeck, P., Marklund, B., Baigi, A., and Fridlund, B. (2004). Evaluation of a health promotion programme to prevent the misuse of androgenic anabolic steroids among Swedish adolescents. *Health Promotion International*, *19*, 61–67.

Ntoumanis, N., Ng, J. Y., Barkoukis, V., and Backhouse, S. (2014). Personal and psychosocial predictors of doping use in physical activity settings: A meta-analysis. *Sports Medicine*, *44* (*11*), 1603–1624.

Pallesen, S. Jøsendal, O., Johnsen, B. H., Larsen, S., and Molde, H. (2004). Anabolic steroid use in high school students. *Substance Use and Misuse*, *41*, 1705–1717.

Petty, R. and Cacioppo, J. (1979). Effects of message repetition and position on cognitive response, recall, and persuasion. *Journal of Personality and Social Psychology*, *37*, 97–109.

Petty, R. and Cacioppo, J. (1986). The Elaboration Likelihood Model of Persuasion. *Advances in Experimental Social Psychology*, *19*, 123–205.

Shekelle, P., Hardy, M. L., Morton, S. C., Maglione, M., Suttorp, M., Roth, L Jungvig, Mojica, W. A., Gagné, J., Rhodes, S., and McKinnon, E. (2003). Ephedra and ephedrine for weight loss and athletic performance enhancement: Clinical efficacy and side effects. *Evidence Report/Technology Assessment (Summary)*, *76*, 1–4.

Stirling, A. E., Cruz, L. C., and Kerr, G. A. (2012). Influence of retirement on body satisfaction and weight control behaviors: Perceptions of elite rhythmic gymnasts. *Journal of Applied Sport Psychology*, *24*, 129–143.

Strauss, R. H. and Yesalis, C. E. (1991). Anabolic steroids in the athlete. *Annual Review of Medicine*, *42*, 449–457.

Šterlinko, G. H., Stubelj, A. M., Besednjak-Kocijančič, L., and Golja, P. (2011). Nutritional supplement use among Slovenian adolescents. *Public Health Nutrition*, *15*, 587–593.

Tanner, S. M., Miller, D. W., and Alongi, C. (1995). Anabolic steroid use by adolescents: Prevalence, motives, and knowledge of risks. *Clinical Journal of Sport Medicine*, *5*, 108–115.

Turrisi, R., Hillhouse, J., Heavin, S., Robinson, J., Adams, M., and Berry, J. (2004). Examination of the short-term efficacy of a parent-based intervention to prevent skin cancer. *Journal of Behavioral Medicine*, 27, 393–412.

Whitfield, C., Jomeen, J., Hayter, M., and Gardiner, E. (2013). Sexual health information seeking: A survey of adolescent practices. *Journal of Clinical Nursing*, *22*, 3259–3269.

World Anti-Doping Agency (WADA) (2009). *The World Anti-Doping Code*. Montreal, Canada: World Anti-Doping Agency. Available at www.wada-ama.org/.

Zelli, A., Lucidi, and Mallia, L. (2010). The relationships among adolescents' drive for muscularity, drive for thinness, doping attitudes and doping intentions. *Journal of Clinical Sport Psychology*, *4*, 39–52.

15 Moving away from penalization

The role of education-based campaigns

Vassilis Barkoukis

> Whenever there are significant sums of money to be won, and glory to be gained, there always will be those willing to come up with new and more cunning ways to cheat.
>
> John Fahey, former WADA President (2013)

In January 2013 a major doping scandal was revealed with Lance Armstrong, a professional cyclist and seven-times-Tour de France winner, publicly admitting prolonged doping use during his athletic career, and also declaring that he did not invent the doping culture, but also did nothing to stop it. Quite interestingly, Armstrong also recalled all the doping controls he managed to circumvent during his career in professional cycling. Shortly after Armstrong's admission of doping, WADA's then President John Fahey declared the need for an even more intensive "war on drugs" in sports, and made the statement used as an opening quote of this chapter. Both Armstrong and Fahey seem to agree on this: athletes (and/or their entourage) can find ways to circumvent doping controls. This raises questions about the efficacy and effectiveness of the existing anti-doping policies and methods, and also calls for attention to alternative doping prevention methods. The present chapter will discuss how and why state-of-the-art doping controls may not meet their targets, why a paradigm shift in doping prevention is needed, and how doping prevention interventions can be informed and developed based on the most recent scientific evidence about the "psychology of doping use" in sports.

Doping controls: the long and the short of it

Currently, the existing doping control paradigm is based on a prohibitionist approach where detection-and-punishment is the prevailing modus operandi (Backhouse *et al.* 2012). Within this framework, practices have been adopted involving more frequent, more thorough (i.e., keeping athletes' samples for eight years to retest with new technologies), random, and out of competition doping controls (see WADA's WHEREABOUT system). In addition, relevant sport authorities, such as the WADA, attempt to discourage doping through punishment, ranging from exclusion from competitions to more harsh sanctions, including ineligibility to participate in competitions for a few months and career termination (WADA 2009). This paradigm is based on the assumption that the fear of sanctions, (e.g., legal prosecution, career termination) acts as a deterrent to doping use.

Nevertheless, the prohibitionist/punitive paradigm has received much criticism over the last decade. Goldberg and her associates (Goldberg et al. 2003, 2007) investigated the effect of a school drug policy (i.e., Student Athlete Testing Using Random Notification; SATURN) on athletes' beliefs and behaviors. More specifically, the authors examined the deterrent effect of SATURN involving random drug testing of the athletes throughout the school year in the experimental condition, whereas in the control condition athletes were subjected to drug testing only during their sport season. The results of the first study (Goldberg et al. 2003) indicated that the application of SATURN reduced the use of illegal recreational and performance enhancement drugs, but increased most psychological risk factors associated with drug use such as social norms and health side effects of drug use. In a subsequent test of the SATURN policy, Goldberg et al. (2007) replicated these findings. Athletes in the intervention condition reported less drug use in the post-intervention and follow-up measurement as compared to those in the control group. However, Goldberg et al. also demonstrated a more maladaptive profile of ability and risk-taking beliefs. In the end, the authors questioned the ability of such deterrent policies in effectively combating drug use.

The ineffectiveness of the existing prohibitionist paradigm in doping control has been also reflected in recent major doping scandals that indicate that these investments do not bring the expected outcomes. Such scandals include Armstrong's doping evasion, Barry Bonds and Jose Canseco's steroid use in the major baseball league in the USA, and the Bay Area Laboratory Co-Operative scandal where scientific knowledge was used by practitioners not to prevent doping use, but, rather, to find new ways to facilitate doping evasion (Fainaru-Wada and Williams 2006). Park (2005) argued that WADA's approach to anti-doping is outdated and resembles a "police" to athlete's bodies. Accordingly, Kayser and Broers (2013) heavily criticized the prohibitionist anti-doping paradigm by arguing that it is fraught with moralistic bias, is highly expensive and ineffective, and cannot meet its goal to eradicate doping from sports.

Another line of evidence suggests that the current anti-doping regime suffers from poor decision-making practices and errors among medical personnel assigned to regulate doping controls and overlook anti-doping policies (Dikic et al. 2012), and that anti-doping policies worldwide were historically concerned with protecting the image of sports, rather than other qualities, such as athlete's health (Hunt et al. 2012). In light of these criticisms, progressively more scientists, mostly from the medical and social sciences, have called for a shift in the anti-doping paradigm toward a better understanding of the driving forces behind doping use, with an emphasis on psychological and decision-making processes (e.g., Backhouse et al. 2012; Ehrnborg and Rosén 2009; Petróczi and Aidman

2008). Drawing on empirical evidence about athletes, doping mindset can provide multiple ways and targets for doping prevention interventions (Backhouse *et al.* 2012; Morente-Sánchez and Zabala 2013).

The empirical basis for doping prevention

Over the last decade, and following WADA's active support of social science research on doping use, there have been more than 100 research articles published in peer-reviewed journals that tackle a broad range of psychosocial processes and risk factors for doping use (Ntoumanis *et al.* 2014). More specifically, the extant literature suggests that attitudes, social norms, and self-efficacy related to doping use consistently predict doping intentions and actual use, across age groups and sporting levels (Barkoukis *et al.* 2013; Lazuras *et al.* 2010; Lucidi *et al.* 2008; Wiefferink *et al.* 2008). Accordingly, self-regulatory processes, like moral disengagement, predict doping intentions and behavior directly, over and above the influence of doping-related beliefs (Lucidi *et al.* 2008). Goal orientations and achievement goals also represent more general dispositions and motivational processes in sports that can further predict the risk for doping use both directly and indirectly (Barkoukis *et al.* 2011; Petróczi 2007). In addition, Barkoukis *et al.* (2013) distinguished between distal-level influences that represent more general dispositions in sports (e.g., achievement goals, moral beliefs) and doping-specific proximal influences on doping behavior, such as pro-doping attitudes and social norms.

In addition to these social-cognitive approaches, several ecological approaches have been developed to describe the psychological underpinnings of doping behaviors with a primary objective to develop effective anti-doping education interventions (Hauw and McNamee 2014). The integrative model of doping use (Barkoukis *et al.* 2013; Lazuras, Chapter 4 this volume), the life-cycle model (Petróczi and Aidman 2008), the drugs in sport deterrence model (Strelan and Boeckmann 2003), the macro analytical model of drugs in sport (Stewart and Smith 2008), the systemic social perspective on doping (Johnson 2012), and the Sport Drug Control Model (Donovan *et al.* 2002) incorporate social-cognitive research on doping and provide a solid theoretical basis explaining the psychological processes associated with doping behavior (for a more detailed presentation see Lazuras, Chapter 4 this volume). It appears that a critical mass of empirical evidence about the psychosocial risk factors for doping use has been reached. The next step is to utilize this knowledge capital for the development of effective, evidence-based anti-doping interventions.

By drawing on empirical evidence about the effectiveness of substance use prevention programs, Houlihan (2008) proposed nine major guidelines that could be usefully applied in the design and implementation of doping prevention interventions. Namely, education-based campaigns vs. punitive approaches are needed, and campaigns should be based on empirical findings about behavior change processes and emphasize counseling rather than exclusion. Furthermore, education-based campaigns should reflect the joint efforts and active involvement of the local community, such as local sports clubs, schools, and the media. The role of family and peer dynamics was also highlighted, and Houlihan (2008) suggested that both peer- and parent-led methods add credibility and increase the likelihood of success. Finally, education-based intervention against doping should start early on, involve interactive learning (vs. one-way delivery of information) and "booster" sessions, and be continuously evaluated in order to ensure success and enable modification if prevention goals are not met as expected. In addition, Backhouse *et al.* (2012) further posited that effective doping prevention interventions should be tailored to fit the needs of the target population; target core life skills, such as effective refusal skills and decision-making); and be delivered by well-trained individuals. Based on these recommendations (Backhouse *et al.* 2012; Houlihan 2008), the following sections discuss existing anti-doping interventions and provide suggestions for further improvements in this area.

Awareness-raising campaigns

WADA has developed several campaigns that target the health side effects of doping use, and accordingly aim to increase athletes' and their entourages' awareness about doping control procedures and anti-doping regulations. The PLAY TRUE GENERATION PROGRAM is an update of the Outreach program and includes a web-based simulation and gaming applications about the consequences of doping use with an emphasis on health, legal, and social consequences (e.g., social stigma following doping-related convictions). These applications also inform target users about the doping control procedures, the therapeutic use exceptions, and the use of healthy alternatives to performance enhancement (e.g., nutrition; www.wada-ama.org/en/what-we-do/education-awareness/play-true-generation). Although WADA's programs have been running for well over five years, and have been adopted by different anti-doping agencies and national anti-doping organizations across the globe, their effectiveness in preventing or reducing doping use remains to be determined by empirical evidence.

Education-based interventions

Another group of interventions aimed to curb doping use by employing a health education perspective, closely aligned to Backhouse *et al.*'s (2012) recommendations about targeting core life skills, such as refusal efficacy. For example, Laure and Lecerf (1999) empirically assessed an intervention that emphasized the adverse consequences and the moral implications of doping use. The intervention targeted individual and team sport adolescent athletes and included: (1) audiovisual information on the prevalence of doping use in competitive sports; (2) a critical discussion about the use of nutritional supplements and other ergogenic aids used to enhance performance; (3) a role-playing activity, where one of the researchers pretended to be the doctor trying to persuade an athlete to use illegal supplements followed by a critical discussion of the arguments in favor of and against doping use; and (4) audiovisual information on self-medication. At the three-month follow-up the athletes who attended the intervention reported significantly weaker intentions to use doping substances and higher resistance efficacy (i.e., self-efficacy to resist pressure), compared to control group participants. In a follow-up study, Laure and Lecerf (2002) further evaluated the effectiveness of their education-based intervention by comparing it with an awareness-raising one that conveyed basic information about the list of prohibited substances, the health consequences of doping use, doping control procedures, and legal sanctions involved in doping use, and a discussion about moral functioning in sports and the importance of sport in athletes' life. The findings of this comparison study verified the effectiveness and superiority of the education-based intervention in modifying the psychosocial risk factors associated with doping use (e.g., reducing doping intentions and improving refusal self-efficacy), compared to the awareness-raising intervention. Similar findings were also reported by Goldberg *et al.* (1990) who suggested that an education-based program was superior to campaigns raising awareness about the adverse side effects and risks from doping use.

Perhaps the most widely studied education-based interventions against doping are the Adolescents Training and Learning to Avoid Steroids (ATLAS) and Athletes Targeting Healthy Exercise and Nutrition Alternatives (ATHENA) programs (Elliot *et al.* 2008; Goldberg and Elliot 2005; MacKinnon *et al.* 2001). As their full titles indicate, ATLAS and ATHENA are interventions that were designed to prevent the use of chemically assisted performance enhancers, including "legal" ergogenic aids (e.g., nutritional supplements) and doping substances, such as anabolic steroids, by targeting different psychological factors between male and female adolescents (Elliot *et al.* 2004, 2008; Goldberg *et al.* 1996a, 2000).

ATLAS and ATHENA are peer-led and coach-facilitated, and delivered through a series of lectures where female and male athletes are differentially targeted (e.g., emphasis on muscularity is given to male participants, whereas the drive for thinness is addressed among females). The full programs consist of ten (ATLAS) or eight (ATHENA) sessions, although in several studies modified versions of the interventions have been used. Target groups receive information about the side effects of doping use, the risks involved in the excessive and careless use of nutritional supplements, as well as alternative and more legitimate performance enhancement methods (e.g., dieting and training regimes; Bahrke 2012; Goldberg and Elliot 2005). ATLAS and ATHENA have been implemented mainly in US high school settings and involved mainly team sports.

Initial studies showed that the ATLAS yielded significant short-term and long-term effects. Specifically, in the short term, athletes who attended ATLAS displayed reduced interest in trying steroids under peer pressure, more negative beliefs about steroids, improved knowledge and positive beliefs toward nutritional supplements, and enhanced body image (Goldberg *et al.* 1996a). With respect to long-term effects, Goldberg *et al.* (1996b) showed that athletes attending the ATLAS intervention demonstrated increased awareness of the effects of steroid use, higher perceptions of health risks associated with steroid use, greater self-efficacy to resist doping, less trust of steroid-promoting messages, improved perceived physical ability and actual healthy behavior, and weaker attitudes toward users and intentions to use steroids as compared to control group participants, who received a pamphlet on the health side effects and moral concerns of doping use. Importantly, most of the effects were retained 9 and 12 months after the end of the intervention.

In a subsequent study implementing ATLAS, Goldberg *et al.* (2000) reported that at the end of the sport season the intervention resulted in lower intentions toward steroid use, more negative beliefs and attitudes toward steroid use, lower use of illicit drugs and nutritional supplements, healthier lifestyle (i.e., nutrition, drinking and driving), as compared to athletes in the control group who received a pamphlet describing the side effects of anabolic steroids and the benefits of a proper athletes' diet. Although the intervention did not significantly influence self-reported steroid use, it was effective in changing adolescent athletes' lifestyle behavior. MacKinnon *et al.* (2001) extended research with ATLAS and investigated the effect of social influences in the promotion of steroid use. This study demonstrated that ATLAS was effective in changing team norms in athletes participating in the experimental group, whereas intentions to use steroids (in the one-year follow-up) were mediated by perceived severity of steroid effects and reasons for using steroids.

ATLAS' sister ATHENA was developed to tackle doping use in females and deal with their self-presentational concerns and overall health behaviors, as they have been considered to be associated with the use of prohibited substances in sport (Elliot *et al.* 2004). ATHENA was also empirically tested in high school team sport athletes and was found effective in reducing female athletes self-reported use of drugs (e.g., diet pills, steroids, and nutritional supplements) and health-harming behaviors (e.g., fastening seat belt, safe sex), and enhancing healthy nutrition. In addition, it was proven effective in lowering intentions in a wide range of unhealthy behaviors (e.g., tobacco use, diet pills; Elliot *et al.* 2004). These findings were further replicated by Elliot *et al.* (2006) who highlighted the importance of peer-led intervention and suggested inclusion of coaches in such interventions. Elliot *et al.* (2008) further investigated the long-term effects of the ATHENA intervention. In this study, the authors followed participants from one to three years after their graduation and indicated that the application of ATHENA resulted in a healthier lifestyle (e.g., less use of alcohol, tobacco, and marijuana).

Despite their intuitive appeal, a recent meta-analysis (Ntoumanis *et al.* 2014) showed that ATLAS/ATHENA have been modestly effective in reducing pro-doping beliefs and attitudes and this can be attributed to several factors. First, ATLAS and ATHENA were developed as harm reduction/health promotion interventions and not as programs aiming to tackle doping use in sport. Hence, they developed curricula and tested their impact by assessing participants' knowledge and attitudes toward steroid use only. The available studies on the doping decision-making process (Barkoukis *et al.* 2013; Lazuras *et al.* 2010; Lucidi *et al.* 2008) suggest that there are more important variables than knowledge and attitudes that shape the doping decision-making process, such as moral disengagement and self-efficacy (i.e., the capacity to resist doping under certain conditions). Second, by the time the interventions were designed and implemented the available research on doping use was rather limited and did not address the range of risk factors that emerged in recent research. Finally, ATLAS/ATHENA were applied in school settings and largely used school-based, peer-led discussions and other pedagogic approaches that can be easily facilitated by educators who have special knowledge on this type of active teaching and learning.

However, several aspects of the ATLAS and ATHENA interventions could be incorporated in a prevention program targeting doping use in sport. Barkoukis *et al.* (forthcoming) proposed such an intervention aiming to develop an anti-doping culture in adolescents. This program involves ten peer-led, cooperative learning sessions which require students to participate in the design, problem-solving, decision-making, or investigative activities. Participants are requested to find information about nutritional supplements and prohibited substances, doping use side effects, safe alternatives to doping use, historical and ethical aspects of doping use, the psychological process underlying doping use, and the development of an end product relevant to doping use. Barkoukis *et al.* (forthcoming) implemented this program in high school students (35.3 percent of students were involved in sport activities) and demonstrated that it was effective in making students' attitudes toward using nutritional supplements more negative, and increasing norm salience with respect to legal/illegal PES use in sports. In addition, the intervention changed evaluations of the values included in the Spirit of Sport statement and identified harms of sport (Connor *et al.* 2011) in a favorable and hypothesized direction.

In contrast to ATLAS/ATHENA and the education-based interventions that utilize information about the health consequences of doping use and doping control procedures Melzer *et al.* (2010) focused on the second important pillar of the anti-doping struggle, morality. They developed a web-based decision-making program aiming to improve athletes' moral reasoning and ethical decision-making. This program was compared with another one providing information about doping use to athletes, but was not successful in altering athletes' attitudes toward doping use (see Elbe and Brand, Chapter 12 this volume). Still, several features of this intervention, such as the online delivery of the program and the ethical decision-making training, could be incorporated into other interventions and provide a more holistic approach in prevention efforts against doping use.

Overall, the aforementioned studies show that education-based anti-doping interventions have been proven effective in changing adolescents' beliefs about doping use and resulted in the development of a healthier lifestyle. However, their implementation requires a lot of time (i.e., many sessions involving athletes and coaches) and specialized personnel (i.e., personnel capable of delivering peer-led interventions). Hence, they are difficult to be implemented in competitive sport settings. Still, the features of these interventions can and should be used in a different format to suit the time constraints posited by competitive sports and influence athletes' doping-related beliefs and behaviors. Also, future research should examine if the education-based interventions reported above can work equally effectively with recreational and competitive athletes across age and gender groups.

Anti-doping interventions for recreational athletes

In addition to competitive sports, there is a growing trend of doping use in amateur and recreational sports (Bojsen-Møller and Christiansen 2010; Sjöqvist *et al.* 2008). Unlike competitive sports, anti-doping prevention in recreational and amateur sports is limited. The subsequent section, thus, will mainly present information about doping use in recreational sport that can be used to inform anti-doping efforts in this setting. One such intervention attempted to prevent doping use in recreational exercise settings involving the use of positive information and messages about healthy nutrition as alternatives to doping use. James *et al.* (2010) investigated the effect of a single exposure to information about using healthy nutrition as a safe alternative to doping, and found that participants in the intervention group displayed increased knowledge about healthy nutrition and more positive attitudes toward healthy nutrition.

Empirical evidence has also shown that a promising, but still underrepresented, way to prevent the use of doping substances among amateur athletes is to focus on the psychosocial risk factors for doping use (i.e., the intra- and interpersonal, and environmental variables that increase the risk to engage in doping). This approach has been widely and successfully used for the prevention of other types of substance use in adolescents and young people (DiClemente *et al.* 2009). Young people often engage in social comparison, and are preoccupied with the way they look to others and with physical attractiveness (Davison and McCabe 2006). Thus, it is sensible to argue that athletes who exercise or engage in amateur sports would be equally at risk of engaging in the use of doping substances in order to improve their physical appearance and/or athletic performance. However, relevant research in the sector of fitness and amateur sports is still scarce.

A few recent studies conducted in fitness centers and among gym members showed that steroid use intentions were predicted by distorted self-perceptions of the body (e.g., a muscular person perceiving himself as skinny and weak), as well as cultural standards about beauty and physical attractiveness (Parent and Moradi 2011). A study with adolescent Italian athletes showed that intentions and actual use of doping substances were associated with the drive for muscularity in males, and drive for thinness in females (Zelli *et al.* 2010). Addressing the need and driving forces behind these practices as opposed to directly targeting the use of specific doping substances may offer a more effective anti-doping prevention.

Anti-doping message content and delivery

The content of anti-doping messages and the method of message delivery can be important features of persuasive appeals in the context of doping prevention. Horcajo and De la Vega (2014) used the Elaboration Likelihood Model (ELM; Petty and Cacioppo 1986) to assess the effects of a persuasive appeal on athlete's attitudes toward doping. According to the ELM, a message can be persuasive and lead to attitude change by using either low cognitive elaboration/ peripheral cues (e.g., emotion-laden cues, heuristics), or high cognitive elaboration/central cues (e.g., evidence-based arguments; Petty *et al.* 2009). Horcajo and De la Vega (2014) found that a single exposure to an anti-doping message decreased athletes' attitudes toward doping. When a high cognitive elaboration message was used attitudes change was more stable and persistent, compared to the low elaboration message. This study is among the first to apply a well-established theory of persuasion in the context of doping prevention, and indicated that the message content can impact athletes' doping attitudes.

Another important issue concerning message content regards the level of threat of the message. According to self-affirmation theory people are motivated to maintain a positive self-image and may process in a self-serving and defensive manner any personally relevant and threatening information, such as warning labels about the negative health effects of tobacco use (Harris and Epton 2009; Steele 1988). Self-affirming (i.e., by reminding people of their core values or their self-worth) is likely to restore self-integrity and, accordingly, reduce defensive processing of health messages (Harris and Epton 2009). For instance, self-affirming an athlete's personal value of being compassionate may make him less defensive in a doping-related message. Barkoukis *et al.* (2015) applied self-affirmation in competitive athletes who admitted doping use, and found that self-affirming their personal values led to less defensive processing of health- and moral-related messages, and weaker intentions and temptation to engage in doping use in the future. These findings may imply that self-affirmation can be effectively used to convey messages in doping preventive efforts.

Anti-doping interventions targeting the athlete's entourage

The communicator of anti-doping information and messages plays an important role in respective interventions (Backhouse *et al.* 2012). Past research on substance use prevention showed that using elite athletes acting as role models had greater persuasive impact compared to other types of communicators, such as parents and doctors (Petersen 2010). Members of the athlete's entourage could be involved as message communicators in anti-doping interventions. In line with this approach, Poussel *et al.* (2013) argued that a greater emphasis should be placed on the proper training of medical staff that may be involved in anti-doping campaigns. This is very important given that serious drawbacks have been documented in the involvement of medical personnel in anti-doping efforts, partly stemming from insufficient training about doping (e.g., Dikic *et al.* 2012).

In their study, Poussel *et al.* (2013) randomly assigned medical students either in an education group, where they received doping-specific information, or in a control group that did not receive doping-specific training. The results showed that the medical students that were exposed to doping-specific training displayed greater efficacy in identifying and effectively managing performance enhancement requests by athletes, and refusing inappropriate prescription requests. Accordingly, their knowledge about doping and doping-related procedures was significantly improved compared to control group participants. Furthermore, Donovan *et al.* (2012) designed an anti-doping intervention that can be implemented by sport psychologists. The intervention included activities and exercises based on research evidence concerning the psychological variables associated with doping use (i.e., motivation, self-presentational concerns, and morality issues). The main objective of the intervention was to reduce athletes' susceptibility to using doping substances. The effectiveness of the intervention is still under investigation, but it is also an important attempt to sensitize and educate another group of people working with athletes about doping use, and, hence, involves the athletes' entourage in fighting against doping in sport. Finally, Dodge *et al.* (Chapter 14 this volume) provide a comprehensive review of the evidence concerning the role of parents in anti-doping campaigns. Taken together, the aforementioned findings suggest that there is a promising start to anti-doping interventions that target the athletes' entourage. Future research may build on this early work and identify best practices in anti-doping training and education.

Implications for future development in doping prevention

The aforementioned interventions were concerned with the content of preventive messages and the carrier of the message. Another important aspect which, however, remains largely underrepresented in the international literature on doping prevention concerns the use of emerging information and communication technologies (ICTs) for doping prevention. More than 80 percent of youth in Europe and other developed countries have access to the Internet, and use online applications and emerging ICTs in their daily activities (Valkenburg and Peter 2007). However, incorporating ICTs in anti-doping efforts means something more than just posting educational material and resources online, and calls for embedding technology in the design and delivery of interventions. Anti-doping authorities across the globe have already responded to that need by initiating various online resources for doping prevention. For example, in March 2014, WADA launched an e-learning resource called "Athlete Learning Program about Health and Anti-Doping" (ALPHA). ALPHA reflects the joint efforts of e-learning specialists, athletes, and behavioral scientists, and targets not only behavior (i.e., doping use), but also other aspects of doping use, such as attitudes and intentions, safe alternatives to doping use, and also empowers athletes to identify the risk factors for doping. In line with Houlihan's (2008) recommendations, ALPHA incorporates the principles of peer-led intervention as anti-doping messages are conveyed by fellow athletes than official authorities.

One important element of ALPHA is that athletes were involved in the development of the program. This is an example of co-creation or shared decision-making that has been usefully applied in other domains, from education to health (e.g., Díaz-Méndez and Gummesson 2012), and is associated with greater satisfaction among end-user target groups. Co-creation can be further integrated in doping prevention strategies as a way to develop tailor-made tools and resources, foster the active involvement of target groups, and increase the likelihood of intervention success.

Finally, so far, anti-doping efforts have largely relied on dealing with the risk factors associated with doping use, whereas relevant research and interventions about protective factors is limited. Petróczi and Aidman (2008) suggested that the joint consideration of risk and protective factors may enhance the effectiveness of anti-doping efforts. Indeed, Rodek *et al.* (2009) indicated that religiousness could serve as a protective factor against doping use. In this line, Chan *et al.* (2015) argued that athletes' autonomous motivation in sport is positively related to anti-doping behaviors. Also, Laure (2011) suggested that educating young athletes on life skills would lower the risk for doping use. Future anti-doping interventions would benefit from the inclusion of protective factors, such as life skills, self-esteem, self-assertion, self-belonging, parental support, and emotion management, which could help athletes avoid doping use in sports.

Conclusions

Both anecdotal and empirical evidence suggests that the prohibitionist/punitive paradigm in doping control and awareness-raising campaigns were not effective in lowering the prevalence of doping use in sport settings. Researchers progressively move toward education-based interventions. The interventions implemented so far have been found to be modestly effective in influencing athletes' psychological risk factors for doping use. Building on these efforts, future preventive efforts should improve the content and delivery of the anti-doping message, involve the athletes' entourage (i.e., coaches, parents, staff) and the athletes themselves (i.e., co-creation of the intervention), incorporate ICTs, and address protective factors against doping use. Doping behavior is a multifactorial and complicated phenomenon and, thus, relevant anti-doping efforts should be multifaceted.

References

Backhouse, S. H., Patterson, L., and McKenna, J. (2012). Achieving the Olympic ideal: Preventing doping in sport. *Performance Enhancement and Health, 1* (*2*), 83–85.

Bahrke, M. S. (2012). Performance-enhancing substance misuse in sport: Risk factors and considerations for success and failure in intervention programs. *Substance Use and Misuse, 47* (*13–14*), 1505–1516.

Barkoukis, V., Lazuras, L., and Harris, P. R. (2015). The effects of self-affirmation manipulation on decision making about doping use in elite athletes. *Psychology of Sport and Exercise, 16*, 175–181.

Barkoukis, V., Kartali, K., Lazuras, L., and Tsorbatzoudis, H. (forthcoming). Evaluation of and anti-doping intervention for adolescents: Findings from a school-based study.

Barkoukis, V., Lazuras, L., Tsorbatzoudis, H., and Rodafinos, A. (2011). Motivational and sportspersonship profiles of elite athletes in relation to doping behaviour. *Psychology of Sport and Exercise*, *12*, 205–212.

Barkoukis, V., Lazuras, L., Tsorbatzoudis, H., and Rodafinos, A. (2013). Motivational and social cognitive predictors of doping intentions in elite sports: An integrated approach. *Scandinavian Journal of Medicine and Science in Sports*, *23*, e330–e340. doi: 10.1111/sms.12068.

Bojsen-Møller, J. and Christiansen, A. V. (2010). Use of performance- and image-enhancing substances among recreational athletes: a quantitative analysis of inquiries submitted to the Danish anti-doping authorities. *Scandinavian Journal of Medicine and Science in Sports*, *20* (*6*), 861–867.

Chan, D. K. C., Dimmock, J. A., Donovan, R. J., Hardcastle, S., Lentillon-Kaestner, V., and Hagger, M. S. (2015). Self-determined motivation in sport predicts anti-doping motivation and intention: A perspective from the trans-contextual model. *Journal of Science and Medicine in Sport*, *18* (*3*), 315–322.

Connor, J. M., Huybers, T., and Mazanov, J. (2011). Sport, integrity and harms: What are the threats to the level playing field? *The Australian Sociological Association 2011 Conference*, Newcastle, Australia.

Davison, T. E. and McCabe, M. P. (2006). Adolescent body image and psychosocial functioning. *The Journal of Social Psychology*, *146* (*1*), 15–30.

Díaz-Méndez, M. and Gummesson, E. (2012). Value co-creation and university teaching quality: Consequences for the European Higher Education Area (EHEA). *Journal of Service Management*, *23* (*4*), 571–592.

DiClemente, R. J., Crosby, R. A., and Kegler, M. C. (2009). Issues and challenges in applying theory in health promotion practice and research: Adaptation, translation, and global application. In R. J. DiClemente, R. A. Crosby, and M. C. Kegler (eds.), *Emerging theories in health promotion practice and research* (185–214). San Francisco: Jossey-Bass.

Dikic, N., McNamee, M., Günter, H., Markovic, S. S., and Vajgic, B. (2013). Sports physicians, ethics and antidoping governance: between assistance and negligence. *British Journal of Sports Medicine*, *47* (*11*), 701–704.

Donovan, R. J., Jalleh, G., and Gucciardi, D. (2012). *Development of a psycho-educational anti-doping intervention program for emerging athletes*. Report to Department of Health and Ageing. Centre for Behavioural Research in Cancer Control, Faculty of Health Sciences, Curtin University, Perth.

Donovan, R. J., Egger, G., Kapernick, V., and Mendoza, J. (2002). A conceptual framework for achieving performance enhancing drug compliance in sport. *Sports Medicine*, *32* (*4*), 269–284.

Ehrnborg, C. and Rosén, T. (2009). The psychology behind doping in sport. *Growth Hormone and IGF Research*, *19* (*4*), 285–287.

Elliot, D. L., Goldberg, L., Moe, E. L., DeFrancesco, C. A., Durham, M. B., and Hix-Small, H. (2004). Preventing substance use and disordered eating: Initial outcomes of the ATHENA (Athletes Targeting Healthy Exercise and Nutrition Alternatives) program. *Archives of Pediatrics and Adolescent Medicine*, *158* (*11*), 1043–1049.

Elliot, D. L., Moe, E. L., Goldberg, L., DeFrancesco, C. A., Durham, M. B., and Hix-Small, H. (2006). Definition and outcome of a curriculum to prevent disordered eating and body-shaping drug use. *Journal of School Health*, *76* (*2*), 67–73.

Elliot, D. L., Goldberg, L., Moe, E. L., DeFrancesco, C. A., Durham, M. B., McGinnis, W., and Lockwood, C. (2008). Long-term outcomes of the ATHENA (Athletes Targeting Healthy Exercise & Nutrition Alternatives) program for female high school athletes. *Journal of Alcohol and Drug Education, 52* (2), 73.

Fainaru-Wada, M. and Williams, L. (2006). *Game of shadows: Barry Bonds, BALCO, and the steroids scandal that rocked professional sports.* New York: Gotham Books.

Goldberg, L. and Elliot, D. L. (2005). Preventing substance use among high school athletes. The ATLAS and ATHENA programs. *Journal of Applied School Psychology, 21,* 63–87.

Goldberg, L., Bosworth, E., Bents, R. T., and Trevisan, L. (1990). Effect of an anabolic steroid education program on knowledge and attitudes of high school football players. *Journal of Adolescent Health Care, 11,* 210–214.

Goldberg, L., MacKinnon, D. P., Elliot, D. L., Moe, E. L., Clarke, G., and Cheong, J. (2000). The adolescents training and learning to avoid steroids program: Preventing drug use and promoting health behaviors. *Archives of Pediatrics and Adolescent Medicine, 154* (4), 332–338.

Goldberg, L., Elliot, D. L., MacKinnon, D. P., Moe, E., Kuehl, K. S., Nohre, L., and Lockwood, C. M. (2003). Drug testing athletes to prevent substance abuse: Background and pilot study results of the SATURN (Student Athlete Testing Using Random Notification) study. *Journal of Adolescent Health, 32* (1), 16–25.

Goldberg, L., Elliot, D. L., Clarke, G. N., MacKinnon, D. P., Zoref, L., Moe, E., Green, C., and Wolf, S. L. (1996a). The Adolescents Training and Learning to Avoid Steroids (ATLAS) prevention program: Background and results of a model intervention. *Archives of Pediatrics and Adolescent Medicine, 150* (7), 713–721.

Goldberg, L., Elliot, D. L., MacKinnon, D. P., Moe, E. L., Kuehl, K. S., Yoon, M., Taylor, A., and Williams, J. (2007). Outcomes of a prospective trial of student-athlete drug testing: The Student Athlete Testing Using Random Notification (SATURN) study. *Journal of Adolescent Health, 41* (5), 421–429.

Goldberg, L., Elliot, D., Clarke, G. N., MacKinnon, D. P., Moe, E., Zoref, L., Green, C., Wolf, S. L., Greffrath, E., Miller, D. J., and Lapin, A. (1996b). Effects of a multi-dimensional anabolic steroid prevention intervention: The Adolescents Training and Learning to Avoid Steroids (ATLAS) program. *Journal of the American Medical Association, 276,* 1555–1562.

Harris, P. R. and Epton, T. (2009). The impact of self-affirmation on health cognition, health behaviour and other health-related responses: A narrative review. *Social and Personality Psychology Compass 3,* 962–978.

Hauw, D. and McNamee, M. (2014). A critical analysis of three psychological research programs of doping behaviour. *Psychology of Sport and Exercise, 16,* 140–148.

Horcajo, J. and De la Vega, R. (2014). Changing doping-related attitudes in soccer players: How can we get stable and persistent changes? *European Journal of Sport Science, 14,* 839–846.

Houlihan, B. (2008). Detection and education in anti-doping policy: A review of current issues and an assessment of future prospects. *Hitotsubashi Journal of Arts and Sciences, 49* (1), 55–71.

Hunt, T. M., Dimeo, P., and Jedlicka, S. R. (2012). The historical roots of today's problems: A critical appraisal of the international anti-doping movement. *Performance Enhancement and Health, 1* (2), 55–60.

James, R., Naughton, D. P., and Petróczi, A. (2010). Promoting functional foods as acceptable alternatives to doping: Potential for information-based social marketing approach. *Journal of the International Society of Sports Nutrition, 7 (1)*, 1–11.

Johnson, M. B. (2012). A systemic social-cognitive perspective on doping. *Psychology of Sport and Exercise, 13 (3)*, 317–323.

Kayser, B. and Broers, B. (2013). Anti-doping policies: Choosing between imperfections. In J. Tolleneer, S. Sterckx, and P. Bonte (eds.), *Athletic Enhancement, Human Nature and Ethics* (271–289). Dordrecht, Netherlands and New York: Springer.

Laure, P. (2011). Doping: reinforce life skills of young athletes. In G. Spitzer and E. Franke (eds.), *Sport, Doping und Enhancement Transdisziplinäre Perspektiven* [Doping, Enhancement, Prevention in Sport, Freizeit und Beruf, Bd. 1, 1. Aufl., S.] (217–224). Cologne: Strauss.

Laure, P. and Lecerf, T. (1999). [Prevention of doping in sport in adolescents: evaluation of a health education based intervention]. *Archives de Pediatrie, 6 (8)*, 849–854.

Laure, P. and Lecerf, T. (2002). Doping prevention among young athletes: Comparison of a health education-based intervention versus information-based intervention. *Science and Sports, 17 (4)*, 198–201.

Lazuras, L., Barkoukis, V., Rodafinos, A., and Tsorbatzoudis, H. (2010). Predictors of doping intentions in elite-level athletes: A social cognition approach. *Journal of Sport and Exercise Psychology, 32*, 694–710.

Lucidi, F., Zelli, A., Mallia, L., Russo, P. M., and Violani, C. (2008). The social-cognitive mechanisms regulating adolescents' use of doping substances. *Journal of Sports Sciences, 26*, 447–456.

MacKinnon, D. P., Goldberg, L., Clarke, G. N., Elliot, D. L., Cheong, J., Lapin, A., Moe, E. L., and Krull, J. L. (2001). Mediating mechanisms in a program to reduce intentions to use anabolic steroids and improve exercise self-efficacy and dietary behavior. *Prevention Science, 2 (1)*, 15–28.

Melzer, M., Elbe, A. M., and Brand, R. (2010). Moral and ethical decision-making: A chance for doping prevention in sports? *Nordic Journal of Applied Ethics, 4*, 69–85.

Morente-Sánchez, J. and Zabala, M. (2013). Doping in sport: A review of elite athletes' attitudes, beliefs, and knowledge. *Sports Medicine, 43*, 395–411.

Ntoumanis, N., Ng, J. Y., Barkoukis, V., and Backhouse, S. H. (2014). Personal and psychosocial predictors of doping use in physical activity settings: A meta-analysis. *Sports Medicine, 44 (11)*, 1603–1624.

Parent, M. C. and Moradi, B. (2011). His biceps become him: A test of objectification theory's application to drive for muscularity and propensity for steroid use in college men. *Journal of Counseling Psychology, 58*, 246–256.

Park, J. K. (2005). Governing doped bodies: the world anti-doping agency and the global culture of surveillance. *Cultural Studies ↔ Critical Methodologies, 5 (2)*, 174–188.

Petersen, T. S. (2010). Good athlete – bad athlete? on the "Role-Model Argument" for banning performance-enhancing drugs. *Sport, Ethics and Philosophy, 4 (3)*, 332–340.

Petróczi, A. (2007). Attitudes and doping: A structural equation analysis of the relationship between athletes' attitudes, sport orientation and doping behaviour. *Substance Abuse Treatment, Prevention, and Policy, 2*, 34.

Petróczi, A. and Aidman, E. (2008). Psychological drivers in doping: The life-cycle model of performance enhancement. *Substance Abuse Treatment, Prevention, and Policy, 3*, 7.

Petty, R. E. and Cacioppo, J. T. (1986). The elaboration likelihood model of persuasion. *Advances in Experimental Social Psychology, 19*, 123–205.

Petty, R. E., Barden, J., and Wheeler, S. C. (2009). The elaboration likelihood model of persuasion: Developing health promotions for sustained behavioral change. In R. J. DiClemente, R. A. Crosby, and M. C. Kegler (eds.), *Emerging theories in health promotion practice and research* (185–214). San Francisco: Jossey-Bass.

Poussel, M., Laure, P., Latarche, C., Laroppe, J., Schwitzer, M., Koch, J.-P., Heid, J.-M., and Chenuel, B. (2013). Specific teaching about doping in sport helps medical students to meet prevention needs. *Science and Sports, 28* (*5*), 274–280.

Rodek, J., Sekulic, D., and Pasalic, E. (2009). Can we consider religiousness as a protective factor against doping behavior in sport? *Journal of Religion and Health, 48* (*4*), 445–453.

Sjöqvist, F., Garle, M., and Rane, A. (2008). Use of doping agents, particularly anabolic steroids, in sports and society. *The Lancet, 371* (*9627*), 1872–1882.

Steele, C. M. (1988). The psychology of self-affirmation: Sustaining the integrity of the self. *Advances in Experimental Social Psychology, 21*, 261–302.

Stewart, B. and Smith, A. C. T. (2008). Drug use in sport: Implications for public policy. *Journal of Sport and Social Issues, 32*, 278–298.

Strelan, P. and Boeckmann, R. (2003). Research notes: A new model for understanding performance-enhancing drug use by elite athletes. *Journal of Applied Sport Psychology, 15* (*2*), 176–183.

Valkenburg, P. M. and Peter, J. (2009). Social consequences of the internet for adolescents: A decade of research. *Current Directions in Psychological Science, 18* (*1*), 1–5.

WADA (2009). *World Anti-doping Code*. Montreal, Canada: WADA

Wiefferink, C. H., Detmar, S. B., Coumans, B., Vogels, T., and Paulussen, T. G. W. (2008). Social psychological determinants of the use of performance-enhancing drugs by gym users. *Health Education Research, 23* (*1*), 70–80.

Zelli, A., Mallia, L., and Lucidi, F. (2010). The contribution of interpersonal appraisals to a social-cognitive analysis of adolescents' doping use. *Psychology of Sport and Exercise, 11* (*4*), 304–311.

16 Next steps in doping research and prevention

Ten big questions

Haralambos Tsorbatzoudis, Lambros Lazuras, and Vassilis Barkoukis

In the preceding chapters, the different aspects of a dynamically evolving scientific field of the psychology of doping use in sports were presented. Although the seed for this growth was planted some 20 years ago (e.g., Anshel and Russell 1997; Laure and Reinsberger 1995), it is within the last decade that the field has flourished and reached one of its first research milestones with over 150 published scientific articles encompassing different theoretical perspectives, methodologies, and concepts (for a meta-analysis see Ntoumanis *et al.* 2014). At this point in time, the direction that needs to be taken is to engage in critical reflection, and develop a strategic vision for research progress for the next phase of research on the psychology of doping use. In the present chapter important aspects of research in the psychology of doping use are discussed, and the relevant themes are outlined in ten big questions that may guide future research in this area. These questions are relevant to theory development, methodological issues in doping research, dilemmas concerning the role of sporting values and the ethics of doping, as well as developments in the design and delivery of evidence-based anti-doping interventions.

Question 1: How important are psychosocial processes?

It has become apparent from the first part of this book that effective and evidence-based doping prevention practices require a sound understanding of the mediation and moderation factors that can predict and explain why some athletes (elite, pre-elite, and amateurs) have increased risk for using doping substances and methods. So far, research on the psychosocial processes underlying doping use has revealed a range of risk factors, including attitudes, motivation, self-regulatory processes, and normative influences (e.g., Barkoukis *et al.* 2013; Lazuras *et al.* 2010; Lucidi *et al.* 2008; Zelli *et al.* 2010). Although this line of research will continue to evolve, there are certain issues that need to be addressed to ensure that drawbacks and limitations that may hinder progression of the field are effectively addressed.

These limitations can be overcome by employing different methodologies, and by developing integrative theoretical models that are relevant to doping use. With respect to methodologies, it is perhaps time to shift from cross-sectional designs to longitudinal ones that will enable researchers to better understand the temporal sequence of risk factors and outcomes (e.g., if certain variables really predict doping use over time). Further, longitudinal designs have a number of other advantages that may be useful in the context of doping research, such as examining cross-lagged effects, reciprocal relationships, trajectories of change or growth, etc. This approach will eliminate reverse causality problems that are apparent in most published cross-sectional studies, allow for a better understanding of mediation effects, and enable researchers to address cross-lagged effects, reciprocal relationships, trajectories of change or growth. Another way is to introduce experimental designs in the field of doping use. Almost all of the published studies about the risk factors (or correlates) of doping use and intentions rely on self-reported measures (see Ntoumanis *et al.* 2014 for a meta-analytic review). A greater focus on experimental designs will allow future researchers to draw conclusions about causality in doping research, and identify the variables that can have a direct impact on doping intention and behavior. For instance, a recent study examined the effects of a self-affirmation manipulation on the decision-making process underlying doping use, and found that self-affirming athletes about their core values has a direct effect on their beliefs and intentions toward using doping substances (Barkoukis *et al.* 2015a).

Regarding model development, Chapter 4 provided an overview of research in this domain. Recently, researchers have moved away from the standard Theory of Planned Behavior (TPB; Ajzen 1991) approach, and have begun to integrate variables from different models, resulting in more advanced models of doping intentions (e.g., Barkoukis *et al.* 2013), as well as doping abstinence (e.g., Chan *et al.* 2015). These developments show us what might be the future of research in the psychology of doping use. It is gradually becoming apparent that a narrow focus on cognitive-affective variables, such as TPB ones, can reveal only part of the picture in doping use. Other correlates of behavior, including motivation, moral values, and personality factors, can play an equally important role, and usefully be integrated in existing models of doping use. However, as Ajzen (2011) noted, it is advisable that such theoretical integrations are made with caution (e.g., using theory-driven criteria), and with extreme care to the overall model's parsimony. Otherwise, we may end up with theoretically sound but impractical models of doping use.

Another important aspect concerns the study of protective factors of doping use. Chan *et al.* (2015) were among the first to introduce this concept and addressed the psychosocial correlates of doping abstinence tendencies. It is important to look further and advance the study of protective factors, as this may lead to an important complement to the ongoing research about risk factors for doping use. Together, these two lines of research can lead to high-quality, evidence-based anti-doping interventions. It is noteworthy that a search for protective factors does not only entail the correlates of "doping abstinence intentions," but may also encompass a more generic protective process that applies to both users and nonusers of doping substances and methods.

Question 2: Which measures should we use?

It is common in the scientific community to react to new changes and advances in a field (e.g., the development of a new method or theory) by throwing (or being really eager to throw) out "the baby with the bathwater." This is an eloquent way to describe the tendency to overlook the advantages of past methods or theories and overemphasize those of new methods or theories. The field of behavioral sciences has numerous examples to show this in quite diverse areas (e.g., Aspinwall and Tedeschi 2010; Dobbins *et al.* 1988; Spector *et al.* 2000). The psychological study of doping use has not yet reached a point of fierce debate over a methodology or theoretical perspective, but there are controversial methodological issues that may provide the basis for debate, such as the distinction between implicit and explicit measures of doping attitudes.

Implicit measures of attitudes are said to yield bias-free findings, but they may also tempt researchers to overemphasize the practical utility or superiority of these measures over other, more traditional, methodologies. That is, to "throw out the baby with the bathwater" for another time. At this point it is noteworthy that automatic attitudes are formed, influenced, or changed in a similar fashion to more deliberative attitudes (Briñol *et al.* 2009; Fazio and Olson 2003). In fact, the use of implicit measures does not always entail higher predictive validity than the use of more explicit measures (e.g., self-reports), except in the case of highly sensitive behaviors, such as racial or sexual bias (Greenwald *et al.* 2009). Doping use is a sensitive issue, and recent studies have shown that doping-specific implicit measures of attitudes may fare better than explicit, self-reported measures (e.g., Brand *et al.* 2011; Petróczi *et al.* 2008). Nevertheless, the merits of novel, bias-free, implicit, or indirect measures should not be taken as evidence that deliberative processes are of inferior importance. Said differently, the development of implicit measures should not be a motive for debate and division within the study of doping use, but rather a call for methodological convergence and integration. As research on novel measurement methodologies evolves, scientists should make the effort to come up with more effective and accurate tools to capture veridical responses, but this task serves the overarching goal of better understanding the processes underlying doping use. When asked, therefore, which measures we should use, it is advisable to keep in mind that the measures are the tools that help us understand a process and address relevant research questions, and the measures that do so more effectively are the ones that should be used.

Question 3: How should doping measures be used?

Following from the previous question about which measures should be used to assess aspects of the psychological processes underlying doping use, another important question is how the measures should be used in the first place – that is to define the scope of using measures of doping behavior. By this time, there have been attempts to commercialize the use of implicit and self-reported measures of doping use as methods to establish "clean" athletes. Such initiatives rest on the assumption that measurement scores, such as reaction times in implicit association tests, can be used as valid indicators of athletes' risk to engage in doping. However, there is still a long way to go before establishing the predictive validity of these measures, let alone to being able to talk about their utility in developing a "doping detection" protocol or method. If anything, explicit and implicit measures of doping attitudes are still in their infancy, and indicate someone's evaluations of doping use as either positive or negative. Individual differences in responding, contextual effects, and a whole host of other limitations, however, currently limit our ability to determine an athlete's tendencies to stay clean and abstain from doping use. Further empirical research is needed to establish the predictive validity of existing measures, and the ecological validity of the psychological processes that these measures presumably reveal (for a detailed discussion see Petróczi 2013a, 2013b). In their present form, implicit and/or explicit measures of doping use should be employed to better understand specific psychological processes – that is, as scientific measurement tools, rather than diagnostic tools. Most importantly, those who have good access to athletes and are interested in doping prevention and control, but do not necessarily possess the knowledge about methods of scientific enquiry and behavioral science, should work together with academics who study doping use to get a synergistic effect.

Question 4: Can sports become doping-free?

The following two questions are concerned with an issue that is not directly applicable to empirical research, but may shape the way we think about future research developments concerning the psychology of doping use. Cleret in Chapter 9 provided an overview of the values that govern modern sports, and explained why doping use is inherently against these values. On the other hand, there is an increased trend in promoting the idea of freeing doping in sports. Advocates of this idea argue that the legalization of doping use can yield more benefits than costs with respect to the athletes' health and to the morality of sports. According to Savulescu *et al.* (2004) when sports authorities ban a group of performance enhancement substances they actually render the use of these substances cheating behavior. Legalizing the use of these substances would eliminate the moral concerns associated with doping use. They also proposed that doping tests be used to identify athletes who may be jeopardizing their health, rather than for detecting individuals who need to be punished for breaking the rules. In line with this view, Kayser and his associates (Kayser *et al.* 2007) argued that medically supervised doping could protect athletes' health and resolve several morality issues pertaining to doping use.

In addition, as Cleret pointed out in her chapter, the motto of modern sports "Citius, Altius, Fortius" is associated with professionalism of competitive sports, and emphasizes performance enhancement at any cost. Although in principle and in theory, this motto may not be directly opposed to the values of sports, in reality athletes may feel the pressure to continuously enhance their performance by any means available, even disputed medical treatments (see Camporesi and McNamee 2014). Since doping substances represent a common, although prohibited, method of performance enhancement, some of the athletes who feel the pressure to perform higher eventually resort to their use. Finally, the prohibition of several substances makes it unethical, and thus impossible, to study their effect on athletes' health. To the best of our knowledge, at the moment there are no clinical trials testing the effects of doping therapies under medical supervision on athletes' short- and long-term health. These arguments indicate that a different view exists about the morality of using (prohibited) performance-enhancing substances in sports. This view is not necessarily antithetical to the existing anti-doping regime and practices. Rather this alternative view may complement existing anti-doping efforts (e.g., the shift from punishment to prevention), and more accurately reflects the context and situations wherein doping takes place. In this sense, future theorizing, and perhaps research in the psychology of doping use, should consider the possibility of freeing doping sports and, accordingly, identify the perceived advantages and disadvantages for athletes' health and the morals of the future sport movement.

Question 5: Are dopers immoral persons?

The prevailing social norms regard athletes who engage in doping as "bad apples" and cheaters that deserve to be put in "tar and feather" and face severe legal and social sanctions (Petróczi 2013a). Morality in sports has often been operationalized as how athletes play their sport, and this may span from respect to authorities and officials, to commitment to fair-play rules. This line of thinking is depicted in measurements of *sportspersonship*, a construct that describes a range of honorable and fair-play behaviors in sports. However, this affective and moralistic view of doping is predominantly shared among anti-doping policy-makers, agencies, and researchers and not necessarily by people who are actively involved in the process, such as athletes and their entourage (Petróczi 2013b).

Defining doping as a form of cheating depends on whether doping is categorized as a violation of constitutive rules (i.e., the specific goals of a sport and the means with which to reach them) or regulative rules (i.e., rules that regulate activities that exist independently of the constitutive rules). If it is perceived as a violation of regulative rules, then doping does not represent a cheating behavior. Loland (2005) argued that a constitutive rule violation can be considered cheating only if it is intentional. Doping use is considered to be an intentional and planned behavior (Petróczi and Aidman 2008) and, thus, it should be considered as a cheating behavior (i.e., a rule violation that aims at gaining advantage over the opponent). However, recent studies have shown that approximately 20 percent of legal nutritional supplements are contaminated with illegal substances and can result in a positive test (Geyer *et al.* 2008; Kohler *et al.* 2010). This implies that at least some of the positive doping tests can be attributed to unintentional doping. By this token, doping use can't be perceived as intentional – and, thus, not cheating behavior. This is consistent with the view that the rules of sport can't determine its application and that for every rule there is a certain interpretation (see Loland 2005). Therefore, doping use shouldn't be considered a priori as a cheating behavior, but rather each positive doping test should be interpreted in light of the certain circumstances in which its test scores were obtained. Having this in mind, dopers should not be considered a priori immoral persons. This is also supported by recent evidence which showed that there were no differences in intention and actual doping behavior between athletes with low and high scores in sportspersonship (Barkoukis *et al.* 2011). Overall, although morality is an important pillar in the anti-doping campaign we should be cautious in labeling a priori doping users as immoral persons, and more evidence is needed in understanding if moral orientations really predict doping use, or a low moral orientation is set as a label after the doping act is evidenced. Future research on the morality of doping use, therefore, might be helped by avoiding using a priory categorization and labeling of athletes as immoral persons – an important issue that may determine the ways scientists think of and approach doping users. Rather, researchers should examine doping use (and anti-doping controls) in relation to the broader context and cultural norms about pharmacologically assisted performance and human enhancement.

Question 6: Nutritional supplements: gateway to doping or safe alternative?

There is accumulating evidence that greater frequency of supplement use is associated with higher chances of self-reporting doping use (e.g., Backhouse *et al.* 2011; Lucidi *et al.* 2008; Ntoumanis *et al.* 2014), and even more positive doping attitudes and beliefs toward the use of doping substances among athletes who have never tried doping before (Barkoukis *et al.* 2015b). Petróczi *et al.* (2011) argued that athletes focus on the functionality of ergogenic aids, such as nutritional supplements. Thus, a common mental representation may underlie the use of both legal performance enhancement substances (nutritional supplements), and illicit ones. This may explain why using nutritional supplements can act as a risk factor for doping use: athletes become acquainted with chemically assisted performance enhancement, without considering the legal implications of their practices. However, other studies (e.g., Barkoukis *et al.* 2015b) show that only a small proportion of those who use nutritional supplements endorse the use of doping substances. In light of the available evidence, what we can safely argue about nutritional supplements is that they tend to co-occur with doping use, and this is likely to happen in a minority of athletes who use them. This raises an important question of how legal nutritional supplements can actually be integrated in the fight against doping use. Rather than viewing nutritional supplements as a potential gateway to doping, we can perhaps use them in doping prevention. In this respect, future research may explore ways to educate athletes about safe performance enhancement methods, including nutritional supplements as safe alternatives to doping use. This is an important (and seemingly counterintuitive) empirical question that may lead both scientific research and anti-doping policies and interventions in the years to come.

Question 7: Is doping use an end-state or a means to an end?

Last decade we experienced a growing interest in doping use with researchers trying to understand the underlying psychosocial processes (Ntoumanis *et al.* 2014). Researchers in the field used prominent theories in mainstream psychology (e.g., TPB) that were originally developed to explain human behavior with respect to drug use, cheating, and unhealthy behaviors. Hence, past evidence has largely focused on the association of attitudes with doping behaviors (Petróczi 2007), the decision-making process underlying doping use (Lazuras *et al.* 2010; Lucidi *et al.* 2004; Wiefferink *et al.* 2008), the association of personal traits and dispositions with doping use (Barkoukis *et al.* 2011, 2013; Donahue *et al.* 2006), the moral explanations of the decision to dope (Lucidi *et al.* 2008; Zelli *et al.* 2010) and the integration of psychological processes for the prediction of doping use (Barkoukis *et al.* 2013; Donovan *et al.* 2002; Lazuras *et al.* (forthcoming). In all these studies doping use was regarded either implicitly or explicitly, as an end-state.

However, doping may represent a means to an end. In line with this view, Petróczi and Aidman (2008) suggested that doping use is a means to achieving higher athletic performance. But even in this case, high performance in competitive sports is not an end-state in itself, but rather another means to an end that helps athletes attain higher goals, such as fame, money, and glory. In this respect doping in sports can be seen as part of a long process of hierarchically organized goals.

Kruglanski *et al.* (2002) proposed a theory of goal systems that can be used to explain such goal hierarchies, and this theory could be usefully applied in the psychological study of doping use. They suggested that in achievement environments people use goal systems that reflect "mentally represented networks wherein goals may be cognitively associated to their corresponding means of attainment and to alternative goals as well" (2002: 333). The theory further assumes that higher-order goals are served by sub-goals. Each sub-goal can be achieved by several means. For instance, consider an athlete who aspires to participate in the Olympic Games (higher-order goal). In order to achieve this goal he/she should improve substantially his/her performance (sub-goal). The means to improve performance may include a wide range of methods spanning from proper training, healthy nutrition, and nutritional supplement use to doping use. Maladaptive self-regulation or a competitive and pro-doping normative climate in the team may explain why some athletes resort to doping use in order to facilitate the fulfillment of their higher-order goals. The means-to-an-end arguments pose a theoretically plausible and compelling question for future research in doping use. It also calls for further research into the type and nature of goals that are more likely to require doping use as a means for goal attainment among different groups of athletes (i.e., elite, sub-elite, recreational. etc.).

Question 8: Should we invest in anti-doping education?

Chapter 15 has clearly showed that the punitive model based on doping controls was not effective in decreasing the prevalence of doping use. It is extremely expensive and the results were not the expected ones. The number of positive tests remains stable at approximately 2 percent of the controls, whereas the prevalence of doping use exceeds 10 percent in studies using self-reports and 30 percent in studies using indirect measures of prevalence. Furthermore, this approach has been employed only in elite competitive athletes, which inherently ignores sub-elite and recreational athletes. In addition, studies testing the effectiveness of random testing in athletes (see SATURN program; Goldberg *et al.* 2003, 2007) were only modestly effective in changing drug use behavior, but increased many risk factors associated with drug use, including doping behaviors. Thus, the punitive approach is rather limited and ineffective in combating doping use on a large scale. Instead, education-based activities can provide a promising alternative.

Past evidence has shown that education-based interventions are effective in changing athletes' beliefs toward doping use. The efforts of Laure and his colleagues (see Laure and Lecerf 2002) and ATLAS/ATHENA (Goldberg and Elliot 2005) demonstrated that an education-based approach can assist in doping use prevention. Still, there is room for considerable improvement of these interventions (Ntoumanis *et al.* 2014). For instance, based on the available evidence the content of education-based anti-doping interventions should incorporate information about the health and moral consequences of doping use (see Question 9) and actively involve athletes in the learning process. Also, the athletes' entourage should be educated on anti-doping. Coaches, medical staff, and parents should be aware of the consequences of doping use and, accordingly, educate athletes. Recently, there have been several efforts toward this end (Dodge *et al.*, Chapter 14; Donovan *et al.* 2012; Poussel *et al.* 2013) that need to be expanded. Future interventions should use the knowledge produced in these efforts and develop education-based interventions that are more targeted to doping, theory-based, and involve more groups of the athletes' entourage.

Question 9: How to craft effective anti-doping messages?

In the context of persuasive health communications there are three important elements to be considered, such as the content of the message, the communicator, and the method of message delivery (Petty *et al.* 2009). In this respect, Barkoukis (Chapter 15) and Elbe and Brand (Chapter 12) indicated that messages focusing only on the health side effects of doping use, on doping control procedures, or only on morality may not effectively influence athletes' beliefs and cognitions toward doping use. In contrast, multifaceted interventions, incorporating information about the health consequences of doping use, the moral hazards, and alternatives to enhance performance could be more effective in changing athletes' beliefs about doping.

In addition, it is important to identify appropriate and suitable communicators to deliver the message. So far, the messages in anti-doping campaigns have been largely delivered by anti-doping authorities. However, athletes may perceive that anti-doping agencies provide biased information in favor of their policies. Hence, alternative types and groups of communicators from the athletes' entourage should be involved in anti-doping interventions. In line with this argument, research has shown that parents should be involved in the anti-doping fight and may be significant communicators of the anti-doping messages (Dodge *et al.* Chapter 14). Other researchers have suggested that sport psychologists (Donovan *et al.* 2012), medical staff (Poussel *et al.* 2013) and physical education teachers (Barkoukis *et al.* under review) should be more actively involved in conveying anti-doping messages.

Finally, another important issue concerning effective intervention is the way the message is conveyed. Research on self-affirmation theory provides a venue to address this issue (Steele 1988). According to the theory, people are motivated to maintain a positive self-image and may process in a self-serving and defensive manner any personally relevant information that is perceived as a threat to their self-image. This explains, for instance, why high-risk groups (e.g., dopers) may react defensively to messages reminding them of the health risks of doping use and subsequently reject the health message (Harris *et al.* 2007). Self-affirming restores self-integrity and reduces the need to be defensive in another less important domain. For instance, self-affirming an athlete's personal value of being compassionate may make him less defensive in a doping-related message. Recent research has shown that self-affirmation can influence the effect of health and moral doping-related messages on doping users' decision-making process (Barkoukis *et al.* 2015a). These findings imply that self-affirmation may influence message acceptance of doping-related messages.

Question 10: Should the study of doping use become more interdisciplinary?

Perhaps one of the most important questions about the future of the psychological study of doping use is whether an interdisciplinary research agenda should be developed. In many occasions, cross-cutting themes in science and/or policy are addressed through an interdisciplinary perspective. As Karl Popper (1963) argued more than 50 years ago, scientists are "not students of some subject matter, but students of problems. And problems may cut right across the borders of any subject matter or discipline" (1963: 88). Indeed, climate change, disease prevention, and healthy and active aging, for example, represent complex problems that are best understood through interdisciplinary research perspectives (Cacioppo and Ortigue 2011; Eisenberg and Pellmar 2000). The increasing trends in doping use among amateur, non-competitive athletes, and even adolescents, as well as studies showing that doping use is a persistent and ongoing threat in sports, suggest that doping represents another major societal and public health challenge that deserves an interdisciplinary look (Laure and Binsinger 2007; Petróczi and Naughton 2011; Simon *et al.* 2006).

Petróczi and Naughton (2011) described the different disciplines involved in doping use and control research, including social and behavioral sciences, education, and biomedical sciences (e.g., biochemistry and epidemiology). In addition to this work, it is possible that anti-doping education and training would greatly advance by the integration of behavioral science, education, and information and communication technology (ICT). Chapter 15 has already discussed how contemporary ICTs are embedded in some of WADA's anti-doping initiatives. Yet, this area is still in its infancy and ICT developments can do more than just contextualize an anti-doping curriculum.

Integrating methodologies used in other scientific areas with the study of doping use is also an important step in encouraging interdisciplinary research. For instance, Zurloni *et al.* (2015) used T-pattern analysis to better understand the non-verbal behavior cues associated with doping use. T-pattern analysis is a method used to discern patterns of behavior that are not easily conceivable with the naked eye, and is commonly used in animal behavior studies (Casarrubea *et al.* 2015). Zurloni *et al.* (2015) applied this method and scrutinized videos of Lance Armstrong interviews, and showed how analysis of non-verbal cues can be integrated in efforts to capture deceptive responding with respect to doping use.

Another area in doping research that would benefit from interdisciplinary studies is the assessment of risk factors for doping use. A growing body of studies in social neuroscience has helped researchers identify the brain mechanisms that may explain aspects of health behaviors, such as failed self-regulation strategies and the occurrence of biased information processing (e.g., Sharot 2011). Similarly, merging social cognition with neuroscience can help researchers in doping use better understand the biological basis of processes that explain doping use across levels of sports. This is not only a call for more basic research in the social science study of doping use, but also an opportunity to reveal a more complete picture of the doping puzzle by utilizing different scientific disciplines and methodologies.

Finally, and perhaps most importantly, interdisciplinary research merging neuroscience (e.g., cognitive and affective neuroscience) with behavior and cognitive sciences can reveal the effects of doping use and nutritional supplement use on the brain. Although it is assumed that doping and nutritional supplement use draw on the same mental representations in the athletes' minds (Barkoukis *et al.* 2015b; Petróczi *et al.* 2011), there is still no evidence about the neural mechanisms that justify this claim. Of course, this is not an extensive list of interdisciplinary research on doping use, but rather an initiative that we hope will generate fruitful discussions among scientists working in the field in the years to come. Doping use is a cross-cutting and ongoing challenge, thus it should be treated accordingly.

Conclusion

The past decade of research into doping use gave us an important intellectual capital about the psychological processes underlying doping use, but also leaves us with important questions that future research in this area should address. In this chapter, we have presented what we consider to be important questions that may be leading the psychological study of doping use in the following years. These questions addressed a wide range of issues, from theoretical integration and novel methodologies, to the utilization of information technology in anti-doping interventions and important dilemmas about moral values and the role of nutritional supplements in the fight against doping. We hope that these questions pave the way for further study in this area and effectively lead us to new research milestones in the psychological study of doping use.

References

Ajzen, I. (1991). The theory of planned behavior. *Organizational Behavior and Human Decision Processes, 50 (2)*, 179–211.

Ajzen, I. (2011). The theory of planned behaviour: Reactions and reflections. *Psychology and Health, 26 (9)*, 1113–1127.

Anshel, M. H. and Russell, K. G. (1997). Examining athletes' attitudes toward using anabolic steroids and their knowledge of the possible effects. *Journal of Drug Education, 27 (2)*, 121–145.

Aspinwall, L. G. and Tedeschi, R. G. (2010). Of babies and bathwater: A reply to Coyne and Tennen's views on positive psychology and health. *Annals of Behavioral Medicine, 39 (1)*, 27–34.

Backhouse, S. H., Whitaker, L., and Petróczi A. (2011). Gateway to doping? Supplement use in the context of preferred competitive situations, doping attitude, beliefs, and norms. *Scandinavian Journal of Medicine and Science in Sports*. doi: 10.1111/j.1600-0838.2011.01374.x.

Barkoukis, V., Lazuras, L., and Harris, P. R. (2015a). The effects of self-affirmation manipulation on decision making about doping use in elite athletes. *Psychology of Sport and Exercise, 16*, 175–181.

Barkoukis, V., Kartali, K., Lazuras, L., and Tsorbatzoudis, H. (under review). Evaluation of and anti-doping intervention for adolescents: Findings from a school-based study.

Barkoukis, V., Lazuras, L., Lucidi, F., and Tsorbatzoudis, H. (2015b). Nutritional supplement and doping use in sport: Possible underlying social cognitive processes. *Scandinavian Journal of Medicine and Science in Sports*. doi: 10.1111/sms.12377.

Barkoukis, V., Lazuras, L., Tsorbatzoudis, H., and Rodafinos, A. (2011). Motivational and sportspersonship profiles of elite athletes in relation to doping behavior. *Psychology of Sport and Exercise, 12 (3)*, 205–212.

Barkoukis, V., Lazuras, L., Tsorbatzoudis, H., and Rodafinos, A. (2013). Motivational and social cognitive predictors of doping intentions in elite sports: An integrated approach. *Scandinavian Journal of Medicine and Science in Sports, 23 (5)*, e330–e340.

Brand, R., Melzer, M., and Hagemann, N. (2011). Towards an implicit association test (IAT) for measuring doping attitudes in sports. Data-based recommendations developed from two recently published tests. *Psychology of Sport and Exercise, 12 (3)*, 250–256.

Briñol, P., Petty, R. E., and McCaslin, M. J. (2009). Changing attitudes on implicit versus explicit measures: What is the difference? In R. E. Petty, R. H. Fazio, and P. Briñol (eds.), *Attitudes: Insights from the new implicit measures* (285–326). New York: Psychology Press.

Cacioppo, J. T. and Ortigue, S. (2011, November). Social Neuroscience: How a multidisciplinary field is uncovering the biology of human interactions. In *Cerebrum: the Dana forum on brain science* (Vol. 2011). Dana Foundation.

Camporesi, S. and McNamee, M. J. (2014). Performance enhancement, elite athletes and anti-doping governance: Comparing human guinea pigs in pharmaceutical research and professional sports. *Philosophy, Ethics, and Humanities in Medicine, 9 (1)*, 4.

Casarrubea, M., Johnson, G. K., Faulisi, F., Sorbera, F., Di Giovanni, G., Beningo, A., Crescimanno, G., and Magnusson, M. G. (2015). T-pattern analysis for the study of temporal structure of animal and human behaviour: A comprehensive review. *Journal of Neuroscience Methods, 239*, 34–46.

Chan, D. K. C., Dimmock, J. A., Donovan, R. J., Hardcastle, S., Lentillon-Kaestner, V., and Hagger, M. S. (2015). Self-determined motivation in sport predicts anti-doping motivation and intention: A perspective from the trans-contextual model. *Journal of Science and Medicine in Sport, 18 (3)*, 315–322.

Dobbins, G. H., Lane, I. M., and Steiner, D. D. (1988). A note on the role of laboratory methodologies in applied behavioural research: Don't throw out the baby with the bath water. *Journal of Organizational Behavior, 9 (3)*, 281–286.

Donahue, E. G., Miquelon, P., Valois, P., Goulet, C., Buist, A., and Vallerand, R. J. (2006). A motivational model of performance-enhancing substance use in elite athletes. *Journal of Sport and Exercise Psychology, 28*, 511–520.

Donovan, R. J., Jalleh, G., and Gucciardi, D. (2012). *Development of a psychoeducational anti-doping intervention program for emerging athletes*. Report to Department of Health and Ageing. Centre for Behavioural Research in Cancer Control, Faculty of Health Sciences, Curtin University, Perth.

Donovan, R. J., Egger, G., Kapernick, V., and Mendoza, J. (2002). A conceptual framework for achieving performance enhancing drug compliance in sport. *Sports Medicine, 32 (4)*, 269–284.

Eisenberg, L. and Pellmar, T. C. (eds.) (2000). *Bridging disciplines in the brain, behavioral, and clinical sciences*. Washington, DC: National Academies Press.

Fazio, R. H. and Olson, M. A. (2003). Implicit measures in social cognition research: Their meaning and use. *Annual Review of Psychology, 54*, 297–327.

Geyer, H., Parr, M. K., Koehler, K., Mareck, U., Schanzer, W., and Thevis, M. (2008). Nutritional supplements cross-contaminated and faked with doping substances. *Journal of Mass Spectrometry, 43*, 892–902.

Goldberg, L. and Elliot, D. L. (2005). Preventing substance use among high school athletes: The ATLAS and ATHENA programs. *Journal of Applied School Psychology, 21*, 63–87.

Goldberg, L., Elliot, D. L., MacKinnon, D. P., Moe, E., Kuehl, K. S., Nohre, L., and Lockwood, C. M. (2003). Drug testing athletes to prevent substance abuse: Background and pilot study results of the SATURN (Student Athlete Testing Using Random Notification) study. *Journal of Adolescent Health, 32 (1)*, 16–25.

Goldberg, L., Elliot, D. L., MacKinnon, D. P., Moe, E. L., Kuehl, K. S., Yoon, M., Taylor, A., and Williams, J. (2007). Outcomes of a prospective trial of student-athlete drug testing: the Student Athlete Testing Using Random Notification (SATURN) study. *Journal of Adolescent Health, 41 (5)*, 421–429.

Greenwald, A. G., Poehlman, T. A., Uhlmann, E. L., and Banaji, M. R. (2009). Understanding and using the Implicit Association Test: III. Meta-analysis of predictive validity. *Journal of Personality and Social Psychology*, *97*, 17–41.

Harris, P. R., Mayle, K., Mabbott, L., and Napper, L. (2007). Self-affirmation reduces smokers' defensiveness to graphic on-pack cigarette warning labels. *Health Psychology*, *26* (*4*), 437.

Kayser, B., Mauron, A., and Miah, A. (2007). Current anti-doping policy: a critical appraisal. *BMC Medical Ethics*, *8* (*1*), 2.

Kohler, M., Thomas, A., Geyer, H., Petrou, M., Schanzer, W., and Thevis, M. (2010). Confiscated black market products and nutritional supplements with non-approved ingredients analyzed in the Cologne doping control laboratory 2009. *Drug Testing and Analysis*, *2*, 533–537.

Kruglanski, A. W., Shah, J. Y., Fishbach, A., Friedman, R., Chun, W. Y., and Sleeth-Keppler, D. (2002). A theory of goal systems. *Advances in Experimental Social Psychology*, *34*, 331–378.

Laure, P. and Binsinger, C. (2007). Doping prevalence among preadolescent athletes: A 4-year follow-up. *British Journal of Sports Medicine*, *41* (*10*), 660–663.

Laure, P. and Lecerf, T. (2002). Doping prevention among young athletes: Comparison of a health education-based intervention versus information-based intervention. *Science and Sports*, *17* (*4*), 198–201.

Laure, P. and Reinsberger, H. (1995). Doping and high-level endurance walkers. Knowledge and representation of a prohibited practice. *The Journal of Sports Medicine and Physical Fitness*, *35* (*3*), 228–231.

Lazuras, L., Barkoukis, V., and Tzorbatzoudis, H. (forthcoming). Towards an integrative model of doping intentions: An empirical study with adolescent athletes. *Journal of Sport and Exercise Psychology*.

Lazuras, L., Barkoukis, V., Rodafinos, A., and Tzorbatzoudis, H. (2010). Predictors of doping intentions in elite-level athletes: A social cognition approach. *Journal of Sport and Exercise Psychology*, *32* (*5*), 694.

Loland, S. (2005). The varieties of cheating – Comments on ethical analyses in sport [1]. *Sport in Society*, *8* (*1*), 11–26.

Lucidi, F., Grano, C., Leone, L., Lombardo, C., and Pesce, C. (2004). Determinants of the intention to use doping substances: An empirical contribution in a sample of Italian adolescents. *Journal of Sport Psychology*, *35* (*2*), 133–148.

Lucidi, F., Zelli, A., Mallia, L., Grano, C., Russo, P. M., and Violani, C. (2008). The social-cognitive mechanisms regulating adolescents' use of doping substances. *Journal of Sports Sciences*, *26* (*5*), 447–456.

Ntoumanis, N., Ng, J. Y., Barkoukis, V., and Backhouse, S. (2014). Personal and psycho-social predictors of doping use in physical activity settings: A meta-analysis. *Sports Medicine*, *44* (*11*), 1603–1624.

Petróczi, A. (2007). Attitudes and doping: a structural equation analysis of the relationship between athletes' attitudes, sport orientation and doping behaviour. *Substance Abuse Treatment, Prevention, and Policy*, *2* (*1*), 34.

Petróczi, A. (2013a). The doping mindset – Part I: Implications of the Functional Use Theory on mental representations of doping. *Performance Enhancement and Health*, *2* (*4*), 153–163.

Petróczi, A. (2013b). The doping mindset – Part II: Potentials and pitfalls in capturing athletes' doping attitudes with response-time methodology. *Performance Enhancement and Health*, *2* (*4*), 164–181.

Petróczi, A. and Aidman, E. (2008). Psychological drivers in doping: the life-cycle model of performance enhancement. *Substance Abuse Treatment, Prevention, and Policy, 3* (*1*), 7.

Petróczi, A. and Naughton, D. P. (2011). Impact of multidisciplinary research on advancing anti-doping efforts. *International Journal of Sport Policy and Politics, 3* (*2*), 235–259.

Petróczi, A., Aidman, E. V., and Nepusz, T. (2008). Capturing doping attitudes by self-report declarations and implicit assessment: A methodology study. *Substance Abuse Treatment, Prevention, and Policy, 3* (*9*).

Petróczi, A., Mazanov, J., and Naughton, D. P. (2011). Inside athletes' minds: Preliminary results from a pilot study on mental representation of doping and potential implications for anti-doping. *Substance Abuse Treatment, Prevention, and Policy, 6* (*10*), 1–8.

Petty, R. E., Barden, J., and Wheeler, S. C. (2009). The elaboration likelihood model of persuasion: Developing health promotions for sustained behavioral change. In R. J. DiClemente, R. A. Crosby, and M. C. Kegler (eds.), *Emerging theories in health promotion practice and research* (215–234). New York: John Wiley & Sons.

Popper, K. (1963). *Conjectures and refutations: The growth of scientific knowledge.* New York: Routledge and Kegan Paul.

Poussel, M., Laure, P., Latarche, C., Laroppe, J., Schwitzer, M., Koch, J.- P., Heid, J.-M., and Chenuel, B. (2013). Specific teaching about doping in sport helps medical students to meet prevention needs. *Science and Sports, 28* (*5*), 274–280.

Savulescu, J., Foddy, B., and Clayton, M. (2004). Why we should allow performance enhancing drugs in sport. *British Journal of Sports Medicine, 38* (*6*), 666–670.

Sharot, T. (2011). The optimism bias. *Current Biology, 21* (*23*), R941–R945.

Simon, P., Striegel, H., Aust, F., Dietz, K., and Ulrich, R. (2006). Doping in fitness sports: estimated number of unreported cases and individual probability of doping. *Addiction, 101* (*11*), 1640–1644.

Spector, P. E., Zapf, D., Chen, P. Y., and Frese, M. (2000). Why negative affectivity should not be controlled in job stress research: Don't throw out the baby with the bath water. *Journal of Organizational Behavior, 21* (*1*), 79–95.

Steele, C. M. (1988). The psychology of self-affirmation: Sustaining the integrity of the self. *Advances in Experimental Social Psychology, 21*, 261–302.

Wiefferink, C. H., Detmar, S. B., Coumans, B., Vogels, T., and Paulussen, T. G. W. (2008). Social psychological determinants of the use of performance-enhancing drugs by gym users. *Health Education Research, 23* (*1*), 70–80.

Zelli, A., Mallia, L., and Lucidi, F. (2010). The contribution of interpersonal appraisals to a social-cognitive analysis of adolescents' doping use. *Psychology of Sport and Exercise, 11* (*4*), 304–311.

Zurloni, V., Diana, B., Cavalera, C., Argenton, L., Elia, M., and Mantovani, F. (2015). Deceptive behavior in doping related interviews: The case of Lance Armstrong. *Psychology of Sport and Exercise, 16* (*2*), 191–200.

Index

Page numbers in *italics* denote tables, those in **bold** denote figures.